TRAUMA AND EXPRESSIVE ARTS THERAPY

Trauma and Expressive Arts Therapy

BRAIN, BODY, AND IMAGINATION
IN THE HEALING PROCESS

Cathy A. Malchiodi

THE GUILFORD PRESS
New York   London

Library of Congress Cataloging-in-Publication Data

Names: Malchiodi, Cathy A., author.
Title: Trauma and expressive arts therapy : brain, body, and imagination in
  the healing process / Cathy A. Malchiodi.
Identifiers: LCCN 2019045197 | ISBN 9781462543113 (cloth ; alk. paper)
Subjects: MESH: Psychological Trauma—therapy | Sensory Art Therapies |
  Emotions | Imagination
Classification: LCC RC489.A72 | NLM WM 172.5 | DDC 616.89/1656—dc23
LC record available at *https://lccn.loc.gov/2019045197*

To the muse and imagination

About the Author

Cathy A. Malchiodi, PhD, ATR-BC, LPCC, LPAT, REAT, is a psychologist, expressive arts therapist, and art therapist specializing in trauma recovery. She is the founder and executive director of the Trauma-Informed Practices and Expressive Arts Therapy Institute, which trains mental health and health care practitioners in medical, educational, and community settings and assists in disaster relief and humanitarian efforts throughout the world. Dr. Malchiodi has given more than 500 presentations in the United States, Canada, Europe, the Middle East, Asia, and Australia, and has published numerous articles, chapters, and books, including *Understanding Children's Drawings* and *Creative Interventions with Traumatized Children, Second Edition.* She has received numerous awards for distinguished service, clinical contributions, and lifetime achievements, including honors from the Kennedy Center and Very Special Arts in Washington, DC. A passionate advocate for the role of the arts in health, she is a contributing writer for *PsychologyToday.com.*

Preface

One of my earliest childhood recollections is of a reparative experience involving the arts and imagination. My maternal grandmother had just died and it was the first time I lost a close and beloved relative. My father somehow sensed that his little girl needed something more than comforting words to help her heal from this loss. He let me use leftover house paint and a wall in our unfinished basement to create whatever I wanted. I used those paints to cover that wall with images of birds, animals, and the dense woods in back of our Connecticut home. I also remember simply taking the brushes and moving the paint rhythmically across the surface, sometimes while listening to music on the radio. After school each day and on weekends, I looked forward to spending time alone with what became a canvas for expressing feelings while dancing to favorite songs.

I never forgot this experience and many others involving the healing capacity of the arts during childhood and adolescence. I always returned to drawing, painting, dance, theater, and music as ways to untangle my emotions and restore a sense of aliveness when experiencing distress or loss. These moments eventually led me to want to become an artist and to study the visual arts and theater in college. But I always carried the belief that the arts were more than an exhibition, recital, or performance. I recognized that imagination and play had another, larger purpose, because when engaged in creative experiences I was able to transcend crises more easily.

Later, when I pursued a doctorate in psychology, it was natural for me to want to continue my quest to understand just how and why the arts and imagination were reparative. In graduate school I bumped up against prevailing "talking cure" approaches that continue to be the dominant ways of treating traumatic stress. Language is, of course, a necessary means of communication, but it is only an approximation of our experiences when it comes to articulating distress. Ultimately, words never quite convey just how the brain and body experience trauma. Sooner or later, they inevitably fail us when it comes to feelings and sensations of anxiety, terror, dissociation, and loss of pleasure in living that come with unresolved trauma's aftermath. Long before the talking cure became a "thing," humans turned to arts-based expression as a way of transforming difficulties when confronted by crisis, tragedy, or loss. As a species we have been turning to the healing rhythms and synchrony of the arts to confront and resolve distress for thousands of years. These actions emerged not only as individual forms of reparation, but also through social engagement, capitalizing on connection with others and community as agents of healing. In recent years, nonverbal approaches, including an emphasis on the body's response to trauma, have emerged as accepted and effective methods to address and resolve traumatic stress. Some of these approaches, like neurofeedback and reprocessing protocols, focus on literally changing the brain's perceptions and responses to traumatic memories and reactions. Others are more somatically based and emphasize the recognition and transformation of the body's response to trauma.

Despite this increase in recognition of the role of nonverbal and implicit communications in the treatment of trauma, expressive arts therapy—the integrative use of movement, music, sound, art, improvisation, theater, creative writing, and play—has often been left out of the array of recognized psychotherapeutic approaches to traumatic stress. One reason for this derives from the marginalization of the arts themselves within modern society; their impact on quality of life, mental health, and general wellness is often misunderstood or devalued. Science is now providing the evidence for what humans have always known, making it increasingly plausible to explain just why the expressive arts may be uniquely effective when it comes to addressing traumatic stress.

Q: psychotherapudic means...?

WHY INCORPORATE EXPRESSIVE ARTS IN YOUR WORK?

The primary intention of this book is to describe the psychotherapeutic benefits of expressive arts therapy in work with trauma. It also explains key frameworks and approaches that all practitioners can apply to their work with traumatized individuals to help them actively address overwhelming reactions and harness the power of the arts, play, and imagination for health and well-being. When speaking to audiences about how to apply expressive arts therapy with children, adults, and families, I often ask them to consider these questions: "What if you could actually enhance your current approach to helping individuals with traumatic stress? What if you could introduce them to approaches that support self-regulation and assist them in experiencing the body's response to trauma in a safe manner? What if you could help individuals learn and practice these skills in playful and enlivening ways? And what if you could help them to use imagination to create new, reparative narratives that transform the traumatic memories that reside in both mind and body?"

Expressive arts therapy is a circumscribed form of psychotherapy grounded in arts-based methodology and "bottom-up" approaches that capitalize on the sensory-based qualities of movement, music and sound, visual arts, dramatic enactment, and other forms of creative communication. However, expressive arts therapy is also "valued added" when combined with effective approaches therapists already use to successfully effect change. These include verbal forms of psychotherapy, somatically based models, mindfulness practices, and even brain-based methods involving reprocessing and neurofeedback. If you are a psychotherapist using one or more of these approaches, this book is an invitation to begin to integrate drawing, movement, music, creative writing, improvisation, and play in your work. These expressive methods will enhance your relationship with your clients and teach them sensory-based approaches that support affect regulation and a sense of safety. These approaches will also help both children and adults identify their bodies' responses to distress, transform trauma-laden stories into resilient narratives, and relearn how to experience pleasure and aliveness once again. Even if you have had minimal arts experience, I hope you will be convinced that these approaches are powerful means of communication that capture not only the brain's explicit imprint of traumatic stress, but also the body's implicit experience that does not translate easily through words alone.

If you are an art therapist, dance/movement therapist, music therapist, or drama therapist, you may already have many of the foundational skills described in this book. But you may not have considered how you can strengthen your approach by strategically including other art forms in your work, ones that you may not have considered, such as drawing, movement, sound, improvisation, play, and storytelling. It is this integrative experience that can make a difference in clients' ability to more quickly and effectively address traumatic stress and engage their own healing processes. For expressive arts therapists, I hope this book becomes a framework for arts-based approaches to traumatic stress that are based not only in neurobiology, but also in our growing understanding of culturally relevant healing practices that are found only in the arts.

HOW THE BOOK IS ORGANIZED

The first three chapters of this book provide an overview of major concepts and frameworks. Chapter 1 explains the origins of expressive arts therapy and its long history as a form of trauma reparation and integration and provides eight key reasons to integrate expressive approaches within psychotherapy. Chapter 2 reviews trauma-informed frameworks, including the role of adverse events, historical and intergenerational trauma, and social justice. It also outlines the basic principles of trauma-informed expressive arts therapy and a four-part culturally relevant model for the arts as healing practices. Chapter 3 explains how the expressive arts can be used to address trauma through a brain–body framework and how to apply a bottom-up or top-down approach to trauma intervention.

Subsequent chapters describe how to integrate expressive arts therapy into psychotherapeutic practice with children, adults, families, and groups. Because expressive arts add a unique dynamic to trauma work, Chapter 4 addresses how they can be used to develop and support safe, resonant, and reparative relationships. Chapters 5 and 6 explain how specific arts-based approaches can enhance an internalized sense of safety and the ability to self-regulate and stabilize trauma reactions. Chapter 7 provides multiple strategies for applying expressive methods to working with the body and helping individuals safely identify traumatic stress in their bodies. Strategies for unpacking trauma narratives are explained in detail in Chapter 8, including how stories are told not only through verbal communication, but also through movement, imagery, and other arts-based expressions. Chapter 9 covers the role of resilience in trauma work and how expressive arts provide unique opportunities to support an internal sense of mastery and competence necessary to overcome distress. Finally, Chapter 10 takes on the topic of meaning making, a critical element in trauma recovery, and explains how expressive arts therapy develops and supports imagination in the healing process.

If you work with traumatized children, adults, families, or communities, you probably know that the individuals you see in your agency or practice often struggle with communicating their experiences through talk alone. You may also recognize that they need action-oriented, participatory, and safe experiences that address immobilizing hyperactivation or dissociation and withdrawal. Effective therapists appreciate and support both their clients' styles of communication as well as strategies that help bring out the best in their clients within the psychotherapeutic relationship. I hope the concepts and practices described in this book help your clients safely express the impact of trauma on their lives and support them in actively mobilizing their own resources to repair, restore, and recover.

Acknowledgments

Once in a while a writer gets lucky and something happens that ignites the creative fire necessary to manifest a vision. It's a pivotal moment that suddenly inspires and makes it possible to articulate what previously felt distant and unattainable. This book is the result of one of those moments and for that reason is particularly special to me. In the process of fanning this creative fire over the course of a year, I have also been extremely lucky to have had the support necessary to sustain the work. That support made it possible to unpack a singular belief I have held for decades—that the expressive arts are uniquely reparative when it comes to healing traumatic stress. And for this reason, there are many individuals to thank for giving me what fueled the energy and audacity to undertake writing this book.

Over months of writing and research, many friends and colleagues heard me say that "I feel like my brain has too many tabs open." As I got increasingly deeper into the actual writing, I found myself digesting and integrating diverse ideas, teachings, and concepts not only from my arts-oriented field but also from many domains, including neurobiology, health psychology, cultural anthropology, and creativity. As it turned out, several "tabs" consistently remained open throughout this project—the contributions of five individuals whose work and publications in the field of trauma guided the construction of theories, models, and approaches described in this book. Thank you to Lenore Terr, my earliest mentor, whose research informed my work with children and families exposed to interpersonal violence. I am also grateful to Judith Herman, whose seminal phase model for trauma recovery forms the overall structure of this book; her work not only has impacted my own thinking, but also has a wide-ranging influence on arts-based therapies in general. I could not have envisioned a brain-wise, expressive arts therapy framework without the contributions of Bruce Perry on neurodevelopment. His seminal work with child survivors of the Waco incident helped me understand the nature of the trauma reactions I encountered in children who experienced violent assault, chronic neglect, and separation from families. Peter Levine explained the role of somatic experiences in traumatic stress, kindling a spark that led to my ongoing investigations of how traumatized individuals communicate distress through movement, art, music, and enactment. And, lastly, I am thankful for the synchronicity of finding Bessel van der Kolk's first paper on how the "body keeps the score" sitting on a table in a medical library 25 years ago. Whether that was an accident or the work of angels, I will never know. But I can say that his ongoing contributions to the somatosensory understanding of trauma made it possible for me to explain the role of brain, body, and imagination in repair and recovery through expressive arts.

While there are many expressive arts therapists to thank, I carried three in particular in my heart throughout this project. One is early mentor Paolo Knill of the European Graduate School, whose wisdom about integrative work laid the foundation for my development as an expressive arts therapist. I thank Shirley Riley, whose work in family art therapy has never been duplicated or surpassed; she taught me the centrality of improvisation in psychotherapy. I miss her every single day but am so lucky to now channel her teachings and love of this work into every client session. Finally, I am grateful to have encountered Gestalt art therapist Janie Rhyne, who taught me the importance of gesture, movement, and sound as forms of communication and dramatic enactment as a way to not only illuminate but also imagine new narratives.

My special gratitude goes to my expressive arts contemporaries Elizabeth Warson, Cornelia Elbrecht, and Laury Rappaport for enduring both my euphoria and what must often have seemed like periods of true insanity during the writing of this book. I only wish I could fully express how much I have learned about the value and uniqueness of this work from each of you.

Writing is impossible without long periods of time for devotion to the process. I thank my husband, David, for allowing me the space to sustain the necessary concentration, for his patience with my frequent dissociative states, and for hearing my repeat performances of Bo-Rhap and Starman through the walls of his office. Thank you also to Emily Johnson Welsh for taking on the day-to-day administrative surprises at the Trauma-Informed Practices and Expressive Arts Therapy Institute. You freed me up to create in ways that would not have been otherwise possible.

The staff at The Guilford Press has been exceptional when it comes to the editorial and production process over the past 20 years. On this round, I don't know if there are words to express my deepest gratitude to Rochelle Serwator for all her support. Rochelle not only was a major source of editorial expertise; she also kept me motivated by patiently pushing me forward and supplying almost weekly support to keep me going during critical junctures. I also thank the following people: Barbara Watkins for early editorial recommendations; Katherine Sommer for her vigilance in pulling together pieces of the manuscript; Robert Sebastiano for handling the wide range of permissions for illustrations, tables, and graphics; Laura Specht Patchkofsky for overseeing the book's production; Paul Gordon for his design advice; and Seymour Weingarten for wisdom that is always greatly appreciated.

The most emotional moments in writing this book emerged as I recalled the countless children, adults, families, and groups I have encountered over more than three decades. My thanks go to them for providing a constant training ground that allowed me to understand how expressive arts and imagination offer possibilities to transform and repair even the most adverse life experiences. Finally, I thank the indigenous peoples of the world who use the arts to address individual and collective trauma. While theories and approaches described in this volume derive from science and the arts, they also come from the traditions handed down throughout cultures for millennia. Contemporary experiential forms of trauma treatment, including expressive arts, have emerged from these uses of movement and gesture, music and sound, visual arts, dramatic enactment, rituals, and storytelling. I express gratitude to those who truly laid the foundations for what constitute healing practices and made possible the manifestation of expressive arts as a form of psychotherapy today.

Contents

CHAPTER 1

• • • • • • • • • •

Expressive Arts Therapy

GOING BEYOND THE LIMITS OF LANGUAGE

Psychological trauma can be a life-changing experience that affects multiple facets of health and well-being. The nature of trauma is to impact the mind and body in unpredictable and multidimensional ways. It can be a highly subjective experience that is difficult or even impossible to explain with words. It also can impact the body in highly individualized ways and result in complex symptoms that affect memory, social engagement, and quality of life.

While many people overcome trauma with resilience and without long-term effects, many do not. Trauma's impact often requires approaches that address the sensory-based experiences many survivors report. Expressive arts therapy—the purposeful application of art, music, dance/movement, dramatic enactment, creative writing, and imaginative play—is largely a nonverbal way of self-expression of feelings and perceptions. More importantly, they are action-oriented and tap implicit, embodied experiences of trauma that can defy expression through verbal therapy or logic.

In the fall of 1980, I began my first work with individuals who had experienced psychological trauma. I had just graduated with a master's degree in art therapy and was immediately hired for my first position as an art and play therapist for children and their mothers from violent homes at a community shelter. I was incredibly happy to get any job where I could use my newly acquired degree, especially since art therapy was very much considered to be a novel approach to treatment and no research yet existed to establish its efficacy. When I interviewed for the position, to my surprise the staff was unexpectedly enthusiastic about my experience and education in art and play therapy methods. As they showed me around the facility, they stopped at a room that a social worker was using to see children for

Q: Implicit vs. explicit?

1

individual and group sessions. On one of the tables there was a set of family puppets that appeared to have been decapitated. When I asked about the puppets, a staff member replied that "the social worker is just not having much luck getting the children to talk. That's the second set of puppets they destroyed this month." It was easy to understand that the children perhaps did not want to verbalize their experiences and feelings and might respond more favorably to a less verbal approach. Although I knew very little about child witnesses to violence and what were then called "battered women," this first impression became the foundation for a personal journey to understand how traumatic events impact us and why less-verbal approaches may be an important piece in trauma reparation (Malchiodi, 1990).

As I anxiously began my first week as a therapist, the first individuals I encountered challenged essentially all of the education and supervision I had accumulated over the previous 2 years. Just about everything I had been taught did not seem to apply to what these children and adults brought into the treatment setting. What I had been taught about art therapy was largely based on psychoanalytic theory, emphasizing interpreting art expressions to achieve insight and resolution of emotional conflicts. With children, art therapy involved evaluation of symbolic content as a way to identify personality traits or defense mechanisms, or it simply became a form of special art education that focused on developmental benchmarks. In reality, none of these approaches appealed to me, and even while I was in graduate school I sought other ways of working with individuals, including Gestalt therapy, Carl Rogers's person-centered and humanistic approaches, and Eugene Gendlin's idea of the "felt sense." I repeatedly returned to the idea that the processes involved in arts-based expression within a psychotherapeutic context contained the healing factor and that interpretation of imagery was not the main source of repair and transformation. What I subsequently learned during my first years as a psychotherapist influenced my worldview of how individuals respond to traumatic events in my current work and formed a crucible that has guided the development of concepts outlined in this book.

The treatment of trauma continues to be a challenge to practitioners, and it requires a variety of approaches. This first chapter begins with some of the clinical experiences that influenced my understanding of expressive arts therapy within the context of psychological trauma. It also provides an introduction to the arts in psychotherapy and an overview of expressive arts, with an emphasis on its role in trauma intervention.

TELLING WITHOUT TALKING

Sandra and her 9-year-old daughter, Sally, and 5-year-old son, Mike, were one of the first families I saw as a new practitioner. They came to the shelter after a particularly violent altercation that left Sandra with numerous

Good Story!

bruises and a swollen eye socket. I soon learned that this was a typical scenario for Sandra who had fled to the shelter on several other occasions when her husband become violently abusive. Sally often took on the role of rescuer, dialing the emergency number and giving the address to an emergency responder and asking law enforcement, "Please come to our house again." When altercations occurred between Sandra and her husband, Mike tried on at least one occasion to stop his father from hurting his mother by using his toy sword to hit and stab "the assailant." During the most recent incident, Mike cowered in a corner behind a chair while Sally screamed the family's location to the person taking her 911 call.

When I asked Sandra to tell me whatever she wanted to about what typically happened at home during a violent episode, she started to speak but suddenly became silent. Because she looked as if talking was painful, I simply nodded empathetically and did not press her to communicate. During the years I worked at this facility and subsequent agencies that treated individuals who experienced assault, I simply came to accept the fact that for some reason language was difficult for many of these abused women. Shelter staff speculated that women and children did not want to say too much because it might endanger them if they had to return to live with the perpetrator; alternatively, some mistrusted staff because giving out sensitive information might lead to a protective services investigation and removal of child custody. While these were plausible reasons for silence, I also felt that something else was interfering with verbal communication. Sandra, like many other women I would meet at the shelter, seemed to try to speak but appeared to actually choke when trying to answer my questions about the incidents that brought her and her family to the facility.

Mike was also remarkably silent. When he first arrived at the shelter with his mother and sister, he was not only mute, but also withdrawn and remote. Later, during his first session in the art and play therapy room, he quickly gravitated to the sandtray, taking various miniature figures from the shelf and moving them methodically in the sand as if I was not there with him. In contrast to my other experiences with preschool children who find joy and laughter in playing with toys in the sand, Mike was just the opposite. His affect only became more depressed and anxious as he rearranged figures in the box, and he did not interact with me unless I initiated contact. While he did not speak during this initial session, in sessions during the following week he described limited scenarios for me about "the police coming to get a bad monster who was hurting and hitting everyone"—represented in the sandtray by a miniature figure of a gorilla (the monster) and miniature police figures, multiple cars, and an ambulance (the rescuers). Despite the numerous responders, none could capture and contain the gorilla, who often ran wild throughout the sandtray, knocking down everything in its path. This story recurred each time Mike came to the playroom; he said very little, moving figures around the sandtray. Although he was likely portraying an actual trauma narrative he had experienced, it was apparent that he was not gaining relief from continually re-enacting the story.

In contrast, Sally was quite responsive and open to verbal communication with me. She showed initiative and even offered to help me organize art supplies, puppets, and toys for "the other children who come to the playroom." On the days when I may have felt a little bit overwhelmed, Sally would quickly sense my fatigue and offer to bring me a snack from the shelter kitchen or insist that I sit down and take a rest. Her composure and positive affect did not make sense to me, given what she had experienced at home on numerous occasions. Her paintings, however, conveyed a very different story and were unlike anything I had seen in art expressions by children Sally's age. At each art therapy session, she methodically included the color black within the center of each image or object (see Figures 1.1 and 1.2). While I do not subscribe to any specific universal interpretations

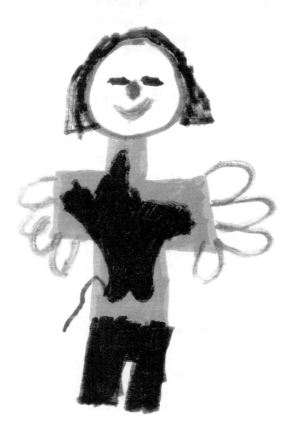

FIGURE 1.1. Sally's self-portrait. From the collection of Cathy A. Malchiodi (not to be reproduced without permission from the author).

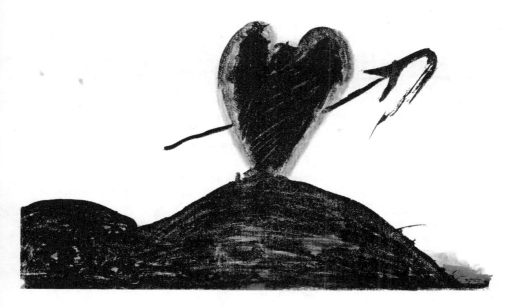

FIGURE 1.2. Sally's depiction of a "heart on an island." From the collection of Cathy A. Malchiodi (not to be reproduced without permission from the author).

of children's drawings (Malchiodi, 1998), her paintings did have unusual idiosyncratic characteristics that communicated something both intriguing and worrisome.

While a psychoanalytic view might simply attribute this repetition to an emotional source, I wondered if this child was conveying something more than just a feeling—that her body was responding in some way to the chronic violence she witnessed through her art products. Several things struck me about Sally. First, she seemed to be able to circumvent any verbalization about her experiences of witnessing family violence by distracting me with chatty conversation, avoiding talking about her experiences that were possibly too overwhelming to disclose. Second, I eventually began to wonder if Sally herself was experiencing a physical impact of repetitive stress in her body. I had been taking a social work course at the local university and was learning about the work of Hans Selye (1976) and other researchers who were just beginning to identify the impact of stress on physical health. Of course, practically nothing in the existing literature mentioned the impact of chronic stress on children, and childhood traumatic stress was not yet a diagnosable condition. But Sally's paintings turned out to be pivotal in my thinking about each child I subsequently saw at the shelter program. Sally, in fact, had a very serious duodenal ulcer that eventually was diagnosed by a visiting physician who was surprised that the child did not complain about the extreme pain she probably experienced on a daily basis.

After working with Sally, I began asking all children and mothers I saw at the shelter what they were experiencing in their bodies. While most mothers did not always have an immediate response to my question, most children did, inevitably telling me about pounding headaches, belly aches, nausea, and generalized body pain. These sensations often turned up in art expressions, especially when they were asked "How do you feel today?" (Figure 1.3). What I learned from these children about how their bodies responded to stress and how they communicated it in nonverbal ways formed a foundation for capitalizing on the embodied qualities of expressive arts to help survivors to "tell without talking" about the somatic experience of trauma.

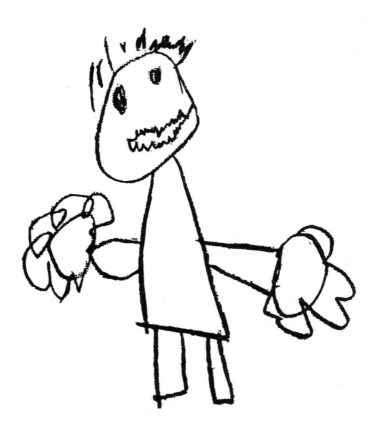

FIGURE 1.3. Child's drawing in response to the question "How do you feel today?" From the collection of Cathy A. Malchiodi (not to be reproduced without permission from the author).

BREAKING THE SILENCE

Of all the families I saw during the first year of working at the shelter, one in particular provided a comprehensive lesson about the wide range of reactions resulting from multiple chronic traumatic events. Joelle, 29 years of age, her 11-year-old daughter, Christa, and her 8-year-old son, Joey, presented a very complicated history to social services on admittance to the shelter. Joelle reported that her husband threatened violence to all family members, although she was unclear about exact details and in general was very guarded and hesitant to provide any detailed information about the family. Christa was selectively mute and appeared distant and withdrawn; she barely could answer any questions the social worker or I asked her on the first day. In contrast, Joey was full of energy, crawling on top of tables in the intake office, playing with pencils and notepads, and crawling into my lap on several occasions. He was spontaneous, talkative, and endearing, presenting more like a 4- or 5-year-old than a boy his chronological age.

During the family's month-long stay at the shelter, I worked with Christa and Joey two to three times a week, seeing them for approximately 10 sessions. Christa, despite all my best efforts, was largely unresponsive to invitations to participate in art making, preferring to remain silently watching Joey engage in play and artistic expression. I quickly realized that, based on his art products and the characteristics of his play activity, Joey was displaying some significant developmental delays. He also clearly had speech problems and was generally quite clumsy in both fine and gross motor skills. In fact, Joey often, for no apparent reason, fell out of his seat while sitting at the art table and had problems with balance when standing. But at least he was engaging with me and the therapy sessions. In contrast, Christa was not forthcoming and generally seemed distant, almost as if she were in a different time and place. One of the only ways I could engage her was through reading storybooks to Joey. Christa would sit right next to me, watching me turn each page of the book and nodding and smiling as I animatedly read a story aloud. Like Joey, her behavior seemed to be that of a much younger child than her chronological age and like a younger child, she seemed comforted by the calming prosody of my voice.

Christa displayed yet another reaction that I would see in numerous children and adults not only in my work with domestic violence survivors, but also in individuals who endured physical or sexual assault during childhood. When introduced to a male therapist who helped me run drama therapy groups for the children, Christa instantly became completely immobile, unable to speak or respond to anything I said to her. Eventually, she began to cry silently; my only option at that time was to put her in the care of another staff member with whom she eventually relaxed. My very gentle and sensitive colleague and I were completely baffled by her reaction, but we recognized that he was the obvious reason for her immobilization.

During the next year, the family returned to the facility; Joelle had now divorced her husband and stated that she had a live-in boyfriend who she reported was physically abusive to her. Although Joey did well during the family's first of three stays at the shelter, he did not display the resilience he previously demonstrated. Intake staff learned from Joelle that both children had been physically assaulted by the live-in boyfriend and that Christa may have been sexually abused; child protective services became involved, concluded that these reports were accurate, and began investigation of the alleged perpetrator.

The physical and emotional maltreatment had taken its toll on Joey, and one day while I was attending a conference near the shelter, he threatened to leap out of a second-story window in the facility. Joelle was at a meeting outside the residence on that morning, so I was called to return to the shelter to literally talk Joey off of a window ledge because he asked for "Mrs. Cathy to please come right away." Although this dramatic moment of being called back to the facility because of a suicidal child gave me some serious anxiety, the instant Joey saw me, he immediately ended his threat and ran to me for a hug. In that moment, I wondered just what was so incredibly powerful in this boy's life that caused him to resort to this action, and, at the same time, I felt reassured that he knew how to seek adult helpers when distressed.

Having no debriefing skills for post-suicide attempts in children, I was compromised as to what to do in that moment, but Joey was very willing to draw a picture for me of what he was feeling at the time (Figure 1.4). His drawing depicts a sad little face with hair standing up straight and loose teeth floating around in his mouth; I did ask him if he would like to include a body, but he declined, saying that "the picture is right this way." At that point, Joey was very agitated while looking at the drawing he created for me, spontaneously commenting that his "mother would finally be sad for me 'cuz I was dead." Obviously, ending his life was the ultimate attention-getting action that he believed would impact his mother and leave her with the guilt of his demise.

Although I was not conscious of the important role of getting the body moving during moments of immobilization, my intuition told me that Joey needed to shift his focus dramatically in the short term. I took him to the shelter's gymnasium, and we ran laps around the perimeter, interspersed with some jumping jacks and playful karate moves. When we returned to the art and play therapy room, we had a nonverbal conversation using toy drums to respond to each other through tapping out various beats, and we did some simple improvisations of characters in storybooks I had read to him during past sessions. The physicality of these activities, coupled with my participation and interaction with Joey, seemed to help him be less frozen and more focused on the current moment rather than on the suicide attempt an hour earlier.

After a period of time, Joey surprised me by telling me that he wanted to draw another picture for me of something he had never drawn

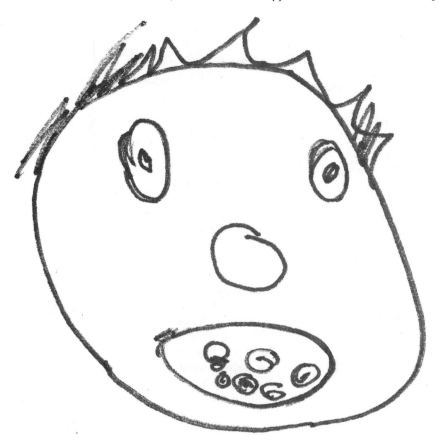

FIGURE 1.4. Joey's drawing in response to the question "How do you feel right now?" From the collection of Cathy A. Malchiodi (not to be reproduced without permission from the author).

before—his family (Figure 1.5). Unlike Christa and despite his challenging speech problems, Joey was anxious to tell me a very detailed story about his worldview of what were typical dynamics within the family system. The drawing clearly illustrated what a typical incident of physical violence looked like through Joey's eyes. Joelle was depicted as the oversized head, mouth open, ominous and angry, and yelling at the other members of the family; Joey felt he was always the target of this verbal barrage, and so he placed himself nearest his mother in the drawing. "Dad" (Joelle's current live-in boyfriend) appeared next to Joey, followed by Christa to the far left. When I asked Joey to explain all the elements in the drawing, he made sure that I understood that his mother "does the yelling" and that Christa "smiles while watching" as an onlooker. Joey included a television at the

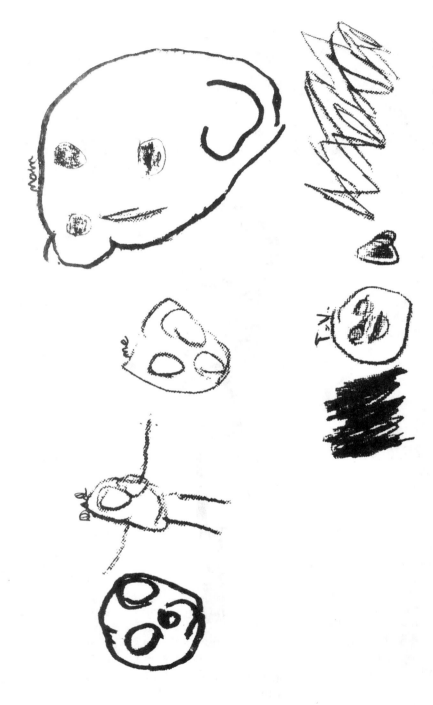

FIGURE 1.5. Joey's drawing of his family. From the collection of Cathy A. Malchiodi (not to be reproduced without permission from the author).

bottom of the drawing, explaining that it was "something to look at" (a distraction) when things got particularly tense or violent in their home.

While Joey's drawings opened up even more questions about how to help him, I was even more curious about what might be troubling Christa. She continued to appear immobilized, and when she did speak, her affect varied from anger to depression; at other times, she would present with a forced smile. On some occasions, she physically clung to me or fell asleep on my shoulder. During this shelter stay, I was finally able to engage her in some expressive work, including drawing a human figure (Figure 1.6). When asked to tell a story about the drawing, the only thing Christa could

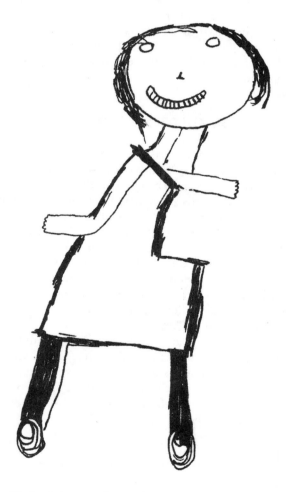

FIGURE 1.6. Christa's human figure drawing titled "Cavewoman." From the collection of Cathy A. Malchiodi (not to be reproduced without permission from the author).

do was to give it the title "Cavewoman." The drawing startled me because of its unsettling affect and characteristics I had never seen before, including distortions of the body and missing elements normally included by children in Christa's age range. In fact, Christa accurately captured her own facial expression, including her vacant stare that I repeatedly witnessed during sessions.

During several more sessions, Christa began to reveal through drawings and verbal disclosures the extent of the severity of her experiences. As child protective services suspected, she had experienced numerous incidents of sexual abuse by different men who lived in their home. As her story unfolded, it became apparent that Christa was also the victim of human trafficking initiated by her mother and various procurers. While traumatic events continued to be a part of her life as described elsewhere in this book, at this point she and Joey were removed from Joelle's custody and placed in a residential psychiatric facility where they could receive more intensive long-term treatment.

FORMULATING A THEORY

When I first began writing about cases similar to Christa and Joey, I noted that "it would be logical to conclude that long-term trauma could dramatically alter cognition and in turn, the content and style of art expressions" (Malchiodi, 1990, p. 152). I also speculated that there were more distinctly different therapeutic challenges for "those children whose abuse has been chronic since early childhood" (p. 152) than for those children who experienced more limited traumatic events. Arts- and play-based expressions of children who endured repeated assaultive incidents were also quite different from those produced by young clients who were exposed to one or two violent episodes at home. Christa and Joey were possibly my first cases of what later became known as developmental trauma (Spinazzola, van der Kolk, & Ford, 2018; van der Kolk, 2005). Countless practitioners have recognized this constellation of reactions in chronically traumatized children, but at the time of my shelter work, we did not have a working definition of developmental trauma or of any specific strategies to begin to address the complex nature of these young clients. My colleagues reported the same wide range of behaviors that tested our clinical skills on a daily basis.

Ultimately, children like Sally, Mike, Christa, and Joey helped me to develop a set of theories and principles identifying why expressive arts strategies should be a key part of trauma intervention. Sally, whose trauma impacted her physical health, completely changed my thinking about trauma's impact to one that included the body's ability to "internalize anxiety, fear and other feelings," resulting in somatic symptoms (Malchiodi, 1990, p. 30). Through play, Mike displayed what was then called post-traumatic play (Terr, 1981), a repetitive engagement with expressive media and toys that never quite brought about positive change or resolution of distress.

Christa and Joey, whose experiences of chronic abuse created what we now commonly refer to as a freeze response, guided me in reframing my application of expressive arts approaches in two basic ways: (1) to pay attention to an individual's gestures and get the body moving when stressed and (2) to help individuals express the body's "felt sense" of trauma through not only art and play, but also music, sound, movement, and dramatic enactment.

Women who had been sexually abused as children also helped me to learn more about the role of expressive therapies with adults, many of whom displayed reactions similar to those shown by children from violent homes. Most of these individuals were challenged by periods of immobilization and/or hyperarousal as a result of multiple traumatic events involving violence, assault, abandonment, and neglect during childhood and adolescence. The majority of the referrals of these women to my practice and outpatient groups actually came because each had kept art or writing journals that they felt were personally reparative in some way. Some explained that making simple drawings or pasting images cut from magazines was the only way to calm themselves when memories of trauma or hyperarousal became overwhelming. Others shared that their images, even when rudimentary or primitive, contained what they believed were the actual stories of what they had survived as children; some women described their drawings as voices from their childhoods that were silenced due to repeated abuse by a parent or other family member (Figure 1.7). These survivors often explained that creating doodles, collages, and painting reduced hyperactivation and other symptoms of physical distress from traumatic memories.

Just as I had done with children from violent homes, I also began introducing movement, sound, music, improvisation and dramatic enactment, and creative writing to help adult survivors of sexual abuse find expressive ways to not only self-regulate and self-soothe, but also to expand beyond "talk only" that did not seem to be consistently helpful. What I began to learn from these individuals was that the action-oriented nature of expressive arts could be a way to cope with what would later be commonly identified as the dissociative episodes many experienced regularly because of traumatic memories. While many of these survivors believed their drawings depicted memories of abuse or violence experienced as children, it was also clear that these were not explicit, chronological memories of events. The implicit "felt sense" of the events continued to be very real and was contained in their drawings, collages, movement, and other nonverbal forms of communication.

THE ARTS IN PSYCHOTHERAPY

As a foundation to understanding exactly how expressive arts approaches can be effective change agents and how they complement current strategies to address trauma, it is important to know a little bit about the use

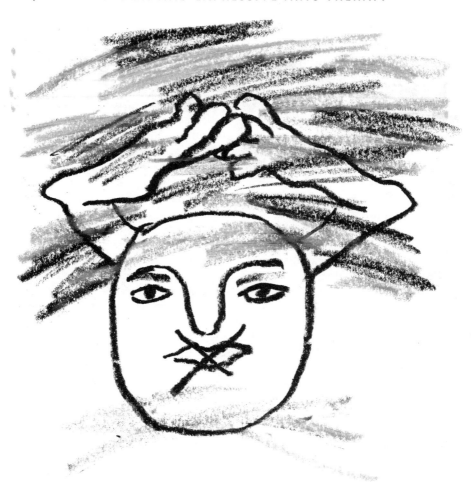

FIGURE 1.7. Participant's drawing of "voices from my childhood and from my abusers and how do we make them stop." From the collection of Cathy A. Malchiodi (not to be reproduced without permission from the author).

of the arts in psychotherapy and their unique role in emotional reparation. Humans have an extensively documented and long history of using the arts for self-expression, self-regulation, reparation, and commemoration, with numerous references throughout medicine, anthropology, and the arts to the earliest healing applications of these forms of communication (Malchiodi, 2007). Image-making, ritual, movement, dramatic enactment, imaginative play, music, and storytelling are repeatedly cited as ways humans make experiences and events special, and address loss, disaster, and traumatic events, even as a form of preventative and reparative treatment

(Dissanayake, 1995). Perry (2015) summarizes these ethnological findings from a modern-day, neurobiology-informed perspective:

> Amid the current pressure for "evidence-based practice" parameters, we should remind ourselves that the most powerful evidence is that which comes from hundreds of separate cultures across the thousands of generations independently converging on rhythm, touch, storytelling, and reconnection to community . . . as the core ingredients to coping and healing from trauma. (p. xii)

Similarly, Botton and Armstrong (2013) note the continual role of art in mediating humans' psychological shortcomings, restoring equilibrium and aspects of the self that can be sensed but often cannot be articulated.

The first formal applications of the arts (visual art, music, dance, drama, and creative writing) in psychotherapy emerged in the 20th century as distinct approaches with a variety of theoretical and methodological frameworks. Some of these applications were unique to the particular art form, and others were hybrids of psychiatry and different art forms. Because these approaches are essentially interdisciplinary, each developed not only from arts-based methods and practices, but also from psychological theories, sociocultural concepts, education, and, more recently, neurobiological principles. Eventually, these applications of the arts as forms of therapy came to be collectively known as the *creative arts therapies* and included specific applications of art therapy, music therapy, dance/movement therapy, drama therapy, and poetry therapy within a variety of psychotherapeutic frameworks (Malchiodi, 2006). These five major domains are defined here.

Art Therapy

Art therapy is the purposeful use of visual art materials and media in intervention, counseling, psychotherapy, and rehabilitation; it is used with individuals of all ages, families, and groups. Within the applications of art therapy, there is a continuum of practice ranging from art as therapy (art making as a reparative, life-enhancing activity) (Malchiodi, 2006; McNiff, 2009) to art psychotherapy (the purposeful, integrative application of arts-based intervention within a variety of psychotherapeutic and counseling approaches) (Malchiodi, 2012a). Most practitioners use a combination of "art as therapy" and art psychotherapy approaches, integrating a variety of psychotherapeutic frameworks, including psychoanalytic, Jungian, humanistic, cognitive-behavioral, and family systems (Malchiodi, 2012c). Many practitioners believe that art expressions communicate aspects of personality, perceptions, and developmental and cognitive characteristics of the art maker. These communications complement or add to the verbal exchange between therapist and client and illuminate the verbal component of talk therapy.

Music Therapy

Music therapy uses music perception, production, and reproduction to effect positive changes in the psychological, physical, cognitive, or social functioning of individuals with physical, behavioral, social, emotional, or educational challenges (American Music Therapy Association [AMTA], 2019; Wheeler, 2016). According to Bruscia (1998), it is a systematic process of "intervention wherein the therapist helps the client to promote health, using music experiences and the relationships that develop through them as dynamic forces of change" (p. 20). In terms of rehabilitation and/or recovery from a variety of disorders or challenges, it enhances integration of sensation and emotions and supports self-regulation through arousal reduction, externalization, containment, and healthy attachment between the individual and therapist (Ghetti & Whitehead-Pleaux, 2015). Music therapy is closely related to other forms of intervention, including *music medicine* (use of music to address physiological status and overall wellness) and *music and neuromusicology* (study of music responses; Wheeler, 2016), two of many areas in which music is used as part of overall health care.

Drama Therapy

Drama therapy is defined as an active, experiential approach to facilitating change through storytelling, projective play, purposeful improvisation, and performance (Johnson, 2009b; National Drama Therapy Association [NDTA], 2019). It uses the body as a medium, capitalizing on voice, prosody, facial expressions, and gestures to help individuals tell their stories and resolve problems, achieve catharsis, extend the depth of inner experience, and strengthen the ability to understand the self and others (NDTA, 2019). While drama therapy has been formalized through education and specific concepts, there are variations found in the practices of psychodrama (Dayton & Moreno, 2004) and acting techniques such as aesthetic distancing and mimetic induction (Ali & Wolfert, 2019). Play therapy capitalizes on imaginative drama as one of many purposeful enactment experiences provided to address children in treatment. Other approaches, such as narrative therapy (Denborough, 2016; White & Epston, 1990), also integrate the power of dramatic storytelling into the experience of psychotherapy. More recently, van der Kolk (Interlandi, 2014) has used variations of role play and enactment to help individuals project their inner worlds into the three-dimensional space inherent to performance.

Dance/Movement Therapy

Dance/movement therapy, based on the idea that body and mind are interrelated, is defined as the psychotherapeutic use of movement as a process that furthers the emotional, cognitive, and physical integration of the individual and influences changes in feelings, cognition, physical functioning, and behavior (American Dance Therapy Association [ADTA], 2019; Gray, 2015). It is grounded in the premise that movement supports brain plasticity (Perry, 2015) and therefore has the capacity with the therapeutic relationship to promote learning, rehabilitation, and well-being. Because it can be both an emotionally and physically restorative approach, dance/movement therapy is not only a creative arts therapy, but also a form of somatic psychotherapy (Gray, 2015). There are a variety of dance-, movement-, and body-based approaches that are not dance/movement therapy per se, but are used in similar ways. For example, yoga is increasingly being employed as a "trauma-sensitive" intervention for self-regulatory and stress-related purposes (van der Kolk, 2014), and Sensorimotor Psychotherapy® (Ogden & Fisher, 2015) incorporates many elements similar to the formal practice of dance/movement therapy.

Poetry Therapy and Bibliotherapy

The terms *poetry therapy* and *bibliotherapy* are used synonymously to describe the intentional use of poetry and other forms of literature for healing and personal growth (National Association for Poetry Therapy, 2019). There is also the broader realm of creative writing and "journaling" (Progoff, 1992), both of which have a long history of application to emotional repair. For example, creative and expressive writing in the form of journaling or written narrative is another important and relevant approach for many individuals, particularly those who have experienced trauma or illness (Pennebaker & Chung, 2011).

Play Therapy

Play therapy, though not defined as a creative art, is another means of expressive communication that has much in common with the arts, particularly the imagination as a source of reparation. It is defined as the systematic use of play to help individuals prevent or resolve psychosocial difficulties and achieve optimal growth and development, and it employs a variety of theoretical orientations, including child-centered, Jungian, Adlerian, cognitive-behavioral, and others (Crenshaw & Stewart, 2016). It is nearly as old as the field of psychotherapy itself and is generally used with children, but it is also employed with families (Gil, 2016). Play therapists use a wide range of creative interventions that include toys, props, games, sandplay, and expressive arts and are very similar in theory and approach to those of arts-based therapists who apply many forms of creative intervention in their work. For example, a play therapist may invite a child to engage in painting or work with clay and then facilitate role play or storytelling through puppets, provide imaginative props, or encourage the use of toy miniatures in a sandbox.

EXPRESSIVE ARTS THERAPY:
INTEGRATING ALL THE SENSES

Humans have historically used the arts in integrative ways, particularly within the contexts of enactment, ceremony, performance, and ritual. However, the creative arts therapies described in the previous section have developed somewhat in isolation from each other over many decades and within their own "silos." There has been relatively little cross-fertilization between creative arts therapies approaches in terms of practice, education, and research because each creative arts therapy has carved out a circumscribed domain and educational standards. In reality, there are many important commonalities across these approaches that complement each other and are necessary to effective applications of arts-based strategies in work with traumatized individuals. To me, it is the integrative synergy of the arts, based on cultural traditions and current trauma-informed practice, that is requisite to addressing traumatic stress with most children, adults, families, groups, and communities.

Expressive arts therapy is a field of practice that emerged in the latter part of the 20th century. In contrast to individual applications of specific art forms described in the previous section, expressive arts therapy is understood as the use of more than one art form, consecutively or in combination and depending on individual or group goals. In other words, one art form may dominate a session, or multiple forms may be introduced in work with a child, adult, family, or group. As mental health and health care have shifted toward more integrative approaches to treatment, expressive arts therapy has gained the attention of a wide range of practitioners interested in applying sensory-based, action-oriented methods within their work, rather than one arts-based approach. In particular, the field of arts in health care has cited the role of expressive arts therapy in hospitals, inferring that it is one of the key strategies currently being used to humanize patient care through the integration of all the arts and psychotherapy (National Organization for Arts in Health [NOAH], 2019).

Shaun McNiff (2009), considered one of the founders of the field of expressive arts therapy, noted, "When art and psychotherapy are joined, the scope and depth of each can be expanded, and when working together, they are tied to the continuities of humanity's history of healing" (p. 259). In brief, he is referring to two basic principles inherent to the use of expressive arts in psychotherapy. First, the arts are forms of self-expression that not only complement the process of therapy, but also can illuminate and extend the value and possibilities for change, reparation, and growth within the therapeutic process. Second, the combined use of the arts for health and well-being, including the amelioration of trauma, is not something new; it is part of humankind's collective history to use art, music and sound, movement and dance, dramatic enactment, and other forms of imagination in response to trauma and loss.

Estrella (2006) provides one of the clearest general overviews of the current practice of expressive arts therapy, underscoring the interrelationship of the arts within treatment and the integrative nature of the approach within the framework of psychotherapy. She observes, "Expressive therapists use a multimodal approach—at times working with the arts in sequence, at other times using the arts simultaneously, and at still other times carefully transitioning from one art form to another within the therapeutic encounter" (p. 183). Estrella emphasizes that expressive arts therapy is not so much media-based, but rather is related to sensory-based expression, aesthetics (beauty, harmony, rhythm, resonance, dynamic tension, and balance), and the creative process itself. In this sense, the approach is similar to integrative psychotherapists who rely on common curative factors among various schools of psychotherapy. This is the foundation, according to Estrella, for making decisions about how to introduce and integrate various art forms into individual and group sessions.

There are many key figures in the development of the field of expressive arts therapy, but three in particular have had a lasting and significant impact in defining theory and practice. One is Natalie Rogers (1993), an early proponent of expressive arts as a humanistic form of psychotherapy. She explains expressive arts therapy as "uses of various arts—movement, drawing, painting, sculpting, music, writing, sound and improvisation—in a supportive setting to facilitate growth and healing." Moreover, Rogers states that "it is not about creating a pretty picture. It is not a dance ready for the stage. It is not a poem written and rewritten to perfection" (pp. 1–2). Rogers also speaks of a *creative connection* between the arts that refers to the use of intuitive expression through different media, individually or in combination. In contrast to diagnostic practices, expressive arts therapy is a humanistic experience that capitalizes on both the imagination and the integrative possibilities inherent to the arts. The goal is to enhance the interplay of the arts to support self-exploration and to "connect" to oneself through arts-based experiences.

Rogers's approach to expressive arts therapy was greatly influenced by her father, Carl Rogers, who is widely known for person-centered counseling that emphasizes the therapist's role as empathetic, open, caring, and congruent. The person-centered philosophy includes the premise that all individuals are capable of manifesting growth and have an innate capacity to reach full potential in life. Therefore, person-centered expressive arts not only summarize Natalie Rogers's approach to therapy, but also her own experience of personal integration via the arts and the philosophy she inherited from her father. In sum, she opened up a conversation within the fields of expressive arts therapy, psychotherapy, and counseling about the integrative nature of the purposeful interplay of various arts-based media for emotional reparation and ultimately health and well-being.

Paolo Knill conceptualized an expressive arts practice known as *intermodal expressive therapy* (Knill, Barba, & Fuchs, 1995). He initially trained as a musician and an engineer and later, as a professor in higher education in both the United States and Europe, he became involved in developing the field of expressive arts therapy. Among other contributions, he originated the concepts of *intermodal transfer* (the shift from one art form to another) and *low skill–high sensitivity* (facilitation of competence in artistic expression in all individuals, regardless of skill or formal training in the arts) (Knill et al., 1995, pp. 147–153). Additionally, the idea of *crystallization* emerged from Knill's teaching and work. In brief, it refers to how various sensory experiences can crystallize into art expressions through the process of expressive arts therapy. For example, sound becomes music; image becomes a drawing, painting, or sculpture; and movement becomes dance and so forth.

Finally, McNiff (2009) is widely recognized for promoting "all of the arts" as a meaningful and effective therapy and as an integrative method for engaging "the whole person in the therapeutic process" (p. 3). Over several decades he established many of the contemporary educational foundations in the field. Primarily a visual artist and art therapy educator, McNiff proposes that the connectedness of the arts in psychotherapy provides the necessary dynamics for personal growth and well-being, and, most importantly, he more accurately addresses the totality of the senses—gesture, body movement, imagery, sound, word, and enactment. In sum, drawing on a number of available creative processes is fundamental to meeting individuals where they are in their own healing. While practitioners may apply a single art form as part of treatment, McNiff, Knill, and Natalie Rogers underscore the interplay of the expressive arts as a key factor in supporting more complete and inclusive opportunities for authentic expression in psychotherapy.

BUT IS THERE EVIDENCE?

Like any emerging set of practices, the evidence for expressive arts therapy, expressive arts, and individual applications of creative arts therapies is at best mixed, and the fields still have a long way to go in establishing a reliable and valid body of evidence. Like many other novel approaches such as massage and yoga, necessary research funding sources to conduct large-scale trials and other forms of investigations have limited investigations. But there are other challenges, too. Many of the basic mechanisms proposed to be healing factors have been difficult to isolate and measure, and actual components (language, relational dynamics, and specific psychotherapeutic frameworks) responsible for reparation are yet to be adequately defined within the context of arts-based approaches. Also, although expressive arts therapy and creative arts therapies have existed for at least 50 years and have produced numerous publications, few specific practices have been clearly documented or standardized. This has made it difficult to measure the efficacy of these practices to identify what actually works to achieve specific outcomes. The vast majority of the literature on expressive arts therapy is philosophical, describing the integrative use of the arts through anecdotal accounts and first-person observations. There has even been some resistance from some practitioners, proposing that the arts therapies cannot be adequately measured due to the nature of the arts themselves.

Although mostly small-scale studies still provide most of the data, fortunately there has been an increase in randomized controlled trials within specific forms of creative arts therapies. While these studies have revealed some promising strategies, the limited results are often confounded by lack of adequate control groups, small sample size, and reliability of instruments or procedures used to measure data. One particularly challenging characteristic of many of the existing arts-based studies is the lack of definition of what constitutes, for example, a creative arts therapy or an expressive arts therapy approach versus a purely arts-based activity. In other words, it is often unclear what is specifically different about a specific arts-based therapy or expressive arts therapy in comparison to arts-based experiences that have therapeutic value.

Three categories of data capture what is currently understood about arts-based approaches: (1) meta-analyses that cull data to identify reparative mechanisms; (2) "value-added" studies that examine arts-based approaches in combination with evidence-based approaches; and (3) individual feedback on the impact of arts-based approaches within treatment. The summaries provided are not exhaustive, but they do capture what is known and what areas remain as challenges for future research.

Meta-Analyses

To date, the majority of research has focused on distinguishing the best creative arts therapies practices through different forms of meta-analyses to attempt to identify the most likely reparative mechanisms in these practices. For example, Landis-Shack, Heinz, and Bonn-Miller (2017) specifically examined existing music therapy literature, summarizing key empirical studies that support its efficacy in the specific treatment of post-traumatic stress, including social, cognitive, and neurobiological mechanisms (community building, emotion regulation, increased pleasure, and anxiety reduction). They concluded that music therapy may reduce symptoms and improve functioning among individuals with trauma exposure and post-traumatic stress. Similarly, a research team interviewed a small sample of dance/movement therapists who had been working with individuals with a history of trauma or post-traumatic stress to ascertain how dance/movement therapy could be an effective intervention with adult populations. This study isolated several core strategies that are key to applying dance/movement therapy to trauma intervention, including a phase model (warm-up, movement themes derived from the warm-up, and ending integrating talk therapy to clarify what transpired during the session). Music, props, mirroring, breathing, and grounding techniques were used to support awareness of where sensations related to trauma are held in the body. Most respondents also recommended that group sessions rather than individual treatment may be more effective in working with trauma in adults.

In the field of art therapy, an analysis was conducted specifically to identify recommendations for targeted art therapy strategies with combat and veteran military. The analysis was conducted by a research team consisting of art therapists Kate Collie and Amy Backos, psychiatrist David Spiegel, and me (Spiegel, Malchiodi, Backos, & Collie, 2006). After a meta-analysis of the existing literature, the team concluded that art-making, especially in the context of post-traumatic stress disorder (PTSD) and the military, enhances feelings of safety and relaxation, generates positive and more regulated emotions, and promotes relational bonding. Furthermore, they proposed that arts-based approaches could help integrate fragmentary and sensory traumatic memories based on what was learned from the data. Since publication of this analysis, progress continues to be slow in establishing and completing studies to examine the findings and recommendations, although a few studies have emerged (Jones, Walker, Drass, & Kaimal, 2018).

One comprehensive meta-analysis of creative arts therapy research focusing on stress management and prevention may provide some reliable clues as to where arts-based approaches might be as effective as mind–body interventions with traumatized individuals. Building on current integrative and embodied stress theories (Payne, Levine, & Crane-Godreau, 2015), Martin and colleagues (2018) sought to identify which creative arts therapies (art, music, dance/movement, and drama) or arts interventions prevented stress and improved stress management. Of the 37 studies they examined, 73% were randomized controlled trials and 81% reported significant stress reduction in participants owing to one of the four art modalities. The researchers rated the evidence level for each of the studies, and while studies of art, music, and dance therapies and interventions did meet the criteria for evidence at varying levels, drama therapy and drama interventions did not. Also, art, music, and dance interventions demonstrated higher evidence levels as forms of stress reduction and prevention than formal creative arts therapies. Music therapy was the only arts-based approach that achieved what could be defined as evidence of efficacy; music interventions also showed evidence of efficacy, in some cases surpassing music therapy in terms of robustness. While the Martin and colleagues study provided more details about each creative arts approach, it also underscored that more often arts-based interventions (art, music, and dance) have been successfully measured in contrast to what are defined as actual creative arts therapies. Also, creative writing was omitted from this analysis, an area that has at least some relevance to trauma reparation;

many studies indicate its usefulness in addressing symptoms and supporting health and well-being (Pennebaker & Smyth, 2016).

"Value-Added" Studies

Another promising way to understand how arts-based approaches contribute to the treatment of trauma is to consider its role as a "valued-added" strategy. In other words, when a specific arts-based approach is added to an existing evidence-based treatment protocol, does it strengthen positive effects? Mindfulness-based art therapy (MBAT; Monti et al., 2006), a series of integrative mindfulness, yoga, and art therapy sessions for cancer patients, is one good example of this. The multimodal design combined these approaches using self-regulation theory and mindfulness-based stress reduction (MBSR; Kabat-Zinn, Lipworth, & Burney, 1985) as the foundation for development of procedures to decrease distress and improve quality of life through health-promoting skills. MBSR has had documented success in reducing stress in cancer populations (Carlson, Speca, Patel, & Goodey, 2004) and is considered one way to enhance self-regulation through cultivation of focused attention and self-acceptance in the present moment. In this particular study, the introduction of art therapy provided a "value-added" component of exploring feelings in tangible and personally meaningful ways while also supporting self-regulation through strategically selected art-making experiences.

Individual Feedback

Finally, simply asking individuals in treatment for their opinions about what they feel works and what treatments keep them engaged in what is often a long process of trauma recovery can tell us a lot about "what works." In other words, just what gets people to come to treatment and stick with it, including those individuals whose trauma is overwhelming and who do not choose to continue standard methods such as cognitive-behavioral therapy (CBT) or prolonged exposure therapy? Fortunately, more researchers as well as treatment facilities are examining this question, providing some consensus on individuals' experiences with various forms of arts-based therapies. For example, a 2012–2014 survey at the National Intrepid Center of Excellence (NICoE), which asked participants to indicate which techniques or tools they found most helpful in improving their recovery, ranked art therapy among the top five most helpful techniques used to treat veterans (Creative Forces, 2018). Similarly, researchers concluded that individuals who may feel stigmatized when asking for more mainstream forms of professional help are more likely to engage in music therapy and thus may be willing to come to treatment (Bronson, Vaudreuil, & Bradt, 2018). While these types of surveys do not verify which treatments are best to ameliorate trauma-related reactions, these results do indicate more patient compliance, thus getting individuals to return to hospitals and facilities rather than completely giving up on psychotherapeutic intervention.

Although cumulative findings are not strong enough to say that expressive arts therapy or any single form of creative arts therapy demonstrates an acceptable level of evidence and outcomes, there is certainly enough data to say that we know that something probably is working for at least some individuals when it comes to trauma. Findings from smaller-scale studies are included throughout this book to explain the rationale for arts-based methods and practices to address trauma. Based on what is known through current data, it is possible to begin to hypothesize about the specific mechanisms that may support reparative and integrative processes when it comes to trauma.

EIGHT KEY REASONS TO INCLUDE EXPRESSIVE ARTS

Although research tells us something about why expressive arts therapy as well as creative arts therapies may be an effective part of the continuum of approaches to address trauma, clinical literature has also helped to clarify best and emerging practices. The International Society for Traumatic Stress Studies (ISTSS; Foa, Keane, Friedman, & Cohen, 2009) created a series of guidelines for the treatment of trauma, including arts-based strategies, noting emerging evidence on art therapy, music therapy, dance/movement therapy, various forms of therapeutic writing, and drama therapy. These ISTSS guidelines underscore how the creative arts therapies often include forms of imaginal exposure, cognitive restructuring, and self-regulation in addressing trauma (Johnson, Lahad, & Gray, 2009) and involve techniques similar to stress management and cognitive-behavioral methods used in talk therapies. Within these ISTSS guidelines, it is evident that some practitioners may focus on one particular art process to address trauma reactions and that others use more than one approach to achieve goals (such as art therapy, dramatic enactment, and creative writing during a session). Although expressive arts therapy by definition involves more than one arts-based approach, an individual may find one form of creative expression more helpful than others.

Since the time these guidelines were published, there has been a shift to incorporate more current brain–body approaches rather than solely cognitive restructuring, exposure therapy, and stress management. Based on current evidence-based and emerging brain–body practices, there are eight key reasons for including expressive arts in trauma intervention: (1) letting the senses tell the story; (2) self-soothing mind and body; (3) engaging the body; (4) enhancing nonverbal communication; (5) recovering self-efficacy; (6) rescripting the trauma story; (7) imagining new meaning; and (8) restoring aliveness. Each of these eight reasons is explained below and in more detail throughout subsequent chapters.

Letting the Senses Tell the Story

Neurobiology research has taught helping professionals that we need to "come to our senses" in developing effective components for trauma intervention. Traumatic reactions are not just a series of distressing thoughts and feelings; they are experienced on a sensory level by mind and body, a concept now increasingly echoed within a variety of theories and approaches by trauma experts. As early as 1990, psychiatrist Lenore Terr observed that individuals' memories of trauma are more sensory, implicit, and perceptional than explicit or declarative. A few years later, van der Kolk (1994) noted that traumatic experiences may not always be encoded as explicit memory and may be stored as nonverbal, sensory fragments. More recently, many trauma specialists have embraced the idea that the "body keeps the score" (van der Kolk, 1994, 2014). This increased acceptance of the implicit nature of traumatic memories and a greater understanding of the body's dysregulation as a result of distressing experiences have led to the development of many sensory-based (Ogden, Minton, & Pain, 2006), body-oriented (Levine, 1997), and "brain-wise" (Badenoch, 2008) methods.

Possibly the most compelling reason for use of the expressive arts in trauma work is the sensory nature of the arts themselves; their qualities involve visual, tactile, olfactory, auditory, vestibular, and proprioceptive experiences. They are also believed to predominantly access the right brain and implicit memory (Johnson et al., 2009) because they include a variety of sensory-based experiences, including images, sounds, and tactile and movement experiences that are related to right-hemisphere functions. Current opinion about trauma supports the idea that trauma is encoded as a form of sensory reality (Rothschild, 2000), underscoring the idea that expression and processing of implicit memories have an important role in successful intervention and resolution. The qualities found in arts-based expression are thought to tap these memories of events (Malchiodi, 2012b, 2012c; Steele & Malchiodi, 2011), releasing the potential of the senses to "tell the story" of traumatic experiences via an implicit form of communication. Some trauma specialists also emphasize that sensory expression found in the expressive arts may make progressive exposure of the trauma story and expression of traumatic material more tolerable, helping to overcome avoidance and allowing the therapeutic process to advance relatively quickly (Spiegel et al., 2006).

Self-Soothing Brain and Body

One of the first things I noticed in work with children exposed to interpersonal violence was how they physically responded to art-making and play activities. While these young clients often remained hypervigilant or withdrawn during therapy sessions, they also actively sought ways to self-soothe, a response we now commonly refer to as "self-regulation." Some children found relief in simply watching paint disperse in a jar filled with water; others seemed to lose themselves in creating repetitive patterns while drawing, doodling, or scribbling. Expressive arts and play activities also served as a form of brief dissociation from anxieties or fears. In most cases, these children found refuge and respite through rhythmic kinesthetic, sensory-based experiences.

Purposeful applications of expressive arts therapy support self-regulation, and for this reason they are often used to help children and adults reduce hyperactivation and the stress responses that result from traumatic events. They can be combined with other standard approaches; for example, art therapy has been combined with mindfulness-based practices to induce and deepen relaxation (Monti et al., 2006; Rappaport, 2015). Similarly, focusing-oriented expressive arts therapy capitalizes on breathing, mindfulness, movement, focus-oriented techniques, and other sensory-based experiences to help traumatized individuals experience a sense of general well-being (Rappaport, 2009). Music therapy has considerable success in reducing hyperarousal, including measurable physiological responses such as heart rate and sympathetic nervous system reactions (Ghetti & Whitehead-Pleaux, 2015). Related studies underscore the role of music, sound, and rhythm in stimulating the senses to mediate depression and anxiety and enhance resilience (Fancourt et al., 2016; Wheeler, 2016). In brief, most expressive arts therapy sessions integrate rhythmic breathing, mindfulness-related practices, and other calming routines into overall intervention, particularly when working with individuals who have experienced traumatic events (Johnson et al., 2009).

Individuals in treatment often note that the structure, containment, and grounding qualities that expressive arts provide feel "safer than words." In contrast to asking individuals to revisit distressful events and emotions that the mind and body try to avoid, expressive arts interventions generally seek to establish an emotional distance from traumatic memories to establish a sense of safety, first and foremost. For example, dramatic enactment and imaginative play capitalizes on distance, allowing the therapist to help participants explore problems or distressing emotions through metaphor rather than reality. The simple act of drawing provides a way to make tangible a sensation or feeling, placing outside oneself on paper. In brief, creative approaches have the potential to support self-regulation by giving individuals ways to separate from what is going on internally while experiencing what is often a pleasurable or novel creative experience.

Engaging the Body

While some therapists believe that body-based techniques are useful adjuncts to treatment, many now view the body as central in the process of trauma reparation. In the 1970s, Pat Ogden (Ogden et al., 2006) started to pay attention to individuals' dissociations from their bodies and their emotions; she developed Sensorimotor Psychotherapy to specifically address the somatic reactions from trauma such as body numbing and inhibitions in movement. Similarly, Levine (1997) identified the body's responses to trauma as key to eventual trauma resolution and integration.

Expressive arts therapy is one of the few approaches to trauma treatment that consistently involves the body in some way. Art forms like dance and drama obviously include physical movement, but we also sense something in our bodies when we make art, play a musical instrument, engage in creative writing, and even when we look at an artwork in a museum, listen to music, or read powerful prose or poetry. Kossak (2015) refers to this phenomenon as *embodied intelligence* and observes that it is one of the foundations of expressive arts therapy. The term *embodied* refers to the body-centered intelligence that informs one of what one knows and experiences in the environment. Traumatized individuals, especially those who have endured chronic traumatic events, find themselves literally cut off from their bodies or, at the very least, are not conscious of how their bodies are communicating or sensing from their surroundings, the embodied intelligence to which Kossak refers. Gardner (1993) identifies a similar *body-kinesthetic intelligence*, and dance/movement therapist Whitehouse (1995) adds that the body ultimately is a source of memory storage, emotions, and associations to oneself, others, and the world.

The same soothing qualities of expressive arts described in the previous section also serve as forms of embodied intelligence, reintroducing individuals to how the body communicates sensations and emotions related to trauma. These body-based experiences may come in the form of anchoring and grounding; transcendence and peak moments of achievement; or focused awareness and presence in the moment where there is a full sense of engagement in the ongoing experience. While investigating the experience of attunement in expressive arts, Kossak (2008) discovered that many participants felt a perceptible change in not only cognitive and emotional awareness, but also somatic sensations. In brief, expressive arts therapy naturally shifts individuals from being "in their minds" to being more fully in their bodies. In cases where individuals are immobilized due to unresolved trauma, arts-based methods can also facilitate a reconnection with the body when frozen due to overwhelming memories, reactions, or sensations.

Enhancing Nonverbal Communication

The practice of psychotherapy is historically based on talking to resolve distress and crises. This tradition goes back to Freud and his contemporaries who proposed that trauma was best resolved through the patient's detailed verbal descriptions of upsetting experiences and through clear recall of the memories that initiated distress. In contrast, survivors of trauma make one common observation about the limits of language when it comes to psychological distress. They say, "If I only could tell you about it with words," "I don't know how to describe it," or "Words are not enough to say what I want to say." Some individuals, depending on the impact of trauma on mind and body, find they cannot speak at all, displaying a freeze response when traumatic memories are stimulated; Sandra, a survivor of domestic violence described earlier in the chapter, is a good example of this type of response. van der Kolk (2014) found that the language area of the brain is impacted in many cases of post-traumatic stress; this inability to express oneself through words seems to occur when articulating "what happened" is overwhelming or reactivates trauma reactions.

Talking about what happened may also bring about powerful sensations of shame in those individuals whose experiences involve guilt or embarrassment, such as a soldier who was unable to protect a friend who was killed in combat, children who believe they caused themselves to be abused or violated, or survivors of disasters who feel at fault when they cannot adequately cope with their emotions. Speaking about these perceptions does not necessarily provide experiences of self-repair for all individuals; they may even fear rejection or additional shaming from those who hear their stories, despite their simultaneous need to be validated for what they have endured and survived. The actual telling of a trauma narrative is often unpleasant not only for the speaker, but also for those who are listening to the story.

As emphasized earlier in this chapter, one key advantage of the expressive arts in trauma intervention is the ability to circumvent the limits of language and to provide additional channels and opportunities for communication when words are not possible. In this sense, these approaches offer the possibility to externalize implicit experiences without words. Creative expression also serves as a nonverbal means for "breaking the silence" (Malchiodi, 1990, 1997) and for "telling without talking" (Malchiodi, 2008) for those individuals who cannot speak publicly about their experiences for various reasons. In *Trauma and Recovery*, Herman (1992) explains that individuals need the opportunity to express their stories in some way in order not only to restore oneself, but also to alter the impact of trauma on the larger community and society. Working with adult survivors of domestic violence and sexual assault taught me that art is one way that individuals find a way to "tell without talking," reinforcing much of what Herman underscores about the essential aspect of expressing personal narratives. Similarly, throughout the United States significant numbers of combat veterans are involved in arts-based communities and various performance groups that provide self-expression, which also breaks the silence about atrocities that "refuse to be buried" (Herman, 1992, p. 1). Although these experiences do not constitute formal therapy, these examples and many other similar ones underscore a consistent drive among humans to seek out ways to communicate "what happened" and not necessarily with words alone or at all.

In therapy with children, language is often not possible for developmental reasons, in addition to the impact of trauma events. In work with children from violent homes and communities over many years, I gradually learned that it was important to find ways for them to express their feelings and experiences that bypassed words or, at the very least, created a sense of safety when talking about distressing or terrorizing memories for both developmental and other reasons. For example, in the cases of Christa and Sally described earlier in this chapter, they knew that their personal safety was critical to survival and that their verbal disclosures might reveal details of interpersonal violence that could put them in danger of retaliation from perpetrators. In these circumstances, nonverbal expression about abuse or violence was the only means of disclosing experiences, often through symbolic art expressions or play activity.

There are various ways the expressive arts can support nonverbal externalization of implicit memories or feelings; in art therapy, for example, trauma memories can be communicated through the creative process of making or constructing an image or object. There is also some emerging evidence that creative activities may actually stimulate language. Drawing, for example, facilitates children's verbal reports of emotionally laden events in several ways: reducing anxiety, helping the child feel comfortable with the therapist, increasing memory retrieval, organizing narratives, and prompting the child to tell more details than is possible in a solely verbal interview (Gross & Haynes, 1998; Lev-Weisel & Liraz, 2007). In brief, when verbal communication is limited after traumatic experiences, it may be that some other form of externalization must be used in addition to verbal therapies such as cognitive-behavioral or other accepted approaches to trauma relief (Malchiodi, 2015b).

Recovering Self-Efficacy

An overarching goal of trauma intervention is to help individuals transform feelings associated with what happened in the past to a here-and-now focus (Ogden et al., 2006). There are many reasons why trauma can appropriate one's sense of efficacy, pleasure, and confidence in life. Being unable to speak about "what happened" may cause a loss of self-efficacy and increase a feeling of disempowerment, particularly when interpersonal violence or chronic trauma is present. One thing trauma can steal from any individual is a sense of confidence not only in one's current sense of mastery, but also in the future; trauma challenges the very core of not only who we are, but what we can eventually be, achieve, and enjoy. Therefore, supporting experiences of personal empowerment and mastery are essential to enhancing resilience through reinforcing an internal locus of control and beliefs that one can successfully address new challenges (Malchiodi, 2015a).

In part, I also believe that any effective intervention helps individuals to regain a feeling of vitality and self-efficacy. In other words, it helps individuals rediscover pleasure in life and a sense of mastery. The expressive arts are action-oriented, experiential approaches that not only make non-verbal communication possible, but also capitalize on active participation. For example, art making, even in its simplest sense, can involve arranging, touching, gluing, constructing, painting, forming, and many other active experiences. Music not only includes listening, but also making sounds, singing, or playing instruments; dance, drama, and just about all forms of play emphasize movement, physical involvement, and active relationships with props, the environment, and other individuals. With reference to dramatic enactment, Haen (2015) shares that children who are struggling to express themselves "begin to speak when given a character to play; kids unable to talk about their past trauma . . . express it through roleplay" (p. 249). Similarly, play therapy is predicated on providing children with experiences that encourage mastery through toys, props, games, and other creative materials and media. In particular, it is often an important aspect of post-traumatic play (Gil, 2017), with mastery being the central benefit of engagement with toys in the play therapy setting. These are experiences of empowerment, a term used to describe a sense of personal self-efficacy as well as within a larger social context, including community and society (Herman, 1992).

Rescripting the Trauma Story

Eventually, revising or "rescripting" the trauma narrative is often part of most forms of trauma intervention. Johnson and colleagues (2009) note that cognitive restructuring is a key factor in trauma intervention and that cognitive reprocessing and reframing are "essential components of the creative arts therapies" (p. 480). In most cases, the goal of expressive arts and play therapy is to help individuals alter their trauma narratives through revising aspects of events, perceptions, and memories. For example, art and play therapy emphasize the capacity of the child to create and explore personal stories through use of images, toys, puppets, and other props. With the therapist's facilitation, the child gradually restructures, reframes, and revises the trauma narrative. Similarly, drama therapy uses role play and other techniques to help individuals act out various aspects of experiences and perceptions, with a goal of changing the perspectives and worldviews and promoting new, healthier endings to problem-laden narratives.

While the expressive arts are action-oriented and hands-on by nature, they are also experiences that emphasize spontaneity, flexibility, and problem solving. Essentially, all expressive arts embrace the use of imagination as a core experience in the therapeutic process. Although many prefer the word "creativity" in describing the expressive arts therapy, it is actually the use of imagination that informs theory and practice. By definition, creativity occurs when self-expression is fully formed and achieves a novel and aesthetic value. In contrast, imagination is really what is at the center of most arts-based sessions. Participants may not always make art, music, or movements that would be considered creative or fully formed expression, but they are encouraged to engage in imaginative thinking and to pretend when it comes to dramatic enactment or play. In this way, individuals not only can verbally rescript trauma narratives, they can also actively practice novel behaviors and corrective experiences.

Imagining New Meaning

Humans naturally want to make meaning about their experiences, including traumatic events that often seem meaningless and random. When we see a painting in a gallery or even a cloud formation in the sky, we tend to immediately want to make some sort of sense out it, associate a theme or subtext with it, or interpret its possible significance. This form of making meaning may tell us a lot about our own worldviews and how our minds work. But in the process of trauma integration, making meaning also takes on a slightly different importance, one of bringing together what can be many painful and senseless events and experiences. It often comes about when there is a sense of resolution of trauma memories, when the mind and body are no longer hijacked by distressful events that occurred in the past.

Expressive arts therapy provides an opportunity for making meaning in ways that perhaps no other current approach to trauma integration offers. It offers a possibility not only to reauthor the dominant narrative of trauma events, but also to transform them in tangible, sensory-based expressions that have the potential of transcendence (Malchiodi, 2016). When making meaning is successful, it often manifests as creative expression of a post-trauma identity of health and well-being and a new and inspirational story of why one's life has been altered but not broken by traumatic events. For some individuals, art forms such as painting, creating music, or creating dance or drama become experiences to be witnessed by others, reaching well beyond the treatment room and to what Herman (1992) observed to be the final stage of trauma integration—the return to community to re-engage with significant relationships and life in new ways.

Restoring Aliveness

With regard to expressive arts, McNiff (2004) observes that "the circulation of energy within the art and healing experience is the most practical and effective feature of the work we do" (p. 212). The success of any therapeutic work we do is intricately connected to how our interventions restore a sense of *aliveness* in individuals, especially those who are experiencing traumatic stress. By aliveness, I mean not just existing and surviving, but living life with experiences of vitality, joy, and connectedness. In contrast, most traumatized individuals report feeling just the opposite of what aliveness feels like in body, brain, and mind. Those who have responded to developmental trauma through freeze responses and dissociation are disconnected from others and the environment, essentially feeling cut off from any sense of joy or vitality. For others, hypervigilance, panic, or anger dominate, cutting off the capacity to play or experience pleasure. If one is afraid of everything, is numb, or is held captive by anxiety, one cannot feel fully alive in one's body.

Joseph Campbell (2011) said, "I don't believe people are looking for the meaning of life as much as they are looking for the experience of being alive" (p. 150). The feeling Campbell refers to is related to energy and a life force, or what other cultures call chi or prana; in fact, it is believed that when this vital energy is disrupted, illness emerges, and intervention is needed to restore the natural flow. My impression about why aliveness is crucial to the reparative potential of the expressive arts comes not only from working with traumatized individuals, but also directly from my own body-based experiences. As occurs with many people, certain pieces of music always send chills throughout my body no matter how many times I hear them; live theater has a similar impact on me, sending a surge of vitality throughout my body. I experience like sensations through painting, singing in a group, dancing with a partner, engaging in play with others, or being part of a performance.

Like most trauma specialists, I know that researchers can explain the sense of aliveness as the amygdala's role in stimulating arousal, resulting in rapid increases in heart rate, breathing, and electrodermal skin conduction (Levitan, 2006; Sacks, 2007) when one hears certain music, has a peak experience of creativity, or is a witness to a powerful dance performance or stage drama. While neuroscience can verify feelings of arousal that are related to aliveness, people engaged in the arts anecdotally provide many more important details, reporting instances of transcendence, connectedness, affirmation of life, and states of energetic flow. These qualities reflect internalized sensations of animation, vigor, and passion; they are affirmations of life.

The expressive arts have a unique role in restoring a sense of vitality and joy in traumatized individuals because aliveness is not something we can be "talked into." Instead, it is experienced in both mind and body and particularly on a somatosensory level. At the same time, we do not know the exact mechanisms for how the enlivening qualities of the expressive arts come about, how they circulate between individuals, groups, and communities, or even how to adequately describe or evaluate them. While aliveness can be experienced in each of the arts, it is most evident in expressive arts groups where there is collective energy among members. It is a type of energy circulation found in singing, dancing, performing, art making, and even laughing together. It is similar to the interpersonal momentum found in team sports where connection with others impacts player performance. In the arts, individuals are influenced by the energy of the group, making possible creativity, imagination, and play, which is not always possible in isolation. It is a synergy that takes on a life of its own, with one expressive movement, gesture, image, or sound leading naturally to others.

THE CHALLENGE OF CREATIVITY AND IMAGINATION FOR TRAUMA SURVIVORS

Because creativity and imagination are core components of expressive arts therapy, they are also central to how arts-based methods are applied to trauma intervention. Expressive arts therapist Stephen Levine (1992) writes, "healing must be understood as the restoration of a person's imaginative capacity" (p. 41). Expressive arts therapy as a field recognizes that creative and imaginal processes are part of human potential and are not only relegated to a special group of individuals, but also are healing and restorative practices possible for all. One of the core goals of expressive arts is to restore individuals' capacity for creativity and imagination because they are believed to be essential to mental health and physical well-being.

Winnicott (1971) noted that getting clients to learn to engage in imaginative play is a primary task of successful therapy. Similarly, expressive arts therapist Natalie Rogers (1993) suggested that discovering one's "creative connection" taps a universal human potential to repair and heal emotional distress. Contemporary psychotherapists such as Marks-Tarlow (2018) underscore the idea that creativity and imagination promote a necessary sense of safety that sets the stage for engagement in treatment, positive shifts in thoughts and feelings, and ultimately, discovery of novel ways to overcome life's challenges.

Leaders in the field of traumatology also echo the importance of imagination and creativity in trauma work. van der Kolk (2014) makes an eloquent statement about the role of imagination in the treatment of trauma:

> Imagination is absolutely critical to the quality of our lives. Our imagination enables us to leave our routine everyday existence by fantasizing about travel, food, sex, falling in love, or having the last word—all the things that make life interesting. Imagination gives us the opportunity to envision new possibilities—it is an essential launchpad for making our hopes come true. It fires our creativity, relieves our boredom, alleviates our pain, enhances our pleasure, and enriches our most intimate relationships. (p. 17)

By all accounts, support for bringing creativity and imagination into trauma treatment is compelling. It is also a challenge for therapists when they are applying expressive arts within the scope of trauma intervention with some individuals. The connections between the capacities to imagine and create remain murky and are still not well understood, especially when adding recovery from trauma into the mix. In the earliest stages of psychotherapy, creativity and imagination may not always be easy for all individuals, particularly for those who have endured multiple or chronic traumatic events. Imagination and creative output are dependent on the person's ability to conceive something beyond one's established thoughts and dominant narratives. An individual with a chronic history of trauma or early attachment disruptions may already have fixed physiological and emotional responses that interfere with the natural ability to be playful, creative, and imagine new possibilities. In both children and adults, these reactions vary from chaotic, hyperaroused states to withdrawn, emotional numbing and rigid responses that interfere with a sense of safety and the focus often needed to engage in fantasy and artistic expression. While some children who are distressed can turn to play to cope with trauma, for children like Mike distressful and recurrent sensations may be hardwired, and these stubborn narratives are not easily transformed. Until Mike was able to recover some sense of self-efficacy and mastery over his reactions, he had difficulties getting beyond a repetitive post-traumatic narrative of domestic violence and physical abuse in his sandplay and other expressive activities.

The constant presence of fear, a common experience in trauma survivors, can be another disruptive factor when it comes to accessing imagination and creative expression. When I was a fine arts student, my instructors often brought up the concept of fear as a key deterrent to my artistic output. Challenging one's fears is often a common denominator taught in art school, which proposes that it separates artists who have the courage to produce art from those who do not (Bayles & Orland, 2001). When extreme fear or terror is a dominant trauma reaction, the ability to imagine is unavailable, repetitive traumatic narratives may be unyielding, and creative output can be frustrating and even stressful for some individuals.

Chronic trauma during childhood impacts creativity in several unique ways. At least one study (Thomson & Jaque, 2017) found that adults who had more than four adverse childhood experiences (exposure to abuse, neglect, or family dysfunction) specified that they had significantly more creative experiences and were more fantasy prone than those who experienced fewer adverse events. Cumulative trauma generated an appreciation of the creative process, although overall more negative psychological effects were present, including anxiety and internalized shame. While much more research is needed, these results may indicate that those individuals who withstood multiple adverse events as children may eventually find creative resilience through arts-based experiences.

The concept of post-traumatic growth (see Chapter 10) proposes that creative abilities may actually increase post-trauma and suggests that individuals may be able to transform negative life experiences and use creativity as a way of coping with adversity. There is also evidence of a strong relationship between the number of adverse lifetime events and perceived creative growth. Forgeard (2013) conducted a study to investigate this idea, measuring post-traumatic growth, rumination related to the event, and growth of creativity. Two measures were used: (1) scores on a measure of post-traumatic growth and depreciation and (2) scores on self-reported measures of creativity in the aftermath of adversity. Forgeard's research concluded that adversity-induced distress indeed predicted self-reported creative growth and breadth, but with qualifications. Intrusive rumination (a process in which an individual is focused on symptoms of distress rather than solutions) about traumatic events was a predictor of perceptions of life-worsening post-trauma. In contrast, deliberate rumination (a process in which an individual engages in reflection about problem-solving possibilities) was a strong factor for post-traumatic growth and subsequent creativity. Two other interesting findings emerged. Individuals who felt more isolated after a traumatic event also reported being more creative. Also, people experiencing physical assault showed the greatest increase in perceived creative growth, significantly greater than sexual assault or accidents.

Conversely, throughout decades of journal articles and books on arts-based approaches, individuals anecdotally report that experiences capitalizing on creativity and imagination provide effective distractions from tenacious physiological reactions and recurrent thoughts related to traumatic events. As more connections between creativity and imagination and trauma are realized, we identify how to adapt creative arts strategies to assist those individuals who may not so easily become engaged in imagination and the creative process.

CONCLUSION

In my experience over decades of applying arts-based approaches in work with children, adults, families, and groups, I have more often used the term *expressive* rather than *creative* to explain and define my psychotherapeutic approach. Creativity is somewhat of a charged word that can be intimidating for many adults in particular. While most children, including those who have experienced multiple traumatic events, may naturally take to one or more of the expressive arts, the immediate response from most adults is, "I am not creative" or "I can't draw (make music, sing, or dance)." As Rollo May (1994) made famous, it really does take courage to create. So when I introduce my approach to individuals who wonder if they can be creative or even imaginative, I remind them that it is true that each of us probably has different capacities for creativity, but in fact, "we all can be expressive in one way or another and there are many ways of being expressive." The core objective of expressive arts therapy is simply to help people discover just what forms of expression will be self-regulating, to communicate their experiences in a reparative way, and to ultimately support recovery, concepts that are explained in more detail in subsequent chapters.

CHAPTER 2

Frameworks for Expressive Arts Therapy and Trauma-Informed Practice

Addressing trauma in children and adults is not a one-size-fits-all endeavor. Effective intervention includes viewing individuals not only through the acute or chronic events they have experienced, but also through the interpersonal, cultural, social, and ecological factors that form the context for their perceptions and trauma-related reactions. These frameworks help provide important guidance in these areas and can direct practitioners, including those applying expressive arts in their work, to current best practices that are inclusive of the multiple factors impacting an individual's experiences of traumatic events.

American psychologist James Hillman (2013) said, "We can't change anything until we get some fresh ideas, until we begin to see things differently" (p. 11). The concept of *trauma-informed practice* marked the formal introduction of "some fresh ideas" based on a growing understanding of the impact of trauma on neurobiology and development. It has notably changed the way practitioners view individuals in treatment and how facilities and institutions provide care. In part, trauma-informed practice emerged in response to existing ways of addressing trauma that often exacerbate distressful reactions or depend on antiquated models that did not address the diversity of individuals' trauma experiences or views of treatment. A growing awareness of needs for cultural competence, individual autonomy and choice, nonpathologizing language, shared power within treatment, and integrative care also contributed to expansion of trauma-informed principles. In brief, trauma-informed approaches recognize that children, adolescents, adults, families, and communities are respected and empowered, informed about the interrelatedness between trauma and the body's response to it, and encouraged to participate as collaborators with helping professionals to formulate treatment (Steele & Malchiodi, 2011).

This chapter presents the basics of the trauma-informed practice model, including precursors that helped shape these currently accepted principles. Because trauma-informed practice is still an evolving concept, the emerging concept of *healing-centered engagement* is included to underscore the importance of cultural and social justice issues that impact clients' perceptions and reactions as a result of traumatic events. Finally, the integration of expressive arts therapy with trauma-informed principles and a culturally based model for arts-based practice are provided to introduce readers to concepts presented in subsequent chapters.

PRECURSORS TO TRAUMA-INFORMED PRACTICE

Trauma-informed practice emerged over the course of many decades from many important models that contributed to the currently accepted concepts. In past decades, these precursors were some of the few frameworks available and were central to the way I provided art and play therapy, particularly with survivors of interpersonal violence and chronic trauma. Even though knowledge of trauma has dramatically expanded and a wide array of approaches have emerged, the basic concepts found in these early models are still consistent with many forms of contemporary methodologies and goals for addressing individuals' distress at various points in treatment.

In the now seminal *Trauma and Recovery*, Judith Herman (1992) outlines a framework for trauma integration that has become a model of recovery based on stages of reparative process for individuals who have experienced interpersonal violence and related forms of trauma. Therapists still frequently use this model to guide intervention, and while some parts of this model have now been challenged by current knowledge about how the brain and body respond to trauma, its concepts are still relevant to current practice. Herman's model is summarized as follows:

- *Stage 1: Safety and stabilization and overcoming dysregulation.* This initial stage involves psychoeducation to help individuals comprehend the effects of trauma, including common symptoms and overwhelming body sensations, intrusive emotions, and distorted cognitive patterns. Safety and stabilization are achieved through establishing an environment that is nonabusive and provides both secure living conditions and adequate social supports; supports body safety, including abstinence from self-injury; and promotes self-regulation (the ability to calm the body, self-soothe, and manage trauma reactions).

- *Stage 2: Remembrance and mourning.* Once a solid foundation for safety and stabilization through self-regulation is established, Herman observes that it may be possible to undertake the work of recalling and talking about painful memories. The focus is on overcoming the fear of trauma memories and beginning the process of integration. In the past, this process generally involved some form of talk therapy, but because trauma is now believed to also be a body-based experience, approaches like eye movement desensitization and reprocessing (EMDR) and mind–body techniques also are employed. During this phase, pacing is particularly important as is sensitivity to the potential for highly distressful emotions emerging and overwhelming the individual.

- *Stage 3: Reconnection and integration.* The final stage in Herman's model focuses on the individual's reinvention of the self, making meaning of what happened and establishing a vision for the future. At this stage, the trauma no longer defines the individual's life and is part of a larger life story; in other words, one is able to gain some closure and experience about what happened with the knowledge that trauma does not define who one is. It is also a time for reengaging with one's community and reconnecting with one's dreams and aspirations or helping others with similar histories of adversity. Herman (1992) summarizes this critical need: "Traumatic events destroy the sustaining bonds between individual and community. . . . The solidarity of a group provides the strongest protection against terror and despair, and the strongest antidote to traumatic experience" (p. 214).

Like most stage models of trauma intervention, Herman's framework is not necessarily linear. In fact, it is more likely that individuals will move in and out of stages and not experience a linear completion of each one; the time each person spends in one or more of these stages is also individual.

A second model, proposed by Bessel A. van der Kolk (2005), is somewhat similar to Herman's phase model but specifically identifies essential areas to address in developmental trauma. Although this model is focused on young clients, it is also easily adapted for use with adults with complex trauma histories. Like Herman's phase model, this three-part framework is not necessarily linear, but rather circular because various issues displayed by children may require attention at any point during therapy. Each area has a specific focus with unique dynamics and goals for treatment, as follows:

- *Establishing a sense of safety and competence.* Habitual fight, flight, and freeze reactions prevalent among young clients with developmental trauma are the initial focus of intervention. Only after children develop the capacity to focus on pleasurable experiences without becoming dysregulated can they engage in successful relationships with others and address more complex aspects of trauma. In brief, this involves redirecting their attention to activities that do not remind them of trauma-related triggers and provide a sense of mastery.

assistance. This principle also takes into account personal responses to stress and sensitivity to an individual's preference and tolerance for disclosure and participation in treatment.

3. *Symptoms and trauma reactions are reframed as adaptive coping necessary to survive, not a pathology.* Concentration camp survivor Viktor Frankl (1997) observed, "An abnormal reaction to an abnormal situation is normal behavior" (p. 20). Rather than defining behavior with pathology-driven words such as *defended* or *repressed,* responses are reframed as normal reactions to abnormal circumstances when it comes to traumatic events. In trauma-informed work, asking individuals, "What happened to you?" is preferable to asking, "What is wrong with you?" In reframing questions to be more objective and less pathology-driven, there is a natural change in dynamics between therapists and clients and their worldviews of trauma, adverse life events and diagnostic labels. This way of speaking of and to individuals in treatment reflects a growing consciousness about how helping professionals define those they seek to serve. Military veterans now embrace the idea that post-traumatic stress is not necessarily a "disorder" but is instead a normal and natural reaction to unique and challenging events because there is nothing normal about war. In all cases, helping professionals provide psychoeducation that reframes reactions and behaviors as adaptive coping skills used to survive.

4. *The individual, family, group, or community is empowered to collaborate in therapy, and intervention reflects cultural preferences and worldviews.* Trauma-informed practice reframes the individual as a participant rather than as a patient. Working in a collaborative manner with survivors of trauma empowers them to become part of their own treatment and facilitates participation and meaningful involvement in planning services and programming. Reparation and recovery are enhanced within relationships in which an experience of choice and meaningful sharing of power and decision making are present. Sensitivity to cultural preferences for treatment and worldviews of health and wellness are also essential. This includes developing collaborative relationships with other systems with the individual's consent (e.g., working with tribal health care systems and healing traditions for Native Americans or including clergy when needed for spiritual support of individuals). Additionally, trauma-informed practice values traditional cultural connections and practices, the importance of gender, age, and socioeconomic influences, and historical and intergenerational trauma.

5. *The individual, family, group, or community is viewed as having the potential not only to survive, but also to thrive.* In trauma-informed practice, enhancing personal resilience and the capacity for post-traumatic growth are as important as addressing the trauma itself. Survivors are

viewed as "thrivers" and are respected as individuals who are given hope regarding their own recovery. Peer support and mutual self-help are viewed as integral to resilience-building and self-empowerment. In all cases, clients' strengths are identified, validated, and encouraged, building on what individuals have to offer rather than focusing on perceived deficits. This translates to creating resilient systems of care (Bloom, 2016) and, as van der Kolk (2005) notes, "Not every child will be a success story, but we should assume everything is reversible until proven otherwise" (p. 408).

Finally, trauma-informed practice asks helping professionals to be knowledgeable about the various definitions and types of traumatic experiences children, adults, families, and groups bring to treatment settings. These include but are not limited to an understanding of what constitutes acute trauma, chronic or complex trauma, and post-traumatic stress. In particular, most trauma-informed practitioners consider individuals' experiences within the context of exposure to distress over the lifespan. The ACE study, developmental trauma (van der Kolk, 2005), and intergenerational and historical trauma are three of the current concepts related to trauma histories and are briefly summarized below.

The Adverse Childhood Experiences Study

The ACE study (Felitti et al., 1998) and subsequent studies (CDC, 2019) continue to be an important part of trauma-informed practice. The ACE study looked at the life histories of over 17,000 people to determine the connections between adverse childhood experiences and health in adulthood. The study found that adverse childhood experiences were vastly more common than recognized, often coexisting and directly linked to later-life substance use, depression, cardiovascular and metabolic diseases, cancer, and premature mortality and mental health problems. Research or ACEs suggests that there are common specific experiences that constitute major risk factors for primary causes of illness and death and poor quality of life in general, not only in childhood, but also throughout the lifespan. Childhood experiences defined as adverse include verbal, emotional, physical, or sexual abuse and the adverse influence of family and community factors, for example, an incarcerated parent, a substance-abusing family member, and interpersonal violence at home or in a neighborhood. In brief, ACEs can be defined as potentially traumatic for most children, and they can continue to result in negative and harmful outcomes during childhood, adolescence, and adulthood.

The findings of this study are summarized by the ACEs pyramid (Figure 2.1), which represents the conceptual framework for understanding how and why adverse experiences in childhood impact multiple areas of functioning and lead to additional harmful behaviors and responses and potentially early mortality. Specifically, the study was designed to identify factors that would help answer the question: "If risk factors for disease, disability,

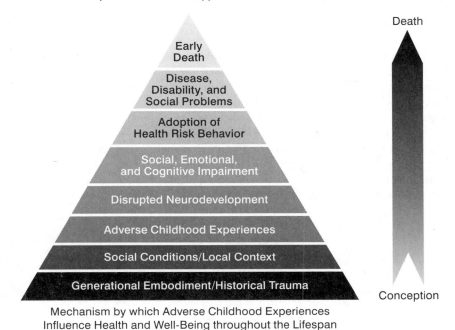

Mechanism by which Adverse Childhood Experiences
Influence Health and Well-Being throughout the Lifespan

FIGURE 2.1. The ACEs pyramid, representing the conceptual framework for the ACE study. The ACE study has uncovered how ACEs are strongly related to development of risk factors for disease and to well-being throughout the life course. From Centers for Disease Control and Prevention (2019).

and early mortality are not randomly distributed, what influences precede the adoption or development of them?" (CDC, 2019). The findings from these studies bring clarity to understanding the consequences of adverse childhood events and their connection to the quality of an individual's emotional, cognitive, social, and physical functioning. This "whole-life perspective" is represented within the pyramid as an arrow leading from childhood to *end-of-life*. As in trauma-informed practice, the ACE study involves viewing how adverse experiences and risk factors that may result from traumatic events can affect developmental progress, psychological and social health, and physical well-being throughout the lifespan.

Developmental Trauma

Developmental trauma is a concept that describes early, repetitive trauma to infants and children and generally involves neglect, physical abuse, assault, sexual abuse, witnessing violence or death, abandonment, and experiences of coercion or betrayal. These events generally occur within the individual's family or caregiving system and ultimately impair healthy attachment and emotional, cognitive, and physical development. Mental health professionals working with children unsuccessfully argued for the need to add the category "developmental trauma disorder" (DTD) to the fifth edition of the *Diagnostic and Statistical Manual of Mental Disorders* (American Psychiatric Association, 2013) listing of childhood disorders. Even though DTD is not an official diagnostic category, most practitioners who work with children who have survived multiple traumatic events use the term *developmental trauma* to describe these survivors' experiences. It is also a framework for understanding current behaviors and functioning. The concept of developmental trauma is intended to redirect helping professionals to the importance of children's trauma histories, thus providing the opportunity for specifically designed trauma-informed interventions.

Cloitre and colleagues (2009) explain:

> Whether or not they exhibit symptoms of PTSD, children who have developed in the context of ongoing danger, maltreatment, and inadequate care-giving systems are ill-served by the current diagnostic system, as it frequently leads to no diagnosis, multiple unrelated diagnoses, an emphasis on behavioral control without recognition of interpersonal trauma and lack of safety in the etiology of symptoms, and a lack of attention to ameliorating the developmental disruptions that underlie the symptoms. (p. 400)

In other words, children who are survivors of multiple traumatic events may be diagnosed with various comorbid diagnoses that may or may not reflect post-traumatic reactions and symptoms. As a result of DTD, children display persistent dysregulation in emotional, somatic (motor and physiological), behavioral, cognitive, or psychosocial functioning; self-attributions may include self-hate, shame, or blame. Additionally, there may be altered expectations, including loss of belief in protection by others and in social justice or a belief in retribution, and a general distrust of family, caregivers, and helping professionals.

The concept of developmental trauma is a focus of Perry (2009), who proposes a Neurosequential Model of Therapeutics® (NMT) as a developmental, neurobiological approach to work with children. It is a way to organize and evaluate children's histories and functioning and, as a result, formulate the goals and objectives of trauma-informed intervention. In brief, the NMT helps practitioners determine therapeutic approaches that are appropriate to the developmental characteristics of the child and to the regions of the brain that are most likely in need of mediation due to developmental trauma and traumatic experiences in general. Because the NMT underscores the recognition of the core developmental factors impacted by traumatic experiences early in the lifespan, it is a popular framework because many practitioners believe that the current post-traumatic stress category does not adequately reflect the influence of multiple traumatic events on children.

Intergenerational Trauma and Historical Trauma

A clinical supervisor once said to me, "Pain moves through families until someone is ready to feel it." That statement captures the essence of what is now referred to as *intergenerational trauma,* a concept based on the idea that trauma's impact does not always dissipate, but rather can continue from one generation to the next and can affect individuals and families in multiple ways. It is central to trauma-informed practice because it may provide an important context for understanding the individual's distress through both interpersonal and cultural lenses as well as the origin of trauma reactions. The concept of intergenerational trauma initially emerged through descriptions of problems in descendants of Holocaust survivors by Rakoff, Sigal, and Epstein (1966), who noted, "The parents are not broken conspicuously, yet their children, all of whom were born after the Holocaust, display severe psychiatric symptomatology. It would almost be easier to believe that they, rather than their parents, had suffered the corrupting, searing hell" (p. 755). At the time, these observations were regarded as stigmatizing the surviving generations, but eventually they inspired more extensive research to better understand just why descendants of survivors might be displaying symptoms and behavioral difficulties.

In taking a thorough trauma-informed history, therapists may find that individuals who have difficulty working through trauma not only may have experienced their own trauma, but may also have come from a family where their parents, and often their parents' parents, experienced trauma that was not acknowledged or treated. Intergenerational trauma also may be present in situations of neglect where children do not develop the necessary resources to flourish because there is a lack of appropriate caregiving. In these cases, therapists may find that the caregivers themselves may not have received necessary parenting skills from their parents; these skills may include imparting to children basic trust and social support resulting from disrupted or inadequate attachment. Intergenerational trauma may disrupt important key experiences necessary for healthy development, affecting how the individual interacts with others and events throughout the lifespan.

Research on intergenerational trauma is clarifying the prevalence and psychological and physical impacts on descendants of those who survived mass trauma. For example, Yehuda and Bierer (2007) demonstrated that an increased prevalence of PTSD in adult offspring of Holocaust survivors was associated with parental PTSD. Yehuda and Lehrner (2018) note, "While some aspects of intergenerational trauma effects remain contested, discussions about whether there are clinically observable intergenerational effects in offspring have become less contentious in the last several years, with the increasing recognition of the universality of this phenomenon" (p. 244). Yehuda also proposes that offspring of people who survived the Holocaust have different cortisol (stress hormone) profiles and may be more likely to have anxiety disorders as a result. These descendants may also be at risk for age-related physical ailments such as obesity, insulin resistance, and hypertension.

The concept of *historical trauma* also emerged from Yehuda's research and other investigators' efforts. Historical trauma is generally associated with events such as colonization, slavery, oppression, and displacement in many cultures, particularly First Nations, Native Americans, African Americans, Australian Aboriginals, and New Zealand Maori. People exposed to genocide and war in many countries and cultures throughout the world have been impacted by what can be defined as historical trauma. In fact, any oppressive actions toward a specific group, such as banning an indigenous language or desecration of graveyards, monuments, or sacred sites, can be associated with historical trauma in an individual or a group and impact the ability to maintain cultural practices that support identity and sense of self. As an example, some of the causes of historical trauma among Native Americans in the United States include early federal prohibition against Native spiritual practices that differ from European practices; views of Natives as savage and unfeeling individuals; prohibition of traditional hairstyles and clothing; and multiple losses of life due to genocide and loss of land. These and other traumatic events have resulted in internalization of ancestral suffering, preoccupation with death, dreams of massacres, suicide, addictions, and even survivors' guilt because vitality in one's own life is perceived as a betrayal to ancestors who suffered during past generations (Braveheart, 2003).

Atkinson (2003) also explains similar impacts of historical trauma on Australian Aboriginal people over decades of invasion, colonization, and patronization by Euro-centric cultures. The multiple violations resulted in anger for which there is no safe outlet and "is therefore stored in the body for expression under duress" (p. 36) in the form of explosive violence and addiction. Similar to Native Americans in the United States, Aboriginal peoples have experienced the removal of children from families, creating generations of individuals with multiple layers of traumatic stress, anxieties and fears, physical illnesses, substance abuse problems, and high incarceration rates. Atkinson emphasizes that these outcomes continue to be disabling, causing a cycle of damage that is difficult to escape without some form of intervention.

These examples of historical trauma are neither quick nor easy to resolve in any clinical session. What is important for practitioners to recognize is that many individuals may also have historical trauma and that this type of trauma may require larger systemic interventions that involve agencies and institutions that provide trauma-informed care as well as the individual's community. According to Atkinson (2003), this includes assisting individuals in understanding their own reactions to reverberating and unresolved historical trauma across generations to initiate the healing process and identify cultural traditions that support eventual reparation.

ILLUSTRATIONS
OF A TRAUMA-INFORMED PERSPECTIVE

The following brief case examples underscore how individuals who seek or are referred for therapy may benefit from a trauma-informed perspective in evaluating current symptoms and behaviors. These examples illustrate that it can be helpful to consider how traumatic events, particularly those that have not been disclosed or have been forgotten or dismissed, can be pivotal in developing effective interventions.

Case Example. Marian

Marian, a 57-year-old woman, was referred for psychotherapy because of chronic depression. Marian reported that she had felt increasingly sad, withdrawn, and anxious for the past 3 years and that prior to the onset of the depressive symptoms, she rarely felt sad or anxious; in fact, she was very energetic, engaged in both her career and various volunteer and social groups. Marian decided to pursue psychotherapy because her family thought that she might be depressed due to aging or medical issues that may not have been diagnosed. In the course of initial assessment, medical illnesses were ruled out through a comprehensive physical examination. Marian was a very healthy individual for her age and, in fact, more vital than many individuals much younger than she.

During initial sessions, Marian and I talked about her preferences for addressing her depression, particularly the anxiety that was interfering with her work and causing occasional panic attacks while she was driving her car. Marian was particularly concerned about her panic attacks because she felt she was becoming less inclined to leave her home and therefore was becoming isolated from friends and family. In one of these initial sessions, I explained a little bit about how the mind and body respond to stress and how depression and anxiety can be signals of distress that can be helped by various strategies. I also explained that her "body was smart" because it might be trying to help her adaptively cope. I also asked Marian to help me understand her worldview about depression and about her family and friends' impact on her. Marian explained that she felt a little "defective" because of the diagnosis, but also a bit angry at her family for thinking her sadness and anxiety were due to "getting older" and being female. This and other information helped me to begin to appreciate the possible cultural, gender, age, and interpersonal aspects of Marian's experiences and perceptions.

Since Marian was not in favor of medications for depression, we co-developed a plan for stress reduction and self-regulation, additional support and resources, and exploration of events and relationships in her life through expressive arts of her choice. After several weeks of weekly expressive arts therapy sessions, while engaged in making a collage with magazine images, Marian spontaneously recalled a bus accident she had survived several years earlier. Several of the magazine images reminded her of a tour she took while on vacation when a large trailer truck hit the bus, causing it to slide off the road and into a wall. She described how she was sitting next to another person on the bus who did not survive and how she fortunately sustained only very minor injuries. What surprised Marian at this juncture was how she had not thought about this incident for a long time and how she consciously tried to forget about it just after it happened. Her family told her to "just forget about it; you are lucky to be alive." Marian said that at the time she felt it was best to just move on, but she also reported in retrospect, "I was one of the lucky ones who survived. But I also felt bad about that, too."

When Marian disclosed this major event, I carefully proceeded with further exploration and with the overall objective of prevention of retraumatization by deeper discussion of the event. The stress-reduction and self-regulatory skills Marian learned in earlier sessions helped to decrease her anxiety while we explored the event and also reinforced the value of these skills in situations outside our sessions. I also introduced the idea that Marian was truly a survivor in many ways in addition to only sustaining a few injuries. In talking more about the incident, Marian recalled her own strengths in being able to help others who were injured and how she was able to resume her work only a week after the accident.

Once we identified these positive resources that Marian had as an individual, we then spent time talking about how it felt to have been so fortunate to walk away from the accident with only a few cuts and scrapes on that day. We explored the idea of "survivor's guilt" and also associated sensory (visual, auditory, tactile, and other senses) memories of the event. Marian realized that her anxiety and panic often occurred when she had specific sensory experiences; for example, the smell of gasoline and a sense of not being in control while driving preceded a feeling of tightness in her chest and increased her heart rate. Marian also started to appreciate that her fears of leaving her home, the need to stay close to home, the withdrawal from friendships and social networks, and panic attacks while driving her car were at least somewhat related to the bus accident she experienced years earlier. While additional challenges were addressed in subsequent sessions, a trauma in the past resulted in many of the reactions that brought Marian to treatment years later.

Case Example. Tanya

Tanya, a 13-year-old girl, was referred to a residential treatment program because of high-risk behaviors, including alcohol abuse, occasional self-cutting, and a possible suicide threat. She had run away from home five times, and her mother and grandmother felt they had tried everything they could to help her. They were concerned that she was now "hanging around with gangs involved in robberies and fighting," as well as "other tough crowds of teenagers who used drugs and alcohol." While her peers escaped the crime scene, Tanya was picked up by the police one evening for vandalizing a neighbor's fence, and she spent the night at the police station. At this point, her mother requested that she see a school psychologist, who in turn referred her to residential treatment for further evaluation and intervention.

Tanya's first week at the facility was extremely difficult for her. In her initial interactions with staff, she repeatedly stated that "nothing was wrong" with her. When I first met with her, she asked if she could draw a picture (Figure 2.2) instead of talking; it was a self-image and, according to Tanya, showed that she was "tough so that people wouldn't mess with her." In individual and group counseling sessions, Tanya was generally

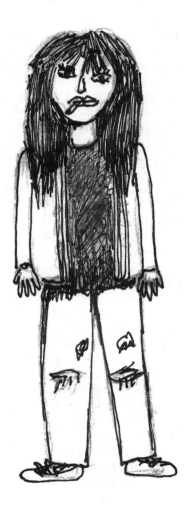

FIGURE 2.2. Tanya's self-portrait. From the collection of Cathy A. Malchiodi (not to be reproduced without permission from the author).

hypervigilant, demanding to be seated where she could see the doorway to monitor who came into the room. She was also easily startled by common sounds such as doors slamming or car noises on the street outside the building. Night staff reported that Tanya often paced the hallway because she had insomnia and, on several occasions, she was found sitting in her closet hugging her bed pillow.

Residence staff, psychologists, and I asked Tanya if she thought something in particular was causing her to worry and to be unable to sleep, but she insisted that being at the residence was the cause of her behaviors. Because all the staff members at this particular residence were educated on trauma-informed practice, every professional attempted to identify any trauma history that Tanya may have had that was not disclosed. Her mother and grandmother stated that they did not know of anything other than the divorce of Tanya's parents and the death of her grandfather when she was about 2 years old. They shared with us that they thought Tanya may have been bullied during one year in elementary school, but that the incident had been resolved and Tanya did not seem to be troubled by it.

A pivotal moment in identifying and understanding Tanya's trauma history came unexpectedly one day when Tanya asked if she could attend play therapy groups for younger children at the facility. Despite being a teenager, Tanya seemed to enjoy the activities, particularly the "story time" when I or another staff member read out loud from children's books to the group as an ending to the session. After the session ended, Tanya stayed to help me clean up the room, which gave me a chance to ask her, "You seem to really understand the 6- and 7-year-olds in our group today. Do you remember anything from when you were in first or second grade? You seem to have enjoyed watching the kids today during their play activities and especially during the story time."

In brief, Tanya actually did remember quite a lot about that time period, including a positive memory of her grandmother reading her stories before bedtime since Tanya's own mother often had to work late. When I asked in a subsequent session if there were any other memories, Tanya finally was able to disclose a memory that she had told no adult before— that her uncle (her mother's brother) had sexually abused her on many evenings after her grandmother read her stories. Tanya was about 7 years old at the time of the abuse, similar in age to the children who attended the play therapy sessions she enjoyed attending. I then asked her an important trauma-informed question that respects an individual's current needs for safety: "Do you ever feel unsafe when you think about what happened?" Tanya quickly answered, "Yes, because he has moved back to our neighborhood a few months ago." She added that she was "a little happy" that she was at the residential treatment facility right now because he had started to visit their home at night and she felt that her mother and grandmother wouldn't believe her or allow her in their home if she told them.

There also was an element of intergenerational trauma within Tanya's family. Tanya's mother and grandmother disclosed in subsequent sessions that each had experienced some form of physical or sexual assault during their childhoods. Neither had ever discussed these incidents with each other, and neither volunteered this information during trauma-informed intake sessions with the residential staff. Both mother and grandmother simply wanted to put these incidents behind them, but now they agreed that it was time to begin the process of healing what was a difficult family story of violence and abuse across generations.

In Tanya's case, there were many additional trauma-informed interventions, some of which used the expressive arts approaches described in subsequent chapters. In both of these case examples, information about earlier trauma exposure was key to understanding current behaviors and distressing symptoms. While not everyone seen in therapy or at treatment facilities has experienced traumatic events, a trauma-informed focus encourages helping professionals to consider that individuals in their care may have been exposed to abuse, interpersonal violence, disaster, complex loss, survivor's guilt, or other previously undisclosed adverse events. For example, the traumatic event Marian experienced was not the only circumstance contributing to her depression; it was also a significant, unaddressed source of distress that was not recognized. In Tanya's case, the reappearance of an extended family member who abused her as a child probably had a relationship to her current alcohol abuse and emotional and behavioral problems. These brief examples underscore many of the principles of trauma-informed practice, including becoming aware of possible undisclosed adverse events; normalizing trauma reactions; depathologizing diagnoses and disorders established at the onset of treatment; co-collaborating with the individual to understand the individual's circumstances and co-creating therapeutic goals; encouraging strengths through enhancing self-regulatory skills; proceeding with caution with respect to possible retraumatization; and identifying resilience behaviors and responses.

TRAUMA-INFORMED EXPRESSIVE ARTS THERAPY

Each of us finds an approach, set of methods, or model that makes sense to us as helping professionals. For me, trauma-informed practice has helped to provide a logical part of the framework I needed to support individuals through the process of reparation and to apply expressive arts therapy to trauma integration. It forced me to clarify the role of body, mind, and brain in treatment and to depathologize intervention by providing expressive methods that most people generally perceive as engaging, pleasurable, and empowering. Most importantly, I found that the principles of trauma-informed practice emphasized individuals' capacities to go beyond surviving to thriving and ultimately make meaning through use of imagination, creativity, and play.

Trauma-informed expressive arts therapy is a model for arts-based approaches that integrates current best practices in trauma-informed care with what is known about how the expressive arts and play assist in trauma reparation and integration (Malchiodi, 2012a, 2012c). Based on the concepts of trauma-informed practice and the characteristics of expressive arts therapy, the following seven points summarize the major components of trauma-informed expressive arts therapy. They are described in more detail throughout the book.

1. *Neurodevelopment and neurobiology inform the application of expressive arts therapy to trauma-informed intervention.* As previously stated, trauma is not just a psychological experience; it is also a mind–body experience. The role of neurodevelopment and neurobiology is central to using the expressive arts to address trauma reactions and to assist individuals in reconnecting implicit (sensory) and explicit (declarative) memories of trauma (Malchiodi, 2003, 2012c). In particular, neurodevelopment provides a framework for determining how to apply expressive arts interventions to various goals of treatment, including when and how to support self-regulation and self-efficacy, positive attachment, and resilience-building.

2. *Expressive arts therapy is focused on supporting self-regulation and co-regulation.* Overactivation, hyperarousal, and general anxiety are common manifestations of not only post-traumatic stress, but also other trauma-related challenges. Expressive arts interventions are used not only to support individuals' own internal resources, but also to provide various creative, action-oriented approaches to self-regulation and co-regulation when applied within groups.

3. *Expressive arts therapy is used to help identify and ameliorate the body's experience of distress.* Individuals who are experiencing trauma-related reactions typically experience the impact of these reactions not only in altered thinking, but also in various somatic experiences. Because the expressive arts are "embodied" experiences, they are helpful in identifying and repairing the body's responses to trauma. In particular, key trauma-informed practices are (a) using expressive arts to support individuals' bodies as resources (Levine, 1997, 2015) and (b) normalizing the body's reactions to trauma as adaptive coping rather than pathology.

4. *Expressive arts therapy is used to establish and support a sense of safety, positive attachment, and prosocial relationships.* Reconnecting with a sense of safety is central to trauma-informed practice. In particular, expressive arts approaches are used to help individuals recover a sense of well-being internally and in relationships with others. This also includes providing various opportunities for the individual to engage in creative experimentation that integrates experiences of unconditional appreciation, guidance, and support, experiences found in families with secure attachment relationships. When applied as group interventions, expressive arts support prosocial interactions and connect individuals through community.

5. *Expressive arts therapy is used to support strengths and enhance resilience.* Trauma-informed practice encourages helping professionals to see all individuals as capable of growth and reparation. It also holds the concept of resiliency as central to recovery. Expressive arts interventions are life-affirming and honor individuals' capacity for resilience and personal strength by encouraging mastery, with a goal of moving individuals' self-perceptions from victim to survivor to "thriver" (Malchiodi, 2012d).

6. *Expressive arts therapy respects the individual's preferences for self-expression, particularly of trauma narratives.* Trauma-informed practice emphasizes the role of individuals in their own treatment and their preferences for participation. These preferences are determined by culture, previous experiences, worldviews, values, and other dynamics. Arts-based approaches offer a variety of ways for expressing "what happened," dependent on the individual's comfort level with self-expression. These therapies also respect the use of personal metaphors and symbols that allow individuals to control how they communicate sensitive experiences.

7. *Expressive arts therapy provides meaning-making experiences and ways to imagine new narratives post-trauma.* As previously stated, expressive arts in particular allow individuals to convey what is often unspeakable. They also allow survivors to explore, restructure, reframe, and restory trauma and loss through nonverbal, asset-driven, participatory, and self-empowering ways.

HEALING-CENTERED ENGAGEMENT: A SOCIAL JUSTICE MODEL FOR TRAUMA-INFORMED PRACTICE

Trauma-informed practice has undoubtedly broadened the scope of how we view the experience of trauma events and has changed the way practitioners and institutions view the individual in treatment. It has improved the way we integrate many important principles within trauma-specific therapy, including the neurobiology of trauma reactions, centrality of the individual in treatment decisions, resilience- and strengths-based concepts, and preference for humanistic language over pathology-driven terminology. While trauma-informed practice is one of the better models for contemporary treatment at this time, it also has its blind spots. For example, neurobiology findings about trauma that currently dominate mental health, explanations of trauma reactions, and psychoeducation of survivors can still place an inadvertent emphasis on "what's wrong," thus reinforcing the idea that individuals are still defined by a set of symptoms rather identifiable strengths and capabilities. Even with trauma-informed principles securely in place in facilities and institutions, many therapists have to fall back on traditional medical models that include pathology-laden, diagnostic language that focuses on the treatment of symptoms rather than on individuals' resilience and well-being. It is difficult for those even with the best trauma-informed intentions to ignore the prevalent brain-disease paradigm and make the shift from "individual as patient" to "individual as participant." This shift allows people to heal from traumatic events through a sense of autonomy and their own capacities for self-regulatory and strength-based actions.

There is also a growing realization that trauma is not just an individual experience, but a collective one that takes place within the context of a complex environment. In other words, how trauma is perceived by an individual is impacted by overarching dynamics and conditions, including socioeconomic status, gender, disability, and race, among other factors. Reparation of the impact of trauma does not solely occur in a therapist's office or treatment facility; it is really only completed through what Herman (1992) identified as a return and reintegration within one's community. Until social conditions that are safe, allow individuals to thrive, and provide environments for successful reintegration into one's community, any trauma-informed intervention will remain incomplete. All efforts to move away from "What's wrong with you?" to "What happened to you" remain limited when it comes to the larger societal and political issues that impact many individuals' experience of traumatic events.

Ginwright (2018) is one of a growing number of voices proposing that the current model for trauma-informed practice is flawed and incomplete because it presumes that the experience of adversity is an individual experience rather than a more global one. For example, people who experience natural disasters such as hurricanes or earthquakes all collectively endure the same danger, destruction, and needs for safety. The vast majority do not encode this type of trauma as an individual event, but as one that they experience as part of a larger community that may include existing socioeconomic challenges and, in some cases, previous historical trauma. Child witnesses to domestic violence, which I described in Chapter 1, may come from violent neighborhoods where all individuals were exposed to similar repetitive trauma, harsh living conditions, and lack of access to necessary services, including law enforcement. Research actually demonstrates that all the children living in these communities often display some form of psychological trauma to varying degrees (Sinha & Rosenberg, 2013).

While trauma-informed practice addresses many important components necessary to effective intervention, most individuals require a more expansive approach that takes into consideration these larger dynamics that impact the experience of trauma. Ginwright (2018) summarizes this requirement as follows:

> What is needed is an approach that allows practitioners to approach trauma with a fresh lens which promotes a holistic view of healing from traumatic experiences and environments. One approach is called *healing centered*, as opposed to *trauma informed*. A healing centered approach is holistic involving culture, spirituality, civic action and collective healing.

A healing centered approach views trauma not simply as an individual isolated experience, but rather highlights the ways in which trauma and healing are experienced collectively. The term *healing centered engagement* expands how we think about responses to trauma and offers [a] more holistic approach to fostering well-being.

A good deal of what Ginwright (2018) proposes about healing-centered engagement is actually part of the existing trauma-informed practice model except for two significant concepts—social justice and intersectionality. Simply put, social justice is based on the principles of human rights and equality and how these are manifested in the everyday lives of people at every level of society. Intersectionality is a more complicated domain to articulate. By its most basic definition, it is defined as the interconnected nature of social categorizations such as race, class, and gender as they apply to a given individual or group. It is also defined as creating overlapping and interdependent systems of discrimination or disadvantage.

Healing-centered engagement brings these two concepts, social justice and intersectionality, into practice to underscore the role of control, power, and inequality in not only the individual's life, but also within systems such as schools, health care settings, mental health agencies, institutions, and other environments. Within this framework, therapists also are asked to become conscious of the multiple intersections of issues and dynamics that impact an individual client such as racism, sexism, ableism, classism, prejudice, and gender as well as hunger, homelessness, poverty, and even environmental stresses, including climate change. In other words, when individuals exist within toxic systems, dynamics, and living conditions, trauma-informed intervention cannot truly be effective if these issues are left unacknowledged. While it makes sense that therapists continue their dedication to resolving symptoms (anger, anxiety, fear), healing-centered engagement moves the pendulum toward a focus on strengthening what supports well-being (hope, imagination, trust, aspirations) inclusive of social justice issues and intersectionality. In brief, it shifts the perspective from "what happened to you" to "what's resilient about you."

EXPRESSIVE ARTS AS SOCIAL ACTION

Healing-centered engagement as a model for trauma intervention is actually present within the foundational principles of expressive arts therapy. Most of the earliest expressive arts practitioners emerged out of the countercultural climate of the 1960s and 1970s in the United States. They were naturally drawn to work in mental health in part out of a desire to be agents of social change, action, and justice in their communities. Natalie Rogers (1993), one of the key founders of expressive arts, expanded person-centered therapy principles of the time period and emphasized that the creative process is inherently linked not only to social action, but also to growth, health, and resilience, concepts resonant with healing-centered engagement. Others, like McNiff (2009) and Knill (Knill, Barba, & Fuchs, 1995), were artists (painter and musician, respectively) before they became therapists. As expressive arts continued to expand into the realm of psychotherapy, these individuals brought conceptual frameworks that included community and social action into the constructs (Heinonen, Halonen, & Krahn, 2018).

As a field, expressive arts therapy has also rejected the idea of the therapist being the sole expert, placing the individual engaged in creative expression as the authority or, at the very least, co-creator. Levine and Levine (2011) note:

> Expressive therapies have followed these dictates: Follow the image. Follow the client and the community. Meet the client and community where they are, and facilitate an environment in which arts-based inquiry and connection can take place, trusting that the process will take you to a place where suffering can be experienced, where feeling can be given form, and where the whole self (personal and collective, body, mind, spirit, and imagination) can be enlisted in the service of healing. (p. 46)

Stephen Levine (in Levine & Levine, 2011) adds that expressive arts therapy is an "experience that gives participants an experience of their own capacities for action" (p. 28), reflecting the central role of individual choice and mastery and resonating the experiences that so many trauma survivors have lost because of the situational and marginalizing conditions in which they find themselves.

Because expressive arts therapy emphasizes the centrality of the person, it is the person who derives meaning from creative expressions in contrast to the therapist providing interpretation. Individual meaning making not only is seen as a function of personality, but also includes the community, culture, and global environment within which the person exists. For several decades I have taken a similar position on how mental health professionals generally view drawings and expressive arts as solely representations of the self. With regard to children's drawings, I (Malchiodi, 1998) said, "Although children bring their own unique thoughts, perceptions and feelings into their creative work, their art expressions may be influenced by the environment in which they draw or the materials with which they create. The impact of the therapeutic relationship is equally important, issues of safety and trust and the therapist's enthusiasm, knowledge and respect" (p. 40). Children's drawings actually communicate a worldview that is also impacted by family and caregivers, neighborhood, and environment. This does not mean that an individual's creative expressions do not represent personal emotional, cognitive, or physical experiences, but it is important to keep in mind that any communication includes elements that are beyond the person and are inclusive of other factors.

Because expressive arts have been applied not only within the context of psychotherapy, but also in communities, the role of place—environment, setting, and way of life—is another concept central to practice. Not all of my work as a psychotherapist has taken place within an office or clinic walls, and occasionally I have had to strategize as to how to apply the arts in nontraditional ways. These settings have included church communities, tribal lands and reservations, disaster sites, and neighborhood centers. In these situations, it is impossible to ignore the role social issues play in the way expressive arts are provided. In addition to mental health professionals, a variety of paraprofessionals apply the principle of expressive arts to transformational work within communities and society; many examples of these applications are described throughout this book. Each highlights the role of arts-based approaches as healing-centered engagement, but also how members of communities being served play an important role in delivery of expressive arts.

Keeping in mind the concepts of healing-centered engagement and trauma-informed expressive arts therapy, here is a basic framework for applying these principles within expressive arts therapy practice with social action in mind:

1. Change is only possible when individuals are supported in their capacity to act and are able to see themselves as being able to impact the world in which they live. Arts-based approaches give participants experiences of their own capacities for action, reflecting the central role of individual choice and mastery, experiences that so many trauma survivors have lost because of the situational and marginalizing conditions in which they find themselves.

2. The goal is not to impose a preexisting set of interventions to direct individuals toward specific outcomes. Rather, the goal is to understand the world in which individuals live and the intersectional challenges they face and then to co-create meaningful experiences that respond to that reality. Expressive arts therapy approaches follow the direction of both the individual and the community.

3. It is essential to shape interventions to support each individual's capacity for imaginative actions that they may have lost due to adversity, while remaining conscious of the impact of the larger communities in which they live and intersectional challenges they face. The goal is to support individuals in transcending perceived limitations and in becoming aware of the unexplored possibilities through self-expression.

4. Oppression, marginalization, poverty, disaster, and other factors may leave individuals emotionally or physically isolated and separated from others. When possible, supporting a sense of solidarity among individuals

within a group or community is essential. The experience of making art together, for example, can provide the sense of community and of being part of a whole that is larger than oneself. It is the collective sense of belonging that manifests tangible change through sharing identity and common experiences, even when those experiences may include shared adversity, marginalization, or oppression.

5. Applying a healing-centered engagement model requires that the therapist possess a humble, curious, and respectful attitude. This attitude includes a willingness to engage in difficult conversations and identify power differentials within society as well as the therapy session.

ARTS-BASED HEALING ENGAGEMENT: A FOUR-PART MODEL FOR CULTURALLY RELEVANT PRACTICE

Because the expressive arts provide a unique context for psychotherapeutic engagement, it is important to have a framework that defines these approaches within the arts themselves. In modifying and integrating principles found in both trauma-informed practice and healing-centered engagement with individuals, families, and groups, I began to consider the historical and particularly the cultural basis for applying expressive arts to trauma intervention. Much of this exploration has come from disaster relief assignments where I have been sent to work with what are often large groups of survivors. In these situations, I have traveled to locations where natural (tornados or hurricanes) or human-made (terrorism or violence) disasters occurred, meeting participants in their own communities. Like many practitioners, I was trained in various forms of crisis intervention and in what has come to be known as various forms of critical incident debriefing. But these models never quite made sense to me when it came to trauma reparation and expressive arts. In particular, these protocols did not integrate the core principles of trauma-informed practice, nor did they resonate culturally relevant approaches that take into consideration the concepts found in healing-centered engagement.

On one particular trip to work with survivors in the aftermath of a tornado that destroyed several small towns and killed several people, I took a risk and tried a different tactic instead of applying a standard disaster relief protocol. After explaining my approach as an expressive arts therapist, I simply asked the group, "What do you do to self-soothe when something bad happens?" I met this particular group of survivors at their church, one of the few buildings in their community that was left standing after the tornadic winds and storms. Given that all the participants were from the same Southern Baptist parish, I added these questions: "Are there hymns or songs that you sing to feel connected as a community? Or are there particular prayers that you say when you want to feel connected to something greater than yourselves?" In addition to trying a new, more empowering way to interact with participants, I sincerely did want to know what strategies they adopted when they collectively confronted trauma and loss.

During this particular encounter, the community quickly let me know all the strategies they had to calm, self-soothe, and connect with each other despite their distress and challenges. They had hymns and prayers, universally known to each person, and they rose to the occasion to teach me what these songs and verses were. I rapidly learned more about how individuals cope using their own internal resources and practices learned within their community through this experience. As a result, I began to ask these questions in other groups, such as first responders to disasters, including violence and other human-made events, cancer patient support groups, and military communities where I was assigned to work with traumatic stress and resilience-building. In each case, it was clear that my curiosity encouraged participants to recognize that they indeed already had some "creative" skills necessary to repair and recovery. These experiences led me to think more deeply about what types of expressive arts were already embedded in various cultural groups and to recognize that these practices often seemed to fall into one or more broad domain.

Rather than use neuroscience as a framework, I decided to look to cultural anthropology for some answers about healing practices within communities. I use the ubiquitous term *healing practices* to show that they originally emerged and evolved within various cultural groups in service of health and well-being. In most cases, these practices materialized in the form of rituals, conventions, procedures, and ceremonies in response to individual and collective experiences of trauma and loss (Malchiodi, 2006, 2013). Ethnologists such as Ellen Dissanayake (1995) define the arts and related activities as processes that have helped humans return to psychological and social equilibrium. She observes, "Art is a normal and necessary behavior of human beings like other common and universal occupations such as talking, working, exercising, playing, socializing, learning, loving, and caring" (p. 18). Cultural anthropologist Angeles Arrien (2013) also defined the arts as having specific reparative functions, noting that the earliest healing practitioners asked, "When did you stop dancing? When did you stop singing? When did you stop being enchanted by stories? When did you stop being comforted by the sweet territory of silence?" (p. 41).

Neuroscience is undoubtedly still an important piece of current investigations of expressive arts to determine best practices. However, the bulk of the neuroscience focus still rests on language and the implicit assumption that human experience resides in the brain; this infers that reparation occurs through the "head" and words. In contrast, for millennia the countless traumatized individuals and groups over decades I have worked with over decades already have identifiable capacities to repair. These are universal approaches found throughout human behavior across all cultures that have yet to be fully acknowledged and integrated into trauma-informed systems of clinical and community practices. I believe that they form as strong a foundation for what we define as "best practices" in addressing traumatic stress in the same way that many of the current methods have been derived from science. To clarify how psychotherapists can apply these approaches, I arrived at a model for clinical practice that places them into four major categories—movement, sound, storytelling, and silence, explained as follows (Figure 2.3).

Movement is a foundation for almost all expressive arts and healing practices and is central to cultures throughout history (LaMothe, 2015). Dance is the expressive art form that is probably most associated with movement for well-being. It has numerous sociocultural and anthropological explanations that support its importance to strengthening not just the individual, but also the social bonds within community throughout history. Some propose that it is, in fact, an experience that has helped humanity to develop empathy and adaptation to the environment because of its emphasis on interconnectedness, rhythm, and synchrony (LaMothe, 2015)

Many cultural groups have specific dances that often go beyond movement to include spiritual and symbolic components such as Polynesian Hula, Australian Aboriginal Corroboree, or Native American Sundance. There are "energy arts" such as tai chi and practices such as yoga that have deeper meanings and significance beyond just movement. Also, there are many other activities and practices, including movement-based sensory integration, bilateral movement via two-handed drawing or clay work and play-based experiences.

Music and music making are arts-based wellness practices across cultures, but they also fall into the broader category of *sound*. Oliver Sacks (2007) summarizes the value of music, noting, "Music can lift us out of depression or move us to tears—it is a remedy, a tonic, orange juice for the ear. But for many of my neurological patients, music is even more—it can provide access, even when no medication can, to movement, to speech, to life. For them, music is not a luxury, but a necessity" (p. 15). Sacks states that music possibly influences and impacts emotions quickly and effectively, encourages movement and speech, and generally enlivens individuals. Singing (whether individually or in a group) and playing musical instruments are core expressive arts approaches. The larger realm of sound reaches beyond music to include chanting, praying, and recital of verse or stories, sound vibrations, and listening.

Storytelling, the third category, is often perceived as a language-driven activity, and often writing or oral storytelling comes to mind. But in fact, stories are communicated in many ways through expressive arts and play-based experiences. Visual art (drawing, painting, clay work, collage, photography, and film) are forms of graphic or symbolic storytelling through images; play, and particularly sandtray work with miniatures, conveys narratives. Any form of dramatic enactment, performance, role play, and improvisation communicates stories. Ceremonies and rituals that include movement,

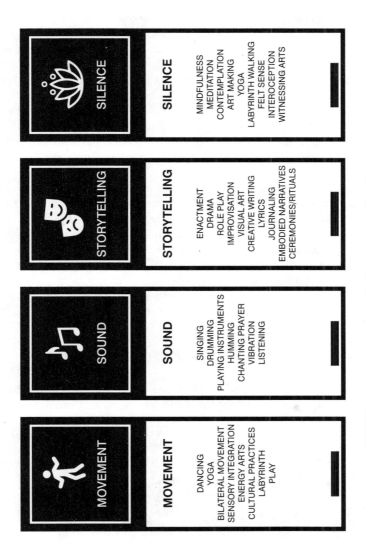

MOVEMENT

DANCING
YOGA
BILATERAL MOVEMENT
SENSORY INTEGRATION
ENERGY ARTS
CULTURAL PRACTICES
LABYRINTH
PLAY

SOUND

SINGING
DRUMMING
PLAYING INSTRUMENTS
HUMMING
CHANTING PRAYER
VIBRATION
LISTENING

STORYTELLING

ENACTMENT
DRAMA
ROLE PLAY
IMPROVISATION
VISUAL ART
CREATIVE WRITING
LYRICS
JOURNALING
EMBODIED NARRATIVES
CEREMONIES/RITUALS

SILENCE

MINDFULNESS
MEDITATION
CONTEMPLATION
ART MAKING
YOGA
LABYRINTH WALKING
FELT SENSE
INTEROCEPTION
WITNESSING ARTS

FIGURE 2.3. Four-part model for arts-based healing practices.

sound, imagery, and language have a similar function. There are also implicit narratives that individuals communicate through movement; even body language, including posture and gesture, tells a story on a sensory-based level.

The final category—*silence*—emphasizes the way many expressive arts can quiet the mind and regulate the body. Arrien (2013) identified silence as an important health-giving experience. We most often think of silence in the form of contemplative practices such as mindfulness and meditation. In particular, art making as a source of mindful focus and mindful movements such as yoga and labyrinth walking fall into this category. Silence is also a factor in how expressive arts enhance the ability to "look inside" oneself through interoception (the sense of the body's internal state) and experience a "felt sense" of what is perceived and sensed in one's body. Finally, attending and witnessing theater performances and art objects in museums often involve silence as a core experience and are a form of focused contemplation.

Although I have identified four distinct categories, there are overlapping functions due to characteristics of the arts themselves (Figure 2.4). For example, *silence* can be found in some forms of *movement* practices such as labyrinth walking or yoga; art making can be a *silent* practice that may eventually communicate stories; and *movement* in the form of dance often takes place with *sound* in the form of music. In using expressive arts to address traumatic stress, these overlapping functions are key to supporting experiences of self-regulation, grounding and anchoring, and the interoception of safety as described in subsequent chapters.

RE-EXPERIENCE, RESENSITIZE, RECONNECT

The four areas that comprise this arts-based and culturally based framework support three key areas of trauma reparation, which are described in

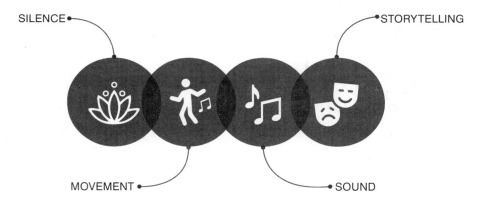

FIGURE 2.4. Overlapping functions of arts-based healing practices.

more detail in subsequent chapters. First, throughout history, the practices within each category have been intuitively used to *re-experience* oneself through sensory-based activities that involve rhythm, synchrony, enactment, and symbolization. They serve as ways to use imagination to develop new stories that will replace what may have become trauma-laden narratives. They also provide experiences that *resensitize* the body to a healthy, embodied experience of enlivenment post-trauma. This enlivenment is found through the multisensory nature of the arts themselves, including tactile, visual, auditory, proprioception, and interoception. For some individuals it involves safe touch and physical proximity with others through expressive arts. Because these practices often occur within groups or communities, they also help *reconnect* people to each other through prosocial and relational experiences. These three "R's" are at the core of how cultures throughout history have used expressive approaches in the service of health and well-being and are foundational to all applications of expressive arts within the context of psychotherapy and trauma reparation.

CONCLUSION

Trauma-informed practice is one of the better overarching frameworks we currently have to guide trauma-specific arts-based interventions that support regulation, stress reduction, body awareness, self-efficacy, and resilience. Though imperfect, it has slowly shifted the prevailing models of care to those that move individuals away from only being patients with a set of symptoms to becoming active participants in their own reparation and recovery. Emerging concepts such as healing-centered engagement have the potential to improve trauma-informed services by making the intersectionality of the individual and global issues of social justice influences consistent priorities in how therapists address traumatic stress. Recognizing the longstanding traditions of arts as healing practices also enhances understanding and application of these approaches within a culturally conscious framework.

Like many other approaches, expressive arts therapy complements the trauma-informed practice model and concepts such as healing-centered engagement. However, neither of these frameworks capitalizes on the unique qualities of the arts themselves and the role of creativity, imagination, and play in psychotherapeutic work. The next chapter highlights the importance of understanding an additional framework for applying arts-based practices—the hierarchical, bottom-up nature of the expressive arts and why it forms a compelling brain-wise and embodied model that can be applied to trauma reparation and integration.

CHAPTER 3

A Brain–Body Framework for Expressive Arts Therapy

Trauma-informed care emphasizes using neurobiology and neuroscience to support reparation and recovery and has become central to current discussions of psychological trauma and best practices with children, adults, families, and communities. It has expanded the focus of intervention to include how the body expresses traumatic stress as well as "brain-wise" ways to address trauma reactions. Like other psychotherapeutic approaches, expressive art therapy and various forms of creative arts therapies have responded to this trend and integrated principles found in neuroscience and neurobiology into treatment over the last two decades. It has become a way to clarify the effectiveness of arts-based methods that appear to have a positive impact on traumatized individuals that have only been intuitively understood until now.

Although neuroscience and neurobiology have helped to give some credence to arts-based approaches in addressing traumatic stress, in some cases these concepts are applied too quickly and unequivocally and without enough evidence. Johnson (2009a) noted that creative arts therapies have hurried to reframe themselves through a "neuroscience paradigm" that specifically correlates the brain with various arts-based applications and outcomes. He proposed that the creative arts therapies may have merely linked arts-based methods to various brain functions as a way of supporting their legitimacy within the mental health and health care domains. The inclusion of indigenous and universal healing practices (movement, sound, storytelling, and silence) described in the previous chapter has not been fully acknowledged within clinical literature and research. The fact that humans have always applied the arts and expressive methods in service of health and well-being is a form of evidence and efficacy that is equally significant.

Although there may be some truth to these observations, it is also impossible to completely ignore the impact of science on the understanding of expressive arts within the scope of trauma intervention. As more is learned from neuroscience and neurobiology, we are finding new ways to measure and identify why expressive arts therapy is both a brain-wise and body-based approach to health and well-being based on current and emerging research in these areas. Additionally, the neuroscience paradigm that Johnson critiques has actually given expressive arts and creative arts therapies support for an emerging brain–body framework and the development of arts-based methods within the context of trauma-informed practice. That uniquely arts-based framework is the subject of this chapter and forms a foundation for subsequent strategies described throughout the rest of this book.

THE DUAL BRAIN

Several decades ago, discoveries about brain lateralization, or the dual brain, generated overly broad conclusions about the functions of its right and left hemispheres. At one point, the two hemispheres were categorized as a dichotomy—the left brain was defined as verbal, analytic, and logical, whereas the right brain was said to contain intuitive, emotional, perceptual, and nonverbal functions. Because creativity, imagination, rhythm, holistic thinking, and the arts have been associated with the right side of the brain, the various arts therapies embraced the notion of being "right-brained" approaches for many years. This idea still appears in discussions about the human brain and expressive arts approaches and often hinders an accurate understanding of how complex brain functioning is.

Although both hemispheres are part of a larger, more complex system, it is true that there are significant and identifiable differences between them. The right brain does play an important role in the creative process and art-related experiences, but, in fact, the expressive arts therapies are whole-brain approaches that emphasize qualities often found in right-brain functions. In other words, these approaches are not relegated to only one hemisphere because engaging in any arts-based activity uses many parts of the brain to participate.

More recently, brain-imaging technology is providing some preliminary information about how the expressive arts may activate various parts of the brain rather than a single hemisphere. Several studies provide emerging data on the relationship of different forms of art making to certain regions of the brain; for example, art processes such as drawing and clay sculpting generate specific brain waves similar to forms of meditation (Kruk, Aravich, Deaver, & deBeus, 2014). A study using fNIRS (functional near-infrared spectroscopy) headbands to measure blood flow in the brain during various forms of coloring, doodling, and drawing revealed increased blood flow to parts of the brain thought to be related to rewards pathways (Kaimal et al., 2017). Music therapy and the related field of music neurology have generated a growing body of research on how various forms of music and sound impact individuals and how music can be applied to trauma reparation and grief and loss interventions (Wheeler, 2016).

Although the impact of trauma on the brain and body is complex, it is widely accepted that highly charged emotional experiences are encoded within the limbic system and the right hemisphere of the brain (van der Kolk, 2006, 2014). The right brain is believed to hold the memories of sounds, smells, and tactile and visual experiences, along with the emotions these memories evoke. Consequently, interventions that address this right-brain dominance are believed to be important for both expressing and processing trauma memories and are an essential part of successful treatment (Steele & Malchiodi, 2011). Similarly, it is speculated that because childhood trauma affects the integration of both sides of the brain (Teicher, 2000), sensory and body-based interventions such as the expressive arts and play are thought to be effective because they do not strictly rely on the individual's use of language for processing.

Despite the complexity of the relationship between the brain's two hemispheres, certain accepted neuroscience theories are relevant to expressive arts therapies and trauma-informed practice. Badenoch (2008) speculates that both hemispheres of the brain are key to a therapist's success, noting, "Whole brain knowing is more apt to make permanent changes in the way any of us do therapy" (p. 4). In applications of expressive arts therapy, practitioners have a similar goal—access to the more embodied, implicit, sensory-based right-hemisphere functions to enhance integration with the more declarative left hemisphere. In other words, from current clinical observations, patient reports, and emerging research, the expressive arts possibility for supporting "whole-brain" integration is not always present in verbal approaches to trauma intervention. This may be due both to the self-regulatory qualities of arts-based, action-oriented experiences and to the process of reconnecting implicit and explicit memories of distressing events (see the next section for more information).

EXTEROCEPTION AND INTEROCEPTION

There are two concepts involving the senses that are foundational to expressive arts and traumatic stress: exteroception and interocepton. *Exteroception* is sensing external stimuli through the five senses (sight, hearing, touch, smell, and taste). These senses are useful in identifying elements of the environment. For trauma survivors, this may determine whether a situation or setting is perceived as safe. Exteroceptive experiences are found throughout all applications of the expressive arts because they involve the senses; that is, these activities can be visual, kinesthetic, tactile, auditory, proprioceptive, vestibular, and even olfactory in some cases. Each art form is multisensorial; for example, music therapy involves not only sound, but also vibration, rhythm, and movement. Dramatic enactment may include vocalization, visual impact, and other sensory qualities. Dance/movement encompasses a variety of body-oriented sensations. Art making is not limited to images; it also provides a variety of tactile and kinesthetic experiences. A visual art experience may include fine or expansive body movements, various smells of art media, and tactile sensations such as fluidity, stickiness, dampness, hardness, softness, or resistance.

In contrast, *interoception* is the perception of internal body sensations (pulse, breathing, pain) and includes proprioception (the sense of position, space, and orientation). Interoception is related to less tangible, but identifiable, perceptions of internal mood or "gut feelings" experienced within the polyvagal system (Porges, 2012) as well as a general "felt sense" (Gendlin, 1982) within the body. The arts themselves include interoceptive moments; when listening to a particularly powerful piece of music or viewing a dance performance or artwork, people often report "being moved." In other words, these are internal feelings not easily articulated with words.

Lanius and colleagues (2005) examined the question of how individuals who suffer from post-traumatic stress perceive interoception. They were able to demonstrate that there is a disruption in the functioning of the part of the brain that might be connected to the emotional disruptions experienced by trauma survivors. Lanius's team (in van der Kolk, 2014) also notes that when comparing the attention to breath in individuals with PTSD and those without, the interoception area of the brain was activated in those individuals without post-traumatic stress, but there was almost no activation of self-sensing in those individuals with PTSD. In brief, those with PTSD had learned to "shut down the brain areas that transmit the visceral feelings and emotion" (van der Kolk, 2014, p. 92). This finding underscores a challenge to just how the expressive arts might be used to actually address the lack of interoception in those with post-traumatic stress.

Individuals who are experiencing distress due to trauma often make determinations about reality based on what they experience internally rather than externally. In other words, a sensory quality of the environment related to the original traumatic event(s) stimulates hyperarousal, anxiety, fear, avoidance, or other responses even when danger is not present in external reality. For example, in initial sessions with Tanya (Chapter 2), the residential staff became aware of her behavioral responses to interoceptively perceived danger; she preferred to sit where she could watch for danger. She slept in the closet of her bedroom at night for safety, even though the original threat (her uncle) was not present. Rothschild (2011) and others who approach trauma resolution from a mind–body framework feel that working with the "dual awareness" of exteroception and interoception is central to intervention. Similarly, one of the key goals of trauma-informed expressive arts therapy is to help the individual identify and express nonverbally both exteroceptive and interoceptive experiences to help reduce distress responses over time. In Marian's case (Chapter 2), arts-based approaches were helpful in differentiating her past experience of trauma (bus accident) from current anxiety and panic attacks when reminders of the original traumatic event stimulated internal sensory responses. With other individuals, expressive arts are useful in supporting awareness of the "here-and-now." They are sensory-based ways of grounding the person in the present and taking focus away from past experiences.

TRAUMA MEMORY

Arts-based approaches are frequently cited as experiences that stimulate memories, particularly trauma memories or fragments of memories (Crenshaw, 2006). While there is wide agreement that music, artistic expression, movement, drama, and imaginative play can stimulate what are referred to as trauma memories, how or why this happens is not exactly known, but it may be related to how these memories are initially encoded.

Lenore Terr (1990) notes that children's memories of trauma are generally more perceptual than declarative in content and, therefore, are often expressed through play and other nonverbal forms of communication. More recently, van der Kolk (2014) explained that when contextual memory cannot accommodate traumatic events, a different memory is created or dissociation occurs; these experiences are often stored as nonlanguage, "sensory fragments." Essentially, psychological trauma is believed to disrupt executive functioning (the prefrontal cortex), causing it to go "offline." Thus, traumatized individuals find they cannot adequately explain what has happened with words or what happens when a reminder of trauma occurs. Similarly, Rothschild (2000) observes that post-traumatic stress responses, in part, may be caused when memory of trauma is excluded from storage as declarative, chronological memory. Perry (2009) reports that trauma interferes with executive function and memory, noting that children whose lives have been disrupted by trauma often hear only about half of the words their teachers communicate in the classroom.

It has also been proposed that memories of traumatic exposure are stored mainly in the brain's right hemisphere, an area noted earlier as preverbal or nonverbal. This observation is based on both brain imaging and accounts from trauma survivors who frequently say that memories are experienced as sensations and images rather than as linear narratives with clear beginnings and endings. These impressions are often felt intensely and may emerge much later and throughout the lifespan. According to Siegel (2012), the right hemisphere is also the more holistic hemisphere and is connected to somatic and sensory systems, including emotional expression.

Additionally, Broca's area in the left hemisphere is deactivated, relegating trauma memory to other forms of information processing such as somatic, sensory, and visual (van der Kolk, 2014).

In sum, trauma's impact on memory is considerable and includes the individual's ability to access declarative memory in many cases. Sensory memories may be more accessible for many survivors, and thus, we can speculate that expressive arts may be one way to tap trauma-related memories. The concepts of explicit and implicit memory may, in part, explain the role of arts-based interventions in trauma recovery. Explicit memory is conscious and is composed of facts, chronological details, and ideas; implicit memory is sensory, affective, and related to the body's memories of events. Rothschild (2000) observes that post-traumatic reactions may be caused when memory of a trauma is excluded from explicit storage. Problems result when implicit memories are not linked to explicit memories; that is, according to Rothschild, an individual may not have access to the context in which the emotions or sensations arose.

One possibility for addressing this disconnect between implicit and explicit memory may involve experiences that help to reconnect the two, resulting in the capacity to form coherent stories. For example, specific expressive arts approaches may help bridge the implicit and explicit memories of a stressful event, helping the person explore and experience these memories through creative expression (Malchiodi, 2003, 2012a, 2013). This may explain in part why individuals engaged in hands-on activities such as drawing have been found to verbally communicate more about emotionally laden events (Gross & Haynes, 1998; Lev-Weisel & Lisz, 2007). If this is true, then expressive arts may help traumatized individuals to think (explicit) and feel (implicit) concurrently (Malchiodi, 2003, 2008) through self-regulatory, relational interventions.

Here is a brief example of how sensory processing and memory are interconnected and how using even a simple arts-based experience can stimulate recall of memories that might otherwise remain unexpressed. As described in an earlier chapter, I once worked at a community mental health agency that provided outpatient groups to adult women who were sexually abused as children and in current need of intervention for trauma-related reactions. The group members and staff developed the theme of "childhood memories" for one session, and I decided to bring each group member a new box of 64 Crayola-brand crayons to use as art material for drawing that day because crayons and paper are familiar media for art activities during childhood. While I had plans to request some specific themes for drawings, the group members' sensory responses to opening the crayon boxes quickly took the session in a different direction than what was planned. As each woman opened the box, each had a spontaneous reaction to the sensory qualities of the box and crayons. Some recalled a favorite childhood moment when a similar box of crayons was received on a special occasion such as a holiday or birthday celebration. For others, the crayon boxes stimulated painful reminders of a childhood cut short and radically changed by sexual abuse; some group members grieved for the lack of a caring adult to provide creative and playful experiences during their earliest years of life. The boxes of crayons stirred sensory memories linked to the familiar crayon brand and box (visual), the smell of new crayons (olfactory), and the excitement of receiving a set of 64 colors as a gift (multiple senses)—even as adult survivors. Because so many strong and important memories emerged during that session, we spent the entire group meeting sharing and talking without ever creating drawings with the crayons. The sensory qualities (implicit memories) of the material were enough to awaken recollections (explicit memories) long forgotten by most of these survivors, and the multisensory qualities of the crayons became a bridge to nonverbal memories.

Movement is another potent sensory-kinesthetic experience that often brings about unexpected recall. Because I start each session with some sort of simple movements (stretches, chair yoga, bilateral moves, and even brief dancing to music), I also check with the child or adult to understand if any feelings or thoughts are arising during the activity. While there are many areas of focus when introducing movement, the throat has particular importance; it is an area of the body that can hold experiences of panic or fear due to its relationship with the vagal system (Porges, 2012). For this reason, in initial sessions I may have individuals focus on hands and feet, parts of the body that are outside the realm of the vagus nerve, until I have a clearer understanding of the individual's distress level.

Although the sensory nature of expressive arts can tap implicit and explicit memories of trauma, recall through art, movement, music, or play may also call forth and release pleasant and enlivening memories. For many years I worked with the HIV/AIDS community at a foundation for patients and their caregivers during a time period when most individuals diagnosed with the illness died due to lack of effective treatments. As the illness gradually debilitated these individuals, most suffered from extreme fatigue arising from multiple opportunistic infections, inability to walk without assistance, and, often, complications such as vision or hearing loss. Working in a sandtray with objects and figures provided not only the experience of self-soothing, but also recollections of pleasure, particularly those related to being in nature. For those individuals who had once walked on a beach, working in a sandtray evoked memories of the sounds of the waves and the feeling of sand under one's feet. Red sand in the tray called up trips to the U.S. Southwest and the independence of hiking among spectacular red rock formations and terrains. While these memories may also bring with them a sense of loss for times past and no longer possible due to illness, for most the sandtray experiences became a way to re-experience pleasurable times through sensory recall. In all cases, they were remembered moments of pleasure, albeit momentary, from being defined solely by the limitations of symptoms, disease, and traumatic stress.

THE EXPRESSIVE THERAPIES CONTINUUM

Many trauma specialists propose phase or stage-by-stage approaches to trauma intervention. Herman (1992), discussed in Chapter 2, provides an example for a framework that involves identifiable stages. Some trauma protocols involve standardized workbooks and other strategies that follow a clearly delineated outline of interventions over a specific time period or number of sessions. Trauma-focused cognitive-behavioral therapy (TF-CBT; Cohen, Deblinger, & Mannarino, 2017) is one such approach that is standardized and supported by evidence-based research.

Art therapists have proposed various stage models to address trauma. Chapman (2014) created a protocol, neuro-developmental art therapy (NDAT), that consists of four phases of treatment over a long period of time and is designed to address relational trauma in children. It is directed at activating and developing the "lower structures of the brain, where relational trauma damage occurred" (p. 50), and it includes art and play activities. Based on Schore (2003) and Perry (2009), NDAT seeks to integrate lower structures of the brain first in order to inform the higher functions later on, with the goal of moving the child to more improved capacities. Chapman's model does not assign a number of sessions to each phase but is designed as a continuum with specific brain-related themes (neural activity, cognition, information processing, psychological reactions, and arts-based processes).

With dance/movement therapy in mind, Dieterich-Hartwell (2017) explains a three-stage model for treatment of post-traumatic stress as follows: (1) safety, (2) reduction of hyperarousal, and (3) interoception. Dieterich-Hartwell emphasizes that this approach, in contrast to other models, is not exhaustive, but rather directly focuses on two basic issues of trauma survivors—disconnection from their bodies and lack of interoception. This type of model is designed to capitalize on one specific form of expressive arts to build a foundation for more complete intervention over time.

While many practitioners find these stage models of trauma intervention helpful, they may not be the most effective way to facilitate expressive arts within the context of psychotherapy. In my experience, individuals who experience traumatic events do not always neatly progress through universal phases of recovery, nor do they fit into sequential steps when it comes to standardized arts-based procedures. The variable impacts of traumatic experiences challenge these methods for many reasons. One person may experience developmental trauma or multiple trauma events across the lifespan, while another individual may be challenged with a specific, acute traumatic event. Some may have experiences of intergenerational or historical trauma in addition to current challenges. Each may have reactions commonly seen in most survivors of trauma, but for the most part, each individual or group has additional, unique responses due to many factors and influences. As Dieterich-Hartwell (2017) underscores in her dance/

movement therapy model, many stage models are designed from a Western perspective and often do not address the individual's needs as part of a larger group or community. Also, most of the existing protocols focus on brain-related functions and do not really incorporate more body-relevant intervention, including polyvagal theory (Porges, 2012) or sensorimotor approaches (Elbrecht, 2014, 2018; Ogden & Fisher, 2015).

Although practitioners often seek out these protocols for phase- or stage-based work, there is another way to organize clinical thinking about how and when to introduce various expressive arts to individuals in treatment that has more flexibility and is more responsive to the needs of individuals in the moment. Like other eclectic methods, expressive arts have historically blended arts and play with various approaches to psychotherapy, including various psychoanalytic, humanistic, cognitive, and developmental approaches to arrive at treatment strategies. But there is one particular model for psychotherapeutic work that fits well with expressive arts as the core approach—the Expressive Therapies Continuum (ETC; Kagin & Lusebrink, 1978; Lusebrink, 1990, 2010). This model is particularly relevant to trauma intervention because it reflects current thinking about the neurobiology of trauma and neurodevelopment (see Table 3.1). Lusebrink (1990, 2010), one of the key figures in the development of the ETC, based her initial concepts on information processing and executive functioning, sensorimotor development, psychosocial behavior, and self-psychology. More recently, she integrated contemporary neurobiology principles within the overall framework of the ETC (Lusebrink, 2010). Graves-Alcorn (formerly Kagin) explained a variety of practical applications of the ETC, underscoring a developmental framework for intervention in clinical and educational settings (Graves-Alcorn & Kagin, 2017).

Lusebrink, Graves-Alcorn, and others who have written about the ETC primarily discuss visual art-based applications. But I see this framework as a way to conceptualize treatment strategies applicable to all the expressive arts and various forms of play as well as some related practices including yoga, mindfulness, and body-based interventions. It is a model for how to define media and methods and the qualities of various approaches with the goal of designing and applying specific interventions based on individual needs.

In a very basic sense, the ETC proposes four levels of experience, moving from simple to more complex processing. Three ETC levels can be loosely associated with Perry's (2009) developmental model of brain function going from brainstem to midbrain to higher limbic and cortical systems. The ETC levels as defined by the original authors are (1) kinesthetic/sensory, (2) perceptual/affective, (3) cognitive/symbolic, and (4) a creative level that may occur at any single level of the ETC or may be the integration of functioning from all levels (Lusebrink, 2010). The following summary provides a basic overview of the ETC levels (summarized from Malchiodi, 2012a).

The *kinesthetic/sensory* level is defined as interaction with the expressive arts in an exploratory way. The kinesthetic experience is characterized

TABLE 3.1. Neurodevelopment and Arts Therapies

Area of brain	General functions	ETC level	Arts therapies interventions
Brainstem	• Focus • Attunement to others • Attachment to others • Stress responses	Kinesthetic/ sensory	• Sensory use of arts materials • Texture and tactile elements • Self-soothing arts experiences (visual, music, movement) • Experiences of connection and approval • Rituals/structure in presentation
Midbrain, diencephalon	• Motor skills • Coordination • Stress responses • Attunement to others • Attachment to others	Kinesthetic/ sensory	• Physically oriented activities (cross the midline; engage body) • Learning skills via art and play • Self-soothing arts experiences (visual, music, movement) • Experiences of connection and approval • Rituals/structure in presentation
Limbic system	• Affect regulation • Pleasure • Relationships • Attunement • Attachment	Perceptual/ affective	• Masks, puppets for projection and relational play • Arts and crafts for creative expression and skill enhancement • Group art therapy/Family art therapy • Self-soothing arts experiences (visual, music, movement) • Rituals/structure in presentation
Cortex	• Cognition • Executive function • Self-image • Social competency • Communication	Cognitive/ symbolic	• Cognitive-based methods possible, but sensory and affective methods may still be needed • Bibliotherapy with arts and play • Arts for skill enhancement and self-esteem • Teamwork in group arts therapy • Problem-solving skills

Note. Based on Lusebrink (2010), Malchiodi (2011), and Perry (2006). From Malchiodi (2012b). Copyright © 2012 The Guilford Press. Reprinted by permission.

by movement and motor activity. For example, spontaneous movement, beating a drum, or a scribble drawing can be defined as kinesthetic in quality; this type of expression can be free-form or even chaotic and disorganized. Sensory simply implies use of the senses in experiencing an art form. A hands-on experience with clay is an example of the sensory level; however, it can also include visual, auditory, olfactory, and gustatory qualities. The vestibular (balance) and proprioceptive (where one perceives one's body in the environment) are also sensory qualities and are part of the experience of dance or movement, for example. In both kinesthetic and sensory experiences, the details of what is created are less important than the actual experience of the expressive arts or imaginative play activity.

The *perceptual/affective* level is defined as engagement with an art form to express perceptions and to communicate emotions. Perceptual aspects have to do with creating a form or pattern, such as using lines and colors with paint or drawing materials. Affective responses involve emotional qualities; using a drum, movement, or sound to convey a feeling state such as anger, happiness, or worry are examples of expression at the affective level. At this level, individuals are able to self-observe and reflect on their experiences with the art form.

The *cognitive/symbolic* level is defined as use of the art form for problem solving, structuring, and, in some cases, meaning seeking. An individual, for example, is able to use analytic, logical, and sequential skills while engaging in the art process. This experience may lead to a symbolic response in which personal meaning can be explored. Clients working at the cognitive/symbolic level of the ETC may demonstrate the use of rational thought and intellect in an expressive arts process and may naturally look for meaning in their images and other creative work.

According to the ETC model, the *creative* level may occur at any of the previous levels, or it may involve the integration of all other levels of the ETC into personal expression. In the case of the latter, all previous levels (kinesthetic/sensory, perceptual/affective, and cognitive/symbolic) are apparent in an art form according to the originators of this framework. Not all individuals or art forms necessarily reach this level, but a form of creativity can be experienced at each of the other three levels of the ETC. For example, someone could experience creativity through spontaneous movement, although the experience would be defined as more kinesthetic on the continuum.

The term *creative* has multiple meanings even within artistic expression, making it difficult to identify and define within a psychotherapy framework. When it comes to trauma reparation, my interpretation of this overarching level is a little bit different from what the originators of the ETC intended. To me, it is the experience of integration that manifests itself when reparative work successfully occurs at all three levels of the ETC. This three-part integration also does not necessarily take place from a bottom-up or top-down process. But because trauma involves sensory, affective, and cognitive experiences, it follows that repair through expressive arts must occur at all three levels in order for integration to occur (see the section below discussing trauma integration for a more detailed discussion). When speaking of trauma recovery, this creative level can be defined as the experience of meaning making through imagining new narratives via the arts (see Chapter 10).

Two other terms are important parts of the ETC: the healing function and the emergent function. A *healing function* is present in each component of the ETC (Kagin & Lusebrink, 1978). Lusebrink (1991) notes that this function "denotes optimum intrapersonal functioning on the particular level" (p. 395). Essentially, it is what is therapeutic about each level or, in the case of a specific intervention, what is helpful in encouraging self-regulation, behavioral change, or insight. Because the term *healing* is somewhat vague, I prefer to use the term *reparative function* because it implies the possibility for positive change in many different areas of functioning, including emotional, social, cognitive, physical, and spiritual. Additionally, according to Kagin and Lusebrink (1978), practitioners can capitalize on the *emergent function* of each component to encourage movement from one level to another within the ETC for therapeutic reasons and individual goals and objectives. For example, a goal of providing specific music, visual arts, or creative writing experiences may help an individual experience a different level of the ETC and thus may support reparation and increase the possibility of integration (Lusebrink, 1991).

Finally, *media variables* are underscored within the conceptualization of the ETC. Media variables are the various qualities of visual art materials as described by the originators of the framework. However, when using the framework with expressive arts therapy and play-based approaches, these variables also describe the characteristics of music, sound, movement, dance, dramatic enactment, props, toys, storytelling, and writing. For most individuals, any expressive arts medium may be predominantly related to a specific level of the ETC, but in most cases expressive arts simultaneously tap multiple areas, including movement, senses, emotion, form, cognition, and/or symbolism. For example, sandplay therapy is an example of what is often a multilevel experience because of the sensory qualities of sand, water, and objects, perceptions and feelings associated with items used in the sandplay process, and storytelling that may occur as a result of the image created in the sand. Additionally, dramatic enactment can include tactile props, kinesthetic movement, and expression of affective and symbolic content.

In order to understand the ETC in an experiential way, I encourage you to be your own arts-based researcher (Malchiodi, 2018). The following three drawing and writing activities introduce the sensory, affective, and cognitive levels of the ETC. These activities are based on some of the original concepts presented by Kagin and Lusebrink (1978) and Lusebrink (1990). For these three activities, you will need some drawing materials (colored pencils, felt markers, or oil pastels), white paper (photocopy paper is appropriate or white sketchbook paper), a copy of the body outline template (see

Appendices 1A and 1B, for adults and children, respectively*), and a pen and notepad on which to write a short story. Be sure to complete these three activities in the order they are presented before reading the rest of this section, and remember, there are no right or wrong responses.

1. "Think of a 'worry' that you have right now. Using colored pencils, felt markers, or oil pastels, make an image of that worry by simply 'making marks' on the paper using colors, lines, or shapes to show your sensory experience of that worry."

2. "Now consider 'where in your body you feel this worry.' Close your eyes if it feels comfortable to do so and scan your body from your head to your feet; notice where you sense or feel this worry. You may feel it in one part of your body or several parts of your body; you may even feel that it extends outside the boundaries of your body. Using a body outline, try to show with color, lines and/or shapes, or mark-making where you experience your worry in your body and what it feels like."

3. "For the final part of this experience, you are going to be engaging in a brief written exercise. Think about the following question: 'If your worry could talk, what would it say?' Write this story from a non-first-person perspective with at least five to six complete sentences to tell a short story about what your worry would say. Do not just think about this story; write it down on a piece of paper. You can give your worry a name, too, if that seems appropriate."

The sequence of these three experiences approximates the ETC and very loosely mimics a "lower-to-higher" brain process (kinesthetic/sensory to affective/perceptual to cognitive). In fact, each experience requires the "whole brain," but in each activity, there is an emphasis on one part of the ETC. For example, the first directive asks you to simply experience and depict your "worry" in a mostly sensory and kinesthetic way by using mark-making. While you may have created actual forms or images as a way to depict an emotional (affective) state, this is generally a sensory/kinesthetic activity. In the second activity, you are asked to perceive where and how you experience the worry in your body, an experience that is a little more perceptual and affective in terms of focus. The final activity asks you to think (cognitive) about your worry and use language to describe it; you may even have experienced it as symbolic in some way at this point. While each activity involves multiple components of the ETC, each emphasizes a level of the conceptual framework. The following brief examples illustrate

---

* Appendices 1A and 1B are two examples of templates that I use in sessions with adults and children. You can find numerous examples by doing an Internet search; it is important to have several different templates, so that individuals can choose the one that appeals to them.

how several adult individuals responded to the three activities through a "worry drawing," body outline indicating the perceived sense of the worry, and a short story about "what the worry would say if the worry could talk."

Example 1

Figures 3.1 and 3.2 are responses to worry drawing and the felt sense of the worry in the body. When asked, "If your worry could talk, what would it say?" the individual wrote the following:

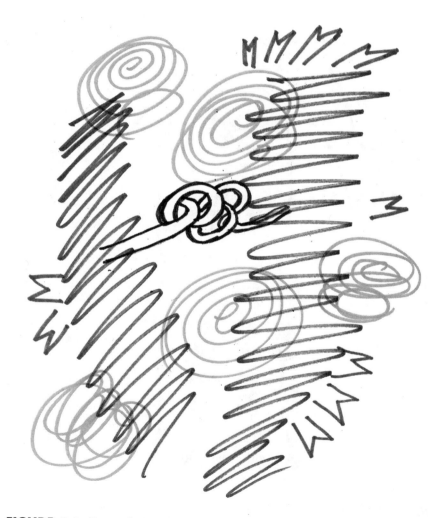

FIGURE 3.1. Example 1: Worry drawing. From the collection of Cathy A. Malchiodi (not to be reproduced without permission from the author).

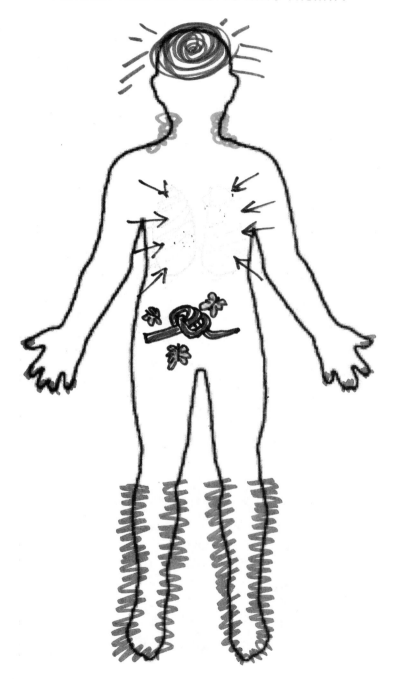

FIGURE 3.2. Example 1: Body outline drawing. From the collection of Cathy A. Malchiodi (not to be reproduced without permission from the author).

"Every night after you go to bed and were getting all relaxed and sleepy, I like to come around. I like to say to you 'look out!' 'Be careful!' 'Don't forget me!' I love to do this when you are just drifting off to sleep. I love to make your body tense all over and make your teeth clench until your jaw hurts. I really love it when you listen to me really closely and remind yourself of all the things you could have done differently. I like to keep you on edge and the more you are on edge, the bigger and more powerful I feel.

"You think you can write about me and get rid of me? I will not be dismissed, and I will make your heart beat faster and sometimes make you feel like you are going to lose your breath. You try turning on some music to appease me, but that does not work. I only work on you even more. Now your neck is tense and you can feel a migraine headache coming on. Sometimes I can even make your eyes twitch. Now you have been awake 2 hours in bed and you are worried that you will not get enough sleep tonight before work tomorrow."

Example 2

Figures 3.3 and 3.4 are another person's responses to the first two directives. In the final part of the process, the individual indicated that her worry says:

"I started to hold you back from doing things since your childhood. I whispered in your ear so that you would be afraid to do what you wanted to do. Now that you are an adult, I am the size of a monster, and I like to shout at you when you are having fun or trying to sleep at night. I will not stay small! Don't try to ignore me! Look at me! Things will never get better and they will only get worse. You can sit around and think 'If I had done things differently.' Or 'If I had done x, y, or z, then things would be better right now.' But you did not because you listened to me and there is nothing you can do now. You are totally trapped and you cannot get away from me.

"Sometimes I enjoy saying to you, 'FREEZE RIGHT THERE! Stop what you are doing or wishing or dreaming.' Seriously, what do you think you are going to do now? You know something bad is going to happen. I am Worry, hear me roar. You cannot get away from me. Are you listening? Do you hear me?"

Example 3

Figure 3.5 represents a worry drawing, and Figure 3.6 is the individual's perception of the worry in the body. The individual wrote the following about what this worry says:

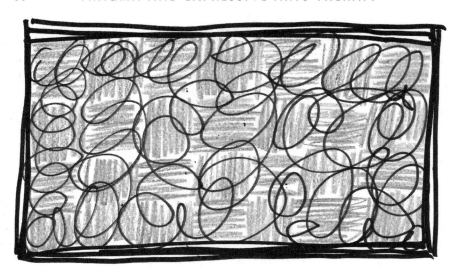

FIGURE 3.3. Example 2: Worry drawing. From the collection of Cathy A. Malchiodi (not to be reproduced without permission from the author).

"When I hit you, I am confronting. I force you to a standstill. You have to reevaluate where you are and what you can do. You have to deal with me, there is no getting around that. You cannot decide what your priorities are right now. I can make you feel flustered by forcing you to pay attention to me. I can scramble your mind and make you look for someone to blame for me causing you pain.

"I can also make you think about the future, and that helps me to make you feel guilty. I am good at helping you to have a racing heart, sweaty palms, breathe rapidly. I can make you focus on trying to gain control of me, but you cannot control me. I make you try to stop the internal chaos I create—good luck on that! When you get flustered, I can grow even more and I make your head feel heavier and your stomach churn. I enjoy that everything feels like a burden to you now and that I create an overwhelming feeling of disempowerment.

"I will not give you an immediate feeling of relief even when I am gone. I enjoy that it takes you a long, long time to get over me, for your stomach to relax and for your headache to go away. I let you put me into a box in the back of your mind, but I never really go away. I love being a reminder that you can lose control any time in the future.

"If Worry gets a little smaller, it says: 'When I am quiet, your world seems calmer. I let you take the time to enjoy life and the qualities of the day. You can admire the warm sun, the smell of coffee and cookies and I let you have a productive day at work. You can really enjoy your life now.'"

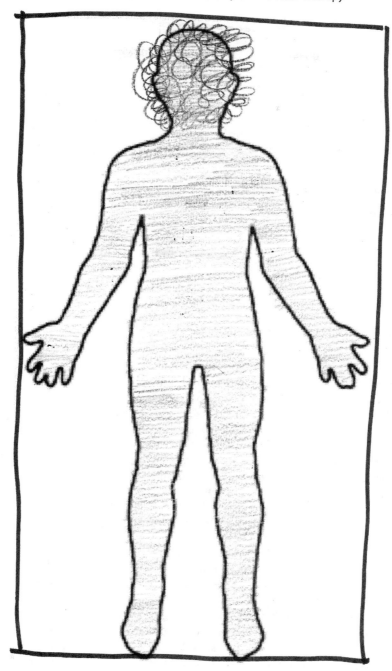

FIGURE 3.4. Example 2: Body outline drawing. From the collection of Cathy A. Malchiodi (not to be reproduced without permission from the author).

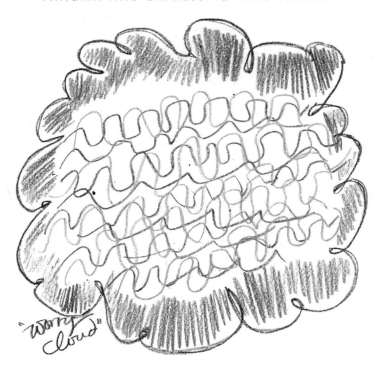

FIGURE 3.5. Example 3: Worry drawing. From the collection of Cathy A. Malchiodi (not to be reproduced without permission from the author).

While this particular ETC exercise is a way to understand the three levels of the continuum, it is also obviously a possible strategy for use in clinical practice. In asking individuals to engage in each of these activities, there are several important considerations when applying it to trauma work. First, in using this three-part experience, I generally ask people to make alterations to their three responses in order to change characteristics of their images and/or story during the session. For example, I may suggest, "If you could help make your worry go away or get smaller, how would your worry look? How would your drawing change?" If it seems appropriate, I may also ask, "Can you show me that change in another drawing or add something to this drawing to show that positive or helpful change?" In Example 3, the individual was not only able to write what the worry would say if it were "smaller" and less obtrusive, she was also about to show on another body outline how her perceived feelings in her body about the worry would change (Figure 3.7). The important point is not only to provide choices to make revisions, but also not to leave the individual with the worry as a session ends, but with an experience that begins to move the individual toward some possible solutions.

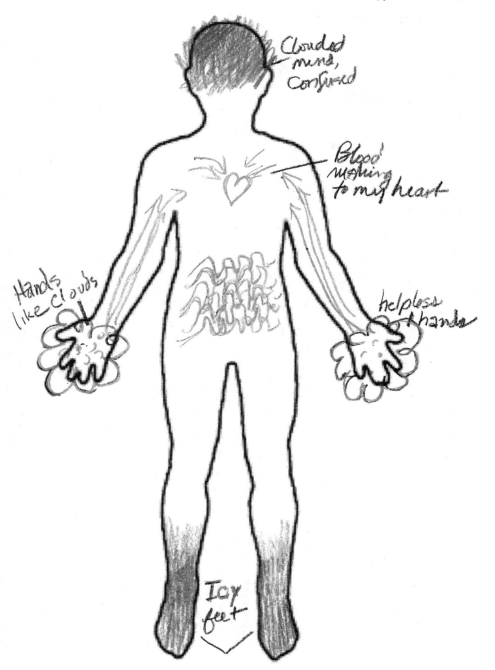

FIGURE 3.6. Example 3: Body outline drawing. From the collection of Cathy A. Malchiodi (not to be reproduced without permission from the author).

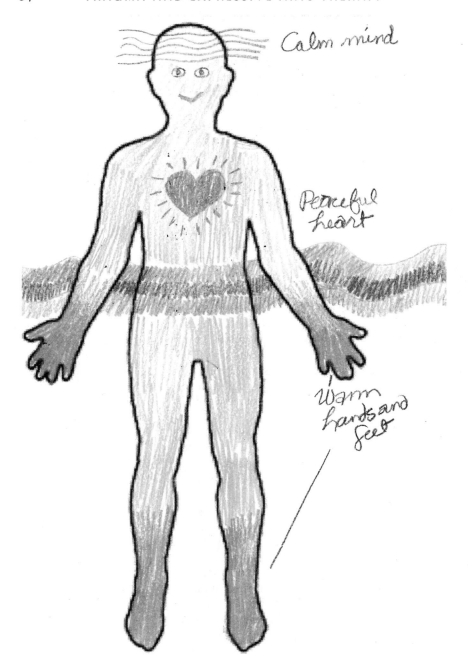

FIGURE 3.7. How the worry would change on the body outline. From the collection of Cathy A. Malchiodi (not to be reproduced without permission from the author).

Not every individual is ready to experience where a worry or distressful sensation is felt. The individual may need to put into place and practice some additional self-regulation supports (see Chapter 6). For example, it may be more appropriate for some trauma survivors first to experience where "relaxation" or "safety" is felt in their bodies and what those feeling states look like in terms of colors, lines, and/or shapes. In the three-part activity, the words *relaxation, inner peace, calm,* or *safety* can be used to substitute for the word *worry* to help the individual identify self-regulatory feelings through art expression, which can later be used as part of stress reduction. For others, gentle physical movement to depict a feeling or mind state may be a better approach than drawing, particularly for individuals who tend toward withdrawal or freeze responses to trauma and need to "get moving."

BOTTOM-UP OR TOP-DOWN?

As discussed in earlier chapters, current theories of trauma intervention emphasize a bottom-up approach to treatment. That is, initial approaches address what are considered lower brain functions, gradually moving toward language and reconstruction of narratives to organize memories into a coherent and cohesive whole. The ETC continuum approximates a model for this application and supports the idea that lower functions must be repaired and form a sort of foundation for moving higher on the continuum to repair and eventually make possible healthy responses in subsequent levels.

There are some situations, however, in which the starting point for ETC is not necessarily a bottom-up affair. The order of the set of arts-based experiences described in the previous section is always open to revision, depending on the person's current needs and status. In other words, it is not necessary to always move from kinesthetic/sensory to perceptions to cognition in an arts-based experience. Consider an anxious parent who is desperately enduring the trauma of a child recently diagnosed with a life-threatening illness; that individual may be uncomfortable with expression of emotions via drawing or movement. Some caregivers feel the need to remain in control, at least for the short term, in order to maintain their focus on their loved one. For these individuals, verbal narratives may feel safer because they maintain a distance from sensations and feelings, even if those narratives are not the ones that will ultimately be helpful or healing as time passes. In contrast, it is not necessarily true that it is better to ultimately function on the cognitive/symbolic level (higher) at the expense of positive or reparation experiences on the other levels. For example, a traumatized teenager might need self-soothing sensory or kinesthetic experiences to self-regulate before working with emotion (affective) or exploring meaning making or problem solving (cognitive). The most appropriate strategy for a distraught caregiver may simply be locating the experience of "relaxation" in the body, especially during times of crises, rather than pursuing the body's more distressful sensations in the short term. In all cases, a trauma-informed approach guides practitioners to carefully consider the individual's needs within the context of current challenges and past trauma events.

APPLYING A TRAUMA-INFORMED EXPRESSIVE ARTS THERAPY CONTINUUM

The practical exercise in the previous section provides a way to experientially understand the basics of the ETC. The ETC is not only a practical construct for understanding, facilitating, and applying various components of arts-based intervention to trauma-informed practice; it also facilitates integrative experiences to address both the brain and body. While the originators of this model saw it as a way to assess art expressions and determine therapeutic interventions, I believe it supports a brain-wise as well as body-based way of understanding and addressing trauma (Malchiodi, 2012b). The multilevel framework roughly corresponds to the lower (sensory), middle (affective), and higher (cognitive) functions of the brain. It is also relevant to the various developmental levels, from young children who engage with their environments on the kinesthetic/sensory level to adults who are generally capable of expression on multiple levels, including cognition and executive functioning.

No one expressive arts experience is completely defined by one ETC level because there is always a degree of overlap with the qualities and characteristics of other levels. However, strategies can be focused on one level more than another and directed to address the individual's needs and objectives in the moment. The following section provides some general guidelines and considerations in applying the ETC as a framework for developing trauma-informed expressive arts therapy.

The Kinesthetic/Sensory Level

Kinesthetic functioning and sensory functioning are closely related principles in trauma intervention, but each also has distinct purposes and approaches within trauma-informed practice. In its simplest form, working with *kinesthetic* functioning is accomplished by getting individuals moving in some way to engage in embodied expression. Because many individuals store traumatic memories in nonverbal ways, action-oriented activities may help individuals feel less immobilized by distressing events. In some cases, movement is thought to be essential to the actual release of trauma memories (van der Kolk, 2014). Among the expressive arts, dance/movement therapy is most clearly kinesthetic, and movement, posture, or muscle tension has an impact on the individual's affect (Gray, 2015). Movement is also an effective outlet for hyperactivation and is helpful in addressing dissociation, two common reactions in post-traumatic stress (Malchiodi, 2015a).

The reparative functions of kinesthetic activities include the discharge of energy and reduction of stress and tension. They also help individuals orient themselves to the present by reinforcing a sense of the body in space (proprioceptive and vestibular senses) through movement and rhythmic breathing. From a somatic perspective, Levine (2015) proposes that people are able to recover more readily from stress by physically releasing the energy that is often accumulated during traumatic events. In contrast to animals that are threatened in the wild and who eventually release the stress they experience, humans tend to replace these natural methods of self-regulation with feelings and thoughts of shame, self-judgment, and fear. These feelings and thoughts inevitably slow down the process of recovery from psychological trauma and sometimes induce post-traumatic stress reactions. Levine believes there are kinesthetically and somatically based ways to help individuals move past them. Movement and action-oriented experiences are helpful when a person is caught in a "freeze" response and is finding it difficult to act when confronted by actual or perceived threats or distress. Rothschild (2011) also agrees that movement is one of several keys to safe recovery from trauma because it is not only an antidote to persistent freeze responses, but also dissipates stress hormones and increases self-control via increased muscle tone.

Perry (2009) highlights the notion that humans need patterned repetitive, rhythmic somatosensory activities and that such experiences originated thousands of years ago as forms of body sensing and self-regulation. Yoga, deep breathing and meditation, singing, dancing, exercising, tai chi, equine grooming, and drumming are among the many expressive activities that are self-regulating, repetitive, and rhythmic. Visual arts, dramatic enactment, and imaginative play emphasize kinesthetic qualities when they are patterned, repetitive, and rhythmic and engage the body in an action-oriented process that is cyclic and recurrent. For example, drawing on large paper to rhythmic music is a kinesthetic experience that may help self-regulation and sensory integration through bilateral movement and gesture by crossing the body's midline. In all cases, patterned repetitions involving rhythm resonate throughout the body and over time can influence neural patterns in the brain. In other words, movement is a direct pathway to promoting brain plasticity and literally revising the brain's response to traumatic memories.

As noted earlier in this chapter, mirroring is a movement experience that is also relational because it is dependent on active attunement to another individual or group. Mirroring can be part of many expressive arts and play experiences, but it is most often a primary component of dance/movement and dramatic enactment. While the goal of mirroring activities is to achieve a sense of connection between the therapist and individual, it is essentially dependent on actions. As a kinesthetic experience, it is a form of nonverbal, right-hemisphere-dominant communication that naturally occurs in secure attachment through movements, gestures, postures, and facial expressions between caregiver and child (Gray, 2015; Malchiodi, 2015b).

The *sensory* component of the ETC is similar to the kinesthetic one but emphasizes multisensory experiences (tactile, visual, auditory, gustatory, and olfactory, along with proprioceptive and vestibular). As described in a previous section of this chapter, expressive arts and play interventions are often defined as sensory-based approaches when it comes to trauma intervention. That is, they capitalize on awareness of the senses and internal experiences and help individuals focus on the body's senses. Ultimately, in applying sensory-based activities as part of trauma intervention, the goal is to help individuals practice and master self-regulation to enhance and achieve relaxation when they are hyperactivated or distressed. Sensory-based experiences also are linked to what Siegel and Hartzell (2003) observe as a "sea of sensation." In other words, during the early years of life, each individual understands and defines caregivers and the environment through the senses.

Hinz (2009) observes that the sensory level of the ETC may be helpful when a person is "caught up with cognition" or "has lost the ability to feel sensations and emotions" (p. 68). In contrast, traumatic events can be so overwhelming for many individuals that the language center of the brain goes offline in an adaptive coping maneuver to perhaps "stop thinking." In this case, sensory approaches, presented at an appropriate pace, can be helpful in assisting individuals to express what essentially is unspeakable or unthinkable. Because traumatic events are believed to include sensory memories of the experiences, many practitioners believe that tapping the senses in various ways is helpful in reparation and recovery from psychological trauma (Malchiodi, 2003, 2012d, 2015b).

Some trauma specialists believe that the sensory nature of expressive arts may make progressive exposure of the trauma narrative and communication of traumatic material tolerable while decreasing avoidance (Spiegel et al., 2006). In particular, sensory-based interventions that enhance self-regulation and decrease hyperactivation can be effective in titrating (allowing a little bit of stress to be expressed at a time) and, as Levine (2015) notes, pendulating (alternating between distress and self-regulation) communication of distressing memories. This is the essence of the reparative function of emphasizing the senses within trauma intervention. Sensory experiences can also stimulate somatic responses related to traumatic memories such as tension, tightness, dizziness, rapid breathing, or other distressing reactions. As described later in this book, when using expressive arts as sensory stimulation, it is essential to also provide sensory experiences that instill an embodied sense of safety as well as strategies for self-regulation via the senses.

Both the kinesthetic and sensory components of the ETC are defined as exploratory in nature (Lusebrink, 1990). In other words, they usually involve experiences and activities that do not necessary lead to a finished product but instead are more process-oriented. However, despite their exploratory qualities, kinesthetic and sensory expressions are just as important as other creative activity found throughout the ETC framework when it comes to trauma. In other words, movement and sensory expressions are valid forms of communication with individuals of any age who are experiencing psychological trauma because nonverbal communication is often a primary form of "language" for many survivors in the early stages of recovery. The expressive arts are essential in this regard because they provide a form of nonverbal communication for what cannot be articulated with words.

Perceptual/Affective Level

The *perceptual* component of the ETC involves use of the expressive arts to convey internal experiences in one or more creative forms. For example, as illustrated in the brief ETC activity in the previous section, a practitioner might ask a person to perceive where an emotion or "worry" is located in the body and to use colors, shapes, and images to depict that perception. A person could also be asked to use a movement or a series of notes on a keyboard to convey a perceptual experience. In contrast to a kinesthetic or sensory activity, the individual is developing a nonverbal language that not only communicates something, but that also produces communication that can be perceived by others.

The perceptual component of the perceptual/affective level is possibly best understood through use of trauma-informed art therapy because art provides tangible, visual representations of experiences, feelings, and perceptions. In Marian's case, being able to communicate her perceptions of her depression, panic attacks, and anger to me became both a meaningful and a hopeful turning point in therapy. Although she had been able to describe these perceptions verbally, she stated that she finally was also able to show what it was really like to live with the heaviness of depression, the chaos of unpredictable panic, feelings of guilt, and anger at her family through drawings. The drawings used to depict these perceptions and the image of where she held her emotions in her body provided a needed structure that helped Marian define these experiences and her response to them somatically.

In Marian's case and that of other trauma survivors, the expressive arts also tap the *affective* component of the perceptual/affective level. According to Lusebrink (1990) and Graves-Alcorn and Kagin (2017), the affective component of the ETC complements the perceptual component by encouraging the amplification of emotions. In contrast, the perceptual component is more concerned with structure and containment of emotions. In terms of trauma intervention, media and modes of expression are key when considering the reparative function of each. The reparative functions of perceptual activities are experiences of containment and structure. When dealing with individuals whose trauma reactions may include hyperactivation and fear, worry, or terror, providing a more structured experience supports expression while creating a sense of safety. For example, a practitioner might ask an individual to use felt markers and a small sheet of paper to express a worry, fear, or other feeling state, thus providing a less expansive and more contained experience of self-expression. In contrast, an individual might be offered the opportunity to use paint, brushes, and a large piece of paper or other surface to freely expand on an emotion through broad gestures of color. Similarly, when working with children and movement, structure can be provided by taping off a confined area (structure and containment) on the floor for movement to communicate emotion or encourage even more expansive and expressive (affective) responses by encouraging free movement within a whole room.

As is true of perceptual activities, the reparative function of affective activities includes communicating the implicit or "felt sense" (Rappaport, 2009) of what one has experienced when it comes to traumatic events. This includes the expression of powerful emotional memories by capturing them in visual, musical, movement or other creative forms. Like the previous level of the ETC, perceptual and affective components often overlap, depending on the expressive arts therapy intervention. Out of all the various components of the ETC, the perceptual/affective level is one of the most complex when determining appropriate expressive arts, trauma-informed interventions because of the centrality of emotional expression. In the simplest sense, it is essential to preserve a balance between containment and structure (perceptual) and less controllable expression and spontaneity (affective). This may mean using more easily controlled art materials (felt markers, colored pencils, collages); providing more structured, regulated experiences of music making, sound, and movement; and titrating (allowing brief experiences over time) less controllable, emotionally expressive experiences to provide an appropriate degree of containment in order to establish a sense of safety and mastery.

Cognitive/Symbolic Level

The *cognitive* component of the cognitive/symbolic level involves problem solving, abstraction, and other parts of executive functioning. Because cognitive development is predicated on age, young children are naturally more sensory and kinesthetic in their interactions with the environment, while school-age children are beginning to develop more concrete thinking and schemas for relationships and the world. Adolescents have more expansive cognitive abilities, including abstract thought and metacognitions (ability to think about one's own thoughts). As Siegel (2012) proposes, brain development, including cognitive capacity, continues well into young adulthood. Cognitive functioning can also be affected by various disorders throughout the lifespan that impact memory, mental processing, and executive functioning. Traumatic events also impact many individuals' executive functioning.

Hinz (2009) emphasizes problem solving, abstraction, comparisons, prioritizing, and complexity as characteristics of arts-based activities on the cognitive level of the ETC. Similarly, Lusebrink (1990) underscores the idea that the development of executive functioning can increase control over behavior. In other words, activities that reinforce cognitive skills may help individuals whose emotions are overwhelming or incapacitating. This is similar to the premise of cognitive-behavioral approaches that provide individuals with strategies to address anxiety and other emotional reactions. For example, TF-CBT (Cohen et al., 2017) capitalizes on the cognitive component when it comes to modifying behavior, particularly in children who are experiencing trauma-related reactions.

Because the cognitive component of the ETC involves more complex operations and processes, it can be challenging to work on this level with many traumatized individuals. For example, language may be compromised by hyperactivation, and cognitive functioning may be unavailable because of distress, dissociation, and dysregulation. If post-traumatic stress responses are disabling, executive functioning, including decision making, problem solving, following directions, and short-term memory, may be significantly affected. As previously mentioned, stage of development and existing barriers to learning also determine cognitive functioning and impact the effectiveness of strictly cognitive strategies with traumatized individuals, especially in the early stages of intervention. In brief, the cognitive level of the ETC depends on addressing the kinesthetic/sensory and perceptual/affective levels in many cases. "Reasoning" (cognition) can emerge only when adequate self-regulation (sensory) and positive, stable relationships (emotional safety) are present.

The reparative function of the cognitive level is related to personal narratives, including the ability to review, redefine, and reframe distressful experiences and traumatic events. Depending on developmental factors, this can include storytelling through play activities or art expression with younger children. For older children, adolescents, and adults, it may involve a variety of creative means to communicate narratives, including trauma narratives about "what happened" in some cases. As previously mentioned, there may also be circumstances when it is beneficial for an individual to "stay in the higher brain" in order to verbalize rather than delve into sensory or emotional qualities of a traumatic experience. Rather than affective interventions, some individuals may need reassurance from helping professionals and cognitively based self-regulation strategies to get through an immediate crisis. In contrast, asking a person to draw an image of painful and confusing feelings has the potential to be overwhelming and counterproductive. Disaster relief work requires similar strategies that allow individuals to engage in self-directed talk; participate in structured, familiar activities and routines; learn simple self-regulating practices; and quiet the mind and body before working with distressing feelings in most cases.

Finally, the *symbolic* component of the cognitive/symbolic level is defined as one of intuition and metaphoric content. It involves creative expression that communicates something that may have one or more meanings and encompass many dimensions (Graves-Alcorn & Kagin, 2017; Lusebrink, 1990). In contrast to the cognitive component, it is less concrete and generally more abstract and may include self-discovery, personal meaning, and universal characteristics. In the fields of psychoanalysis and depth psychology, dreams and their contents are still seen as symbols of both conflicts and healing. The nature of arts expression is directly related to symbolization and includes personal, cultural, and collective connotations (Jung, 2009) that are externalized in the form of images, music, movement, performance, stories, and play.

From a trauma-informed, expressive arts perspective, the symbolic level of the ETC is about helping individuals find or make meaning from what they have survived. The experience of meaning making through concrete narratives or through symbolic communications is an important part of the reparative process in trauma recovery. While self-regulation and resolution of distressing emotional memories are key factors, expressive arts approaches also provide unique processes and opportunities for individuals of all ages to tell their stories through largely nonverbal narratives in the form of art, music, movement, and dramatic enactment or in combination with the written word or storytelling. Historically, symbolic content in the expressive arts is defined as a creative product that may contain many facets of personality, including negative and positive (Lusebrink, 1990; Malchiodi, 2007).

The process of creating personal symbols and metaphors within trauma-informed expressive arts therapy is defined as adaptive, transformative, and, ultimately, a naturally reparative process rather than a compensatory, regressive, or otherwise defended response. For example, even though children's post-traumatic creative expressions may contain symbols or metaphors indicating distress, from a trauma-informed stance they also represent attempts to make meaning of worries and fears. They are efforts to find ways, with the help of the therapist, to repair the self and resolve traumatic memories. Encouraging and supporting meaning making through creative expression, post-trauma, is a central goal in the overall process of intervention. It is the culmination of therapeutic intervention that hopefully results in the integration of traumatic memories as well as the emergence of a more resilient self after trauma. This integration and increased resilience may also be a function of the *creative* level of the ETC, which proposes that authentic creativity includes the ability to synthesize and the experience of self-actualization (Graves-Alcorn & Kagin, 2017; Kagin & Lusebrink, 1978; May, 1974).

THE QUESTION OF TRAUMA INTEGRATION

The role of trauma integration in expressive arts therapy is an intriguing unanswered question and is often the subject of speculation and clinical observations. In my experience with children and adults, one cannot just talk one's way out of traumatic memories; something more is needed to resolve the body's survival responses and trauma reactions. For this reason, the body's implicit memory has become an additional focus in treatment. Similarly, the capacity of various creative art forms to express what words cannot suggests that these approaches might have an integrative role (Malchiodi, 2003, 2012c; Steele & Malchiodi, 2011).

Various expressive arts are currently being employed with the goal of trauma integration, offering a continuum of experiences that address multiple levels found in the ETC. For example, Elbrecht's (2014, 2015) work with the Clay Field® (a process of working with potter's clay within a confined space over time) and sensorimotor art therapy (2018) reflect many of the somatic approaches proposed by Levine (2012). These processes eventually lead the individual to address feelings and perceptions associated with traumatic memories and to arrive at narratives (language) and symbols (meaning making) for experiences. Gray (Gray & Porges, 2017) explains trauma reparation and integration through dance/movement and body-based processes. Their methods demonstrate how integration can occur by addressing neuroception and social engagement with children who do not have the full capacity to verbally communicate trauma narratives. Applications of dance/movement may help these individuals resolve the body's responses to traumatic memories as well as support healthy expression and resolution of emotions and thoughts.

Working with the various levels of the ETC though expressive arts engages individuals in addressing multiple components of traumatic memory, supporting trauma processing, and allowing both brain and body to realize that a trauma is not only over, but also resolved. In particular, this continuum addresses a component of trauma that is not generally targeted in strictly cognitive approaches—sensory-based processing that is related to lower parts of the brain. Future research may show us that introducing traumatized individuals to effective and relevant arts-based experiences, inclusive of the sensory, emotional, and cognitive levels of the ETC, helps at least some survivors in the process of integration, reparation, and recovery.

NEURODEVELOPMENT AS A TRAUMA-INFORMED EXPRESSIVE ARTS THERAPIES FRAMEWORK

The concept of neurodevelopment is an important component of trauma-informed intervention with children. The growing understanding of neurobiology is beginning to clarify developmental approaches to applications of the creative arts and play therapy. Siegel (2012), Chapman (2014), Malchiodi and Crenshaw (2014), and Perry (2006, 2009), among others, stress the importance of neurodevelopmental approaches in trauma treatment and resolution. As previously mentioned, Perry (2006) provides a framework for neurosequential development that informs the application of expressive arts therapy and play therapy (Gaskill & Perry, 2014, 2017) to children from infancy through adolescence. It is founded on the principle that the brain is organized in a hierarchical fashion, beginning with the development of the brainstem to the midbrain to limbic and cortical systems (Perry, 2009; see Figure 3.8). As noted earlier, the ETC is organized on levels that can be loosely associated with Perry's model of neurodevelopment and the premise that any intervention must first be relevant to the individual's needs

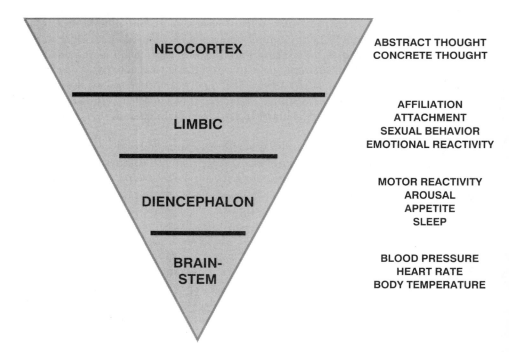

FIGURE 3.8. Neurodevelopment and hierarchy of brain function. From Malchiodi (2012a; adapted from Perry, 2006). Copyright © 2012 The Guilford Press. Reprinted by permission.

rather than chronological age. In particular, this framework is particularly useful in applying expressive arts therapy to young clients who have experienced chronic or developmental trauma. Gaskill and Perry (2014) highlight that any approaches such as play therapy must match the developmental stage of the individual. Although he is referring to children, this framework applies to adolescents and adults, especially those who have survived multiple traumatic events or who have complex trauma histories.

When applying neurodevelopmental principles to intervention, expressive arts therapy generally focuses on the lowest part of the brain affected and moves forward sequentially as improvements emerge. For example, intervention might begin with repetitive, relational, and rhythm-oriented activities fundamental to early development, attachment, and self-regulation. Ultimately, the goal is to help individuals achieve improvements in cognitive, emotional, and social functioning, including positive attachment, self-regulation, attunement to others, and affiliation (Perry, 2009). The following two case examples illustrate some of the basic principles of neurodevelopmental applications of expressive arts therapies and play therapy with an emphasis on concepts of the ETC explained in the previous sections. Both cases involve children who have experienced multiple traumatic and adverse events during childhood and are summarized from Malchiodi (2012c).

Case Example. Kristie: Addressing the Lower Brain and Midbrain

Kristie was 5 years old when she was referred to play therapy because of problems she was having with impulsive behavior and attention span in preschool. Her teachers reported that she bit another child on at least one occasion and frequently had extreme outbursts of anger. She was also unable to make eye contact with adult caregivers at preschool. Her parents reported that they felt Kristie was having trouble bonding with them and struggled with her tantrums and withdrawn behavior. Kristie also was having some problems with toilet training, something that should have been resolved at an earlier age. In addition, she also had difficulty with fine and gross motor skills during art and play sessions, and her drawings were more like those of a 2- or 3-year-old. She was having difficulties manipulating toys appropriate for her age and stage and using art tools such as paintbrushes, pencils, and markers; she was just as likely to try to eat various art and play materials as to use them appropriately despite prompting from adults.

Kristie experienced physical neglect and abuse for at least the first 6 months of her life and lived in several foster care placements before she was adopted at about age 3. From the time of her adoption, her parents felt she was a difficult child who was "fussy," frequently cried, and was impulsive; in a neurodevelopmental approach, these responses may indicate a need to address lower and midbrain functioning. In Kristie's case, sensory-stimulating activities, combined with experiences supporting self-soothing and self-regulation, were provided. For example, the therapist offered her structured opportunities to use tactile materials such as shaving cream, pudding, and sand to recapitulate earlier art and play activities Kristie may have missed experiencing due to a disrupted childhood. Interventions emphasized all the senses (smell, touch, sound, and taste) through listening to various rhythms and lullabies while drawing in sand and pudding, making cookies, and using felt markers with different smells of familiar foods. Developmental goals for Kristie included improving coordination and motor skills through learning to use a paintbrush, glue stick, and toys that involved simple repetitive construction. She was also encouraged by her therapist to talk about her scribble drawing, which would in turn encourage her to begin to tell stories, associate language with drawings, and enhance verbal skills more appropriate to her chronological age.

The therapist also capitalized on attachment-building strategies, inviting Kristie's adoptive parents to weekly sessions so that they could learn art and play activities they could practice at home with Kristie as well as expressive arts therapies and play therapy methods to enhance attachment, such as rocking and cuddling with soft toys to soothing music and singing lullabies. Play and expressive arts therapies were provided weekly for a little more than a year, as a result of which Kristie did make considerable progress and entered kindergarten with her peers. At the same time, she participated in a special classroom that continued to help her practice self-regulation and other developmentally relevant skills.

Case Example. Tommy:
Addressing the Middle and Higher Brain

I first met 12-year-old Tommy in a children's residential treatment program. He had experienced two divorces and three long-term separations from his mother from the ages of 1 to 3. When he was 8 years old, he was in a car accident and was hospitalized for a short time. After several reports were made to child protective services concerning abuse and domestic violence in his home, Tommy spent close to a year in residential treatment. He received regular visits from his biological mother, Anna. He recently had been placed on medications for attention difficulties because of his erratic and disruptive behavior; residential treatment staff reported that he had frequent short-term memory lapses. He also often fought with other children in the program, was overly anxious in new situations, had a sleep disorder and occasional nightmares, and experienced difficulty understanding others' feelings.

Tommy had obviously been exposed to multiple traumas during his lifespan that possibly accounted for his current cognitive and behavioral problems. While Tommy could benefit from activities to help him learn self-regulation like Kristie, his trauma reactions also indicated lower and midbrain reactions such as hyperarousal (sleep problems, nightmares, and anxiety), lack of empathy and attunement with others, and poor social skills. From a neurodevelopmental perspective, he could most benefit from interventions that addressed emotional reactions and stress responses, created a sense of safety, and increased empathy and social awareness.

I began with helping Tommy gain skills to calm his emotions and respond appropriately when he was feeling threatened or upset. Activities included construction with Legos® and building with clay because Tommy particularly enjoyed the tactile, self-soothing qualities of these materials. He also responded positively to repetitive, engaging art activities. In order to help Tommy communicate and learn more about what caused his anger reactions to other children, I asked him to use a gingerbread outline to identify "how your body feels when you are upset" and "where you experience the feelings in your body." In particular, I asked him to show me how "fear" and "anxiety" looked in colors, shapes, and lines. For Tommy, fear meant a pounding headache and a wish "to punch someone," while worries often caused his chest to "feel like it has a rope around it." I also asked Tommy if he could show me through movements and sounds what these experiences felt like and then to show me what he would feel like when he did not have the headaches or tight chest. The latter took some coaxing, but after several sessions Tommy was able to recall times at the program when he felt calm (during arts and crafts and when the therapy dog came to visit with the children) and when he felt happy (when his mother came to visit and brought him a present). Repeating these activities over the course of expressive arts therapy was extremely helpful to Tommy, and with the staff's help, he was able to begin to recognize how he felt various emotions in his body and when certain situations caused him to become anxious, angry, or fearful.

In both case examples, expressive arts and play therapy interventions were selected for Kristie and Tommy to specifically address their needs in terms of their neurodevelopmental status. In Kristie's case, she benefited from activities that helped her to develop motor skills, reduce impulsivity, and increase attachment; for Tommy, a structured approach to reducing emotional activation, increasing attunement to the feelings of others, and self-regulation were helpful. A neurodevelopmental approach to expressive arts therapy focuses on areas of development that allow individuals of any age to grow, thrive, learn new skills, improve interpersonal responses, and achieve a sense of self-worth in the process. In particular, these brief vignettes also emphasize the role of kinesthetic/sensory components with Kristie and perceptual/affective components and some cognitive work with Tommy, providing developmental examples of the ETC described in previous sections.

CONCLUSION

Emerging research from neuroscience and neurobiology continues to influence how practitioners view psychological trauma. Similarly, it has helped to inform the understanding and growing base of knowledge about the expressive arts as forms of intervention and treatment of children and adults. In this sense, neuroscience and neurobiology represent the most current way of explaining just how expressive arts and play methodology supports trauma reparation and recovery. However, it is also important to remember that the fields of neuroscience and neurobiology are always evolving, not only as new information derived from brain imaging emerges, but also as reports are collected from those who have experienced traumatic events. We are only at the very beginning of conceptualizing just how the expressive arts may be part of a larger brain-wise framework for effectively addressing the multitude of trauma-related reactions experienced by survivors.

CHAPTER 4

. . . .

The Reparation
Is in the Relationship

In part, humankind has survived for millennia because of a neurobiological drive to achieve safe and lasting relationships. Bruce Perry (in Perry & Szalavitz, 2017) explains three main functions for all animals: the brain must help them to stay alive, procreate, and nurture and protect offspring. However, he also notes that we humans are a "social species that is dependent on the brain's capacity to form and maintain relationships" (p. 70). Within these relationships, we have not only been able to move forward as a species, but also maintain a sense of resiliency even when exposed to the most distressing of experiences. Positive attachment, social support, and a sense of belonging to a community are all significant factors in perception of quality of life, reparation from loss and illness, and general health and well-being. They are also essential experiences in recovery from traumatic events. In the field of psychotherapy, all forms of transformational change propose that healing is consistently found through reparative relationships.

I have been more fortunate than most of the individuals I see in practice with regard to reparative relationships. I have had positive, secure relationships at various points in my life that have changed me in significant and growth-producing ways. My parents and extended family did the best they could to instill in me a sense of safety and hope, even though they had numerous challenges in their lives; in addition, partners have provided affection and devotion that opened me to deeper emotional levels of trust and courage. My closest friends have been patient, generous, and caring during times of loss and distress. Many teachers and mentors throughout my childhood, adolescence, and adulthood helped me to develop various capabilities, intelligence, and creativity. Other individuals have almost miraculously appeared during my life at what seemed like synchronistic moments, imparting advice and introducing life-changing experiences. Of course, there were also therapists who skillfully and empathetically moved me through difficult memories of childhood and inevitable traumas throughout life. It is easy for me to say that all truly healing moments have occurred through the presence of relationships with others in my life.

While I have been fortunate, many individuals I have seen over the years in practice have not been so lucky. Their experiences have not been as rich, supportive, or positive. In particular, those who have suffered trauma at the hands of family members or other people may no longer feel secure in any relationship, including the one we are trying to initially establish through expressive arts therapy. Their worldviews and internal maps of life have been formed around experiences of assault, verbal abuse, neglect, ostracism, and abandonment and even as a result of the failures of mental health professionals and agencies to acknowledge their struggles and pain.

While relationships may heal us, it is also true that trauma almost always impacts and alters our perceptions of relationships not only with others, but also ourselves. While we haven't identified one single universal method or approach that universally heals all individuals who suffer the effects of trauma events, we do know that recovery does involve one significant element—a reparative relationship. Establishing safety and providing strategies for self-regulation form the foundations of effective trauma-informed intervention, but the psychotherapeutic relationship remains the central factor in reparation. Although I am proposing that expressive arts therapy can impact trauma recovery in positive ways, any approach to health and well-being is predicated on the type of relational dynamics the therapist creates with the individual.

Transformation and reparation of trauma through relationships is not a singular event; it involves multiple moments that support the unfolding of trust, safety, and co-regulation. Psychotherapy is one such corrective experience because it includes a consistently empathetic relationship with another individual who can respond empathetically to anger, fear, and mistrust from the traumatized person. Verbal therapy contains valuable and effective relational qualities such as well-chosen prosody, gesture, and eye contact. Expressive arts therapy, however, adds something uniquely important to work with traumatized individuals by naturally bringing implicit sensory and body-based elements to psychotherapeutic dynamics that are not always available through even the most skilled verbal exchanges. In some cases, introducing expressive arts may be the only possible entry point to developing and restoring connection to others for those activated by personal narrative or unable to talk about any details even remotely related to their experiences. This is particularly true for individuals who have endured developmental, relational, and interpersonal trauma, which is described through a case example in the next section.

RELATIONSHIPS MATTER

Christa, described in Chapter 1, taught me much of what I know today about the psychotherapeutic relationship formed through expressive arts therapy. Christa's experience of developmental trauma did not resolve with her stay at an inpatient psychiatric unit for intensive treatment of multiple challenges. During the two occasions she resided at the shelter with her mother and brother Joey, I truly believed I had failed miserably to help Christa in any meaningful way because of her lack of responsiveness to my many attempts to establish trust and communication. Her experiences of interpersonal violence and assault continued into her adolescence with prostitution instigated by her mother Joelle, despite the attempts of child protective services workers to remove Christa and her brother from the home. At age 15, Christa finally decided to run away from home to escape more sexual assault and prostitution. Her dissociative disorder and depression became so overpowering that by age 16 she contemplated suicide. But Christa consciously decided not to take her life when she remembered what she later called a "life-saving memory" of time spent at the shelter with her brother, Joey, in our art and play therapy sessions. That memory really did save her life; because of it, she managed to get herself to a university neuropsychiatric hospital, where she presented herself for inpatient treatment by reporting her symptoms and intentions to end her life to the hospital staff.

Once Christa became a psychiatric patient in the hospital's adolescent unit, she insisted that the social service workers assigned to her case contact "Dr. Cathy" to let me know that she remembered to "get help" if she felt in danger from others or herself at any time in the future. At first the social workers were at a loss for who this person might be until Christa added, "You might know her. She is the one with the really funny last name. She was my art therapist when I was younger. We stayed at a big shelter for mothers and children in the city." At that point, the social workers easily guessed that it was me, given my unusual last name, art therapist identity, and previous work with domestic violence.

Of course, I was extremely curious and concerned about Christa's condition, but also greatly relieved that she was safe from further assault and prostitution. The social workers who were handling her case agreed to meet with me, and Christa gave them permission to share her status and more detailed information about her current treatment. But what most intrigued me at this time was what really brought Christa to arrive at the doorstep of the neuropsychiatric hospital, which was not an easy journey for her due to its location. What she wrote in a short note to me has stuck with me to this day: what Christa said convinced me that how we relate to individuals, both through words and nonverbal cues, always matters even when individuals do not acknowledge in the moment that we therapists are indeed making an impact on them. She wrote:

"I know Dr. Cathy really cared about my brother [Joey] and me. She let me sit right next to her while she read stories to Joey and did not mind if I held her hand or laid my head on her shoulder sometimes. She always had time to play and draw with my brother. I couldn't draw at the time and I couldn't talk much. She really wanted me to have fun when she and Joey played games and danced to music. But she was patient and let me just sit and watch Joey draw and play. I always knew that she loved both of us, and I want her to know that."

Christa included an image that she said only I would understand; it was the small collage about "what I need," which she had struggled to make during one of our sessions (Figure 4.1). I remembered that, in addition to the basic needs depicted (food and a house), Christa searched through many photos for an image of a face. While she could not say anything about the face she chose, I always felt she was trying to communicate her internal emotional pain that was impossible for her to articulate out loud. It was obviously an important art expression for Christa, so much so that she managed to keep the collage in her possession for the several years after her last stay at the shelter program.

Reading the last sentence of Christa's statement brought me to tears; seeing the collage image once again brought back many memories of what she and Joey had endured and survived. The fact that Christa also chose to communicate with me through that image affirmed that even during the times when she was too overwhelmed or dissociative to draw or create, she did feel that there was value in relating to me through art. Most of all, I was stunned that Christa recalled so many of the simple interactions I had initiated to establish a relationship, despite any identifiable responses from her at the time when she was at the shelter in sessions with me. Her message, image, and ability to seek out help convinced me that we never really know how meaningful our psychotherapeutic interactions may be and that we can build purposeful relationships even with the most severely impacted individuals. The fact that Christa used the word "love" let me know that she not only remembered, but she also felt something quite powerful within our relationship. Fortunately, she had been able to retain that feeling over the course of not only sexual assaults, but also her struggles to stay alive.

Children are not the only individuals who have taught me the importance of relational moments during expressive arts. Over the years, many adults have come forward with similar memories that not only recall the psychotherapeutic relationship, but also the sensory, implicit qualities that expressive arts added to the experience. Christa's story reminds me that one of the most powerful and life-changing feelings one can have is to know that both one's presence and absence mean something to someone else. Relational work, at its best, is reflected in both the individual's belief that the therapist values the person not only in the session, but also long after the therapy has ended. In this case, I was fortunate to receive the gift of

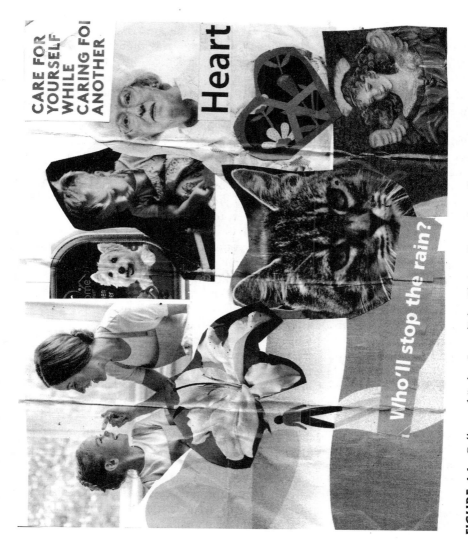

FIGURE 4.1. Collage of "what I need" by Christa. From the collection of Cathy A. Malchiodi (not to be reproduced without permission from the author).

being valued for the help I tried to offer during treatment as well as being remembered long after therapy had concluded.

TRAUMA CHANGES RELATIONSHIPS

Over the course of my first 10 years as an art and play therapist, I worked with approximately 5,000 children similar to Christa and her brother, Joey. Most came from abusive families, learning to exist in personal war zones of unpredictable violence and constant threats to safety that ruptured their capacities to trust any adult. Like many individuals who have endured years of traumatic stress, Christa experienced situations that altered her interactions with others, including helping professionals. For most of her life, she lived with intense fear of repeated assaults and numerous threats; psychological withdrawal and dissociation were her adaptive coping strategies in order to survive. Although these responses made it possible for Christa to tolerate unbearable situations, they also prevented her from engaging with other adults and, on many occasions, expressive arts and play.

As a matter of full disclosure, until I began to understand the nature of traumatic stress experienced by these young clients, attempting to develop relationships with them often brought me to the point of exhaustion. Terr explained to me one reason for my fatigue: Traumatized children in particular also may have experienced a disruption in their capacities to play and spontaneously create early in life (Terr, 1990), largely owing to their inability to regulate arousal. James (1989) also provided a well-needed reality check for me, saying, "This work is not for the faint-hearted or those who become therapists to make themselves feel good. This is work that is exhausting, physically, morally and spiritually" (p. 17). I would often remark to colleagues that, while I might often feel exasperated, I was never bored because every day brought a new surprise in terms of behavior. In shelters, safe houses, and psychiatric hospitals, I regularly encountered children who either could not remain still long enough to pay attention to what I was saying or demonstrating to them or, in contrast, could not engage with me because of dissociative episodes, depression, or extreme fatigue due to stress or physical neglect. On some occasions, I would slowly realize that a child was not responding to me and instead was masturbating under the art table. No matter how I structured a session, children spontaneously started fights or played games in destructive ways that ended with me taking them on a trip to the main office for first aid. There were girls who were extremely accommodating, offering to help me clean up the art and play therapy space, just as they assumed care of younger brothers and sisters when their mothers were emotionally unavailable. I admit I secretly appreciated their empathy after what often felt like a marauding group of hooligans regularly took the room apart and left it in shambles, post-session. But often these girls were also emotionally remote or highly anxious, and I sense that they were unable to truly feel safe with me, nor could they tolerate the presence of a male therapist, becoming frozen or excessively anxious until at a safe distance. They intensely watched my every move in the art and playroom, with some fearing reprisal or punishment. Others simply wanted to stay aware of my needs and feelings, just as they did with their own unpredictable parents and family members.

Bruce Perry explains just how deeply fear, extreme threats, and traumatic stress influenced relationships during time spent with children in 1993 at the Branch Davidian compound in Texas. The compound was the eventual site of a catastrophic raid (also known as the Waco Siege) by law enforcement, which resulted in the deaths of 80 people, including 23 children. When Perry first met with a group of the children from the compound, as he walked into the room one of the children looked up and asked, "Are you here to kill us?" (Perry & Szalavitz, 2017, p. 64). In his subsequent work with these children, Perry quickly realized that they seemed as if "they were from a completely alien culture" (p. 68) and had an altered worldview of adults, defining Perry as an outsider and a threat to their safety. In the aftermath of the Waco Siege, Perry established that the youngest of these children's developing brains were at the greatest risk for lasting effects of trauma and continued to be susceptible to negative experiences throughout childhood.

Like Perry, I realized that the children I was attempting to assist did not hold a belief that "helpers" existed, including this benevolent expressive arts therapist who was often perceived as a possible menace. In fact, they had far different views of relationships and generally did not see most adults as sources of support or relief. While observing their art expressions and spontaneous play, I rarely encountered images, symbols, or stories about helpers or successful rescues during early sessions. Even if these children had positive encounters with first responders or medical personnel, they did not seem to readily internalize those experiences as ones that could be relied upon in the future. I also learned that even though I was a consistent provider of art making, play activities, and other expressive arts, they felt that I was not to be depended on, just as previous adult caregivers who abused and neglected them were not to be trusted.

Establishing relationships with the children's mothers or caregivers came with its own set of challenges, who had their own trauma histories. While they were not as chaotic as the children, they often preferred to remain detached and noncommunicative, often mistrustful and overwhelmed by their own experiences with violence and chronic trauma. Like their children, they also had short attention spans, could not engage due to dissociative episodes, anxiety, or depression, or simply were exhausted due to stress and multiple violent incidents. Years later, when I began to work with individuals who survived wars, terrorism, and multiple disasters as well as with returning combat military service individuals and veterans, it became obvious how traumatic stress inhibits the capacities to be in the here-and-now and to tune in to others, including the therapist. From these experiences, I learned to accept that establishing a relationship with someone who is struggling with trauma reactions is a complex process, particularly those who have endured interpersonal trauma of sexual abuse, physical assaults, and constant verbal threats.

INTERPERSONAL AND RELATIONAL TRAUMA

Play therapist and art therapist Eliana Gil (2010) summarizes the impact of interpersonal trauma in the following short, yet compelling, vignette:

> After 4 months of therapy, 6-year-old Miranda came into my office with a Ping-Pong paddle in her hand, announcing, "Here, this is for you!" "Oh, what is it?" I asked, and she said, "It's a paddle." When I then inquired what the paddle was for, she said, "For you to hit me," in a matter-of-fact way. "Why would I want to hit you?" I replied with shock, and she earnestly replied, "You like me, don't you?" (p. 3)

Most therapists who have worked with children who have been physically or sexually assaulted have heard similar and often shocking statements from young clients. Trauma at the hands of significant others inevitably changes expectations and worldviews; if left unresolved, beliefs that the world is filled with dangerous and unpredictable people persist throughout childhood and into adulthood. For some individuals, punishment becomes an anticipated part of relationships with caregivers; others may expect negative responses based on the therapist's most benign gesture, body language, or prosody. Children in chronically abusive or violent environments develop the capacity to scan their surroundings for warning signs of anger, sexual arousal, drug or alcohol intoxication, or mood swings. Eventually, an individual automatically responds outside of conscious awareness to what are encoded as threats and danger even when not actually present (Herman, 1992).

All traumas have the potential to alter one's abilities to relate to others, but traumatic stress from ruptures in relationships due to violence, assault, abuse, and neglect is the most tenacious and often the most difficult to address. *Interpersonal* or *relational trauma* (Schore, 2003) are terms that are commonly used to clarify the complex traumas resulting from abuse and neglect from caregivers or other individuals. Mental health is now finally recognizing the significant impact of trauma on relationships at all stages along the lifespan, including developmental trauma (van der Kolk, 2005), a descriptor that includes the adverse effects of childhood trauma on interpersonal and neuroaffective development in young children (Perry, 2009). Whether the individual suffers assaultive events directly or is a witness to them, experiences have the potential to impact brain, mind, and body in wide-reaching psychological and physical ways.

The impact of interpersonal and relational trauma is not limited to ruptured connections in need of repair between individuals. These types of traumas also alter interpersonal relations (relationship with one's mind, body, and spirit) and community relations (group membership). When we work with individuals who have sustained psychological trauma, we also often encounter changes in their relationships to these areas, too. We may find that people whose religious beliefs previously sustained them now lack faith in those spiritual teachings. Because trauma alters the body's responses to everyday life, other individuals may feel that their sense of physicality is altered and their body is betraying them through uncontrollable sensations and distressful reactions. Also, because of trauma's impact on body, mind, and brain, individuals may suddenly feel isolated from family, the workplace, and communities that were once sources of social support. All of these dimensions are also part of the relational disruption caused by traumatic stress and are in need of focused intervention as much as the capacity to feel safe and co-regulated within interpersonal relationships.

Several concepts are key to how expressive arts therapy supports critical relational transformation during the course of treatment and provides helpful frameworks for understanding the uniqueness of the expressive arts/psychotherapeutic relationship. These frameworks include (1) interpersonal neurobiology, (2) polyvagal theory and social engagement, (3) mentalization, and (4) attachment theory.

Interpersonal Neurobiology

Interpersonal neurobiology (IPNB; Siegel, 2012) is an overarching theory based on attachment research, neurobiology, and developmental and social psychology. The concept of neuroplasticity (the formation of new neural networks and responses) is central to IPNB approaches to treatment. The idea is that social relationships shape how our brains develop, how our minds perceive the world, and how our bodies adapt to stress throughout the lifespan. IPNB is grounded in evidence indicating that the brain is capable of change, especially through positive attachments and relationships, and this may be relevant to trauma recovery and other conditions that were once believed to be irreversible. Siegel (2012) cites the importance of "critical micromoments" of interaction with clients that include the client's tone of voice, postures, facial expressions, eye contact, and motion that he believes provide clues to the individual's psychobiology. These sensory-based cues become particularly important in identifying and formulating strategies for therapy, including expressive arts therapies.

In their work with trauma, attachment disorders, and other problems, practitioners often use the phrase "right-mind-to-right-mind" or "right-brain-to-right-brain" to underscore the importance of addressing implicit memory and experiences through a positive, sensory-based relationship (Badenoch, 2008). Schore (2003) identifies the right brain as the implicit self and the central mechanism in psychotherapeutic change. Additionally, the right hemisphere of the brain is particularly active during early interactions between very young children and caregivers, and it stores the internal working model for attachment relationships and affect regulation (Schore, 2003; Siegel, 2012).

While this concept is often mentioned as a rationale for use of expressive arts therapy throughout the lifespan, there is not enough evidence that right-mind-to-right-mind actually applies beyond the early years of life that Schore proposes. However, the concept is a good representation of what an expressive arts psychotherapeutic relationship constitutes within an IPNB framework because of the role of sensory-based methods predicated on modeling, imitation, and reflection. For example, the therapist using arts-based approaches is a provider of materials (nurturer), an assistant in the creative process, and a participant in facilitating visual self-expression. These experiences emphasize interactions through experiential, tactile, and visual exchanges, not just verbal communication between the therapist and the individual. Music therapy provides similar experiences through interaction with music making; it also has the potential to tap social engagement and communication when collaborating or playing instruments together. Vocalizations, music, and rhythm are particularly effective in stimulating a sense of affiliation and relationship. For example, experiences involving specific music inherently can calm, entrain, and self-regulate. Dance/movement therapy also capitalizes on rhythm to establish relationships between individuals and to apply kinesthetic approaches such as mirroring to reinforce connection and positive attachment.

More importantly, the concept of right-mind-to-right-mind is central to *attunement*, which is generally defined as a central feature of every positive caring relationship as well as secure attachment. For example, well-attuned parents or caregivers are capable of detecting what their children are feeling, and they reflect those emotions back through sensory means such as facial expressions, vocalizations, touch, and other behaviors. These forms of attuned behavior help children recognize their own feelings and develop the ability to self-regulate through expressive arts and play-based experiences (Malchiodi, 2015b). Siegel (2010) refers to this as *mindsight,* a capacity for insight (knowing what one feels) and empathy (knowing what others feel). Perry (2009) echoes the importance of attunement through repetitive, relational experiences found in movement, music, and play-based interventions, underscoring their positive impact on development and on establishing secure attachment. Additionally, Perry's neurodevelopmental perspective emphasizes the essential role of sensory-based experiences in early childhood and how they enhance secure attachment, affiliation with others, empathy, and self-regulation. He observes that our history as a human species has always included wellness practices for self-regulation that include relational dynamics such as holding each other, engaging in dance, song, image creation, and storytelling, and sharing celebrations and family rituals. According to Perry, these activities are effective in altering the neural systems involved in stress responses as well as developing secure attachment.

Expressive arts approaches may address IPNB principles in two additional ways. First, they encourage the individual to be *active* within the therapeutic process rather than a passive recipient, reinforcing mutual interaction between the individual and therapist. Second, while listening is a key component of talk therapy, expressive arts therapy provides experiences that are *witnessed* because they are implicit, sensory-based, and often tangible communications that are central to each session. The therapist takes on the role of a witness who is not only authentically interested and attentive to the individual's arts-based communications, but also provides unconditional positive regard for these creative expressions.

Although a right-hemisphere dominance may be involved in creativity, imagination, and play, any applications of expressive arts are actually "whole-brain" endeavors. Practitioners of expressive arts therapy have a similar goal—gaining access to the more embodied, implicit, sensory-based right-hemisphere functions to enhance integration with the more declarative left hemisphere. In other words, current clinical observations, patient reports, and emerging research show that expressive arts therapies may support "whole-brain" integration, which is not always possible in verbal approaches to trauma intervention. This may be due both to the self-regulatory qualities of arts-based, action-oriented experiences and to the process of reconnecting implicit and explicit memories of distressing events.

Polyvagal Theory and Social Engagement

Polyvagal theory (Porges, 2012) explains the role of the autonomic nervous system in guiding relationships between humans and between humans and the environment; it mediates safety through a process labeled *neuroception*. Neuroception (Porges, 2004) is an unconscious, neural process that allows the body to rapidly shift the autonomic state in response to environmental cues. Neuroception is part of an ancient survival system that detects danger and life-threatening conditions. It adjusts physiology and emotions to assess risks, determine safety, and allow connection with others. Polyvagal theory continues to provide new insights into the relationship between attachment and safety, a foundation that supports meaningful relationships, including those established in therapeutic relationships.

Polyvagal theory also informs the *social engagement system,* a specific neural circuit that is found only in mammals (Gray & Porges, 2017). These physiological, biological, and neurological processes guide interactions with the environment via the vagus nerve, a nerve that runs from the brain through the heart, lungs, and digestive track in the body. The sound of a voice or facial expressions communicate an individual's physiological state to others. For example, a high-pitched voice might convey anger, fear, or distress, causing others who hear it to feel unsafe and become concerned. Additionally, internal body awareness influences how individuals track, respond, or engage with others. In particular, people who are impacted by traumatic events may feel disconnected from this ability to sense what is going on with their bodies or, in contrast, feel a perpetual state of fear.

Many principles and practices found within the expressive arts support social engagement and build the sense of safety within relationships necessary for trauma reparation. For example, the concept of kinesthetic empathy proposed by dancer and dance therapist Marion Chace (in Reynolds & Reason, 2012) describes the nonverbal, sensory-based expression of empathy between therapists and clients. Through mirroring and attunement, it promotes social engagement. This is demonstrated through posture and movement in dance and movement (Gray & Porges, 2017); sounds and musicality; becoming the "third hand" to support art making (Kramer, 1986); and a variety of kinesthetic and sensory actions such as prosody, gesture, and facial expression. Other practices are found in expressive arts approaches that support experiences of safe social engagement. They include entrainment (using rhythmic gestures, movements, sounds, music, prosody, and breathing) and grounding (establishing self-regulating rituals through creative arts). These approaches are particularly useful with trauma survivors, who may benefit from downregulating hyperactivation or shifting away from states from dissociation. Therapist-initiated sensory-based interventions in treatment can teach and reinforce the self-regulation necessary for development of reparative interpersonal relationships.

Mentalization

Mentalization, a term coined by Peter Fonagy and Mary Target, is another framework relevant to relational work and expressive arts approaches. Fonagy uses this term to refer to the ability to see oneself from the outside and others from the inside (Allen, Fonagy, & Bateman, 2008). He proposes that this capacity is connected to empathy, self-regulation, self-preservation, expression of affect, self-efficacy, impulse control, and understanding how actions impact others. Being able to mentalize is thought to reduce the impact of traumatic stress; additionally, early exposure to developmental and interpersonal trauma may compromise mentalization. The latter is a challenging aspect in applying mentalization when individuals have learned to turn off their thoughts if traumatic stress is activated, making it difficult to mentalize because of highly emotional states.

Mentalization is developed at least in part through the capacity for imaginative play, a necessary capacity when engaging in expressive arts. Verfaille (2016) notes that "arts therapists who work with clients with attachment problems, children with developmental problems . . . will find points of reference in the concept of mentalization" (p. xv). In relational work with trauma, Bateman and Fonagy (2006) frame expressive methods as alternate ways of promoting mentalization, allowing what is internal (experience and feeling) to be communicated externally, placed outside the self. "An aspect of the self is outside and so less dangerous, controlling and overwhelming. Feelings become manageable and the understanding of oneself and others is more tolerable" (p. 174). All forms of expressive arts also can be adapted to support mentalization. The experiences of using colors, shapes, and lines in a drawing or musicality to communicate the feelings of another individual are essentially expressive arts-based mentalization exercises.

Mentalization is really a stance (an art) as opposed to an actual technique (a science) when it comes to addressing trauma: "The patient has to find himself in the mind of the therapist and, equally, the therapist has to understand himself in the mind of the patient if the two together are to develop a mentalizing process. Both have to experience a mind being changed by a mind" (Bateman & Fonagy, 2006, p. 93). This stance reflects the key principles embedded in applying expressive arts to relational work—the therapist follows the individual's pace and is curious, sometimes playful, and often active in motivating the individual's creativity and imagination. When engaged in imaginative play, individuals are invited to mentalize through taking on other's perspectives, thoughts, and feelings, particularly within the process of dramatic enactment or role play. For example, puppet play is a natural mentalization strategy with children; with adults, facilitating the role play of a person who may have a different personality or quality than the individual is another strategy to support mentalization. Haen (2015) suggests the psychodrama technique of doubling to encourage mentalization. In this technique, participants are asked to speak as if they are another individual in order to give voice to something that individual is feeling or thinking. Haen gives this example:

> An avoidant child might say, "I'm not talking today." When group members double, with permission of the child, they stand behind the child and say things like, "I'm bored," or "I'm afraid to talk," or "I'm not sure I like this group." The child is then encouraged to share with the group which doubles came closest to articulating his true feelings. (pp. 246–247)

According to Haen, dramatic enactment may be the most effective expressive arts approach in tapping mentalization as a way to help traumatized individuals safely explore intrapersonal (self) and interpersonal (others) experiences.

Attachment Theory

During the last several decades, attachment theory has significantly influenced the practice of psychotherapy; this has resulted in the acceptance of early bonding experiences as essential to well-being later in life. Attachment theory is not an approach in and of itself, but it has generated a whole range of therapeutic practices and models focused on increasing an insecurely attached or traumatized individual's ability to form secure relationships and emotionally and physically attune to others. Attachment research emphasizes the psychobiological characteristics of communication between caregiver and child, including interactive speech, vocalizations/sounds, body language/gestures, and eye contact. Healthy attachment between caregivers and infants achieves a consistent body-based state of reciprocity, connectedness, synchrony, and mutual delight (Schore & Schore, 2008).

Individuals in secure attachment relationship can feel safe and confident, including gaining the ability to co-regulate themselves with others. Secure attachments are a core component of resiliency in individuals exposed to distressing experiences. Schore (2003) clarifies this co-regulation as appropriate and nurturing preverbal communication between caregiver and infant that impacts the maturation of the infant's right brain. When all goes well in healthy attachment, caregiver and children learn each other's rhythms and co-create a shared rhythm. In brief, the caregiver focuses on the child's face, prosody, and gestures, establishing moment-to-moment attunement. As a result, the child learns how to regulate emotions through the caregiver's responses to the child's reactions.

In contrast, responses from an abusive or neglectful caregiver are not comforting and are not perceived as protective or nurturing by the infant and may instead be encoded as chaotic or rejecting. This forms the basis for early relational trauma that impacts an individual's right-brain development, dysregulating the body's ability to respond to others and the environment and reducing the capacity to adaptively cope with emotional stress. Schore (2003) notes:

> Instead of modulating, she induces extreme levels of stimulation and arousal, and because [the caregiver] provides no interactive repair the infant's intense negative states last for long periods of time. Prolonged negative states are toxic for infants and although they possess some capacity to modulate low-intensity negative affect states, these states continue to escalate in intensity, frequency and duration. (p. 124)

In other words, the child may experience hyperarousal or hypoarousal and a reduced ability to function flexibly.

The overall goal of attachment work in therapy generally involves recreating experiences that recapture what the individual may have missed in early relationships. Bowlby (1988) emphasized the necessary foundation of a "secure base" that allowed children to crawl away from the caregiver and explore the world and return to the safety of the attachment to a responsive adult. Tronick (2007) conducted "still-face" research suggesting that when a caregiver withdraws interaction with an infant, the infant responds by attempting to reestablish connection through a variety of tactics. We are wired to connect with others, even when reciprocal communications are absent. When these important attachment systems are compromised through multiple and chronic missteps by caregivers, crucial neural systems can be altered (Gaskill & Perry, 2014, 2017), contributing to a variety of psychiatric problems and resulting in social and emotional difficulties across the lifespan, including disruption of healthy relationships. Strategies designed to help individuals cope and self-soothe rather than withdraw from relationships are essential, but also difficult when the earliest secure base has not manifested itself.

In all cases, attachment research underscores how the caregiver–infant relationship is predicated on making meaning through a series of nonverbal cues, including movement, gestures, and affect. This suggests that the first sense of security within relationships develops through body-based communications and that these communications produce the basis of self-regulation and co-regulation throughout life. Principles found in attachment theory and research also form the foundations for applications of expressive arts with individuals whose relationships with others have been ruptured by traumatic events. In the following example, these principles are addressed not only through individual expressive arts therapy, but also through an important additional relational strategy—dyadic expressive arts with parent and child.

ESTABLISHING ATTACHMENT THROUGH EXPRESSIVE ARTS

Joanne, age 10, was referred to therapy after she witnessed her father beating her mother, Diana, on three occasions and for repeated physical abuse to Joanne and her brother by her father. Diana declined to report the incidents of physical abuse or domestic violence until child protective services removed Joanne and her younger brother, Mark, age 5, from the home when Diana became unconscious due to a drug overdose. Joanne found her mother lying on the floor of their apartment and called the police to come to their home while Mark knelt screaming next to his parent's lifeless body. Although Diana recovered, social services felt it was in the children's best interest to stay at a residential treatment facility for the short term.

When I first visited Joanne at the facility, she was hypervigilant and unable to concentrate for very long. But she was able to sit beside me for short periods of time, allowing me to soothe her through singing favorite songs together. Joanne eventually told me that she did like to draw and paint and wanted to "make a picture of her family" because she missed her mother due to the separation initiated by social services. When I asked Joanne to tell me more about the drawing, she said it was a picture of herself, Mark, and her mom. There were three human figures in the picture, each drawn appropriately for Joanne's age range (Figure 4.2). Because in my experience family drawings are often incomplete, I asked, "Is there anyone else in the picture?" Joanne indicated that she left out her father because "he was mean to us" and "we probably won't see him anymore."

In Joanne's case, in order to resolve her difficult relationship with an abusive father, she simply chose to leave him out of the picture. In contrast to many children who have been assaulted by a parent or caregiver, Joanne was forthcoming about her father. Her statement did not surprise me because interpersonal and domestic violence affects attachment relationships. Most children generally do not want to talk about the abusive caregiver, feeling fearful that a parent will cause injury or put them in danger and may even side with the perpetrator, out of loyalty or fear of

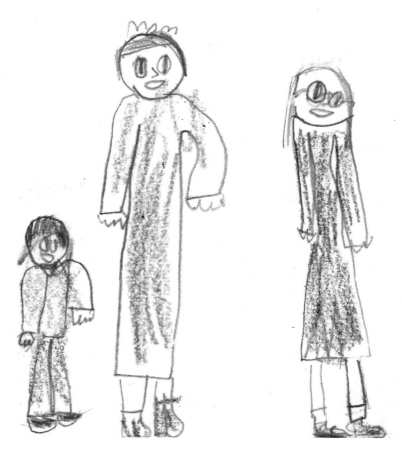

FIGURE 4.2. Drawing by Joanne of her family without her father. From the collection of Cathy A. Malchiodi (not to be reproduced without permission from the author).

reprisal. In subsequent expressive arts therapy sessions with Joanne, I also learned more about the complexities of her relationship with her mother and how Joanne had increasingly become frightened and often angry at her mother, feeling abandoned during numerous incidents when Diana passed out from drug overdoses. In Joanne's case, attachment was also disrupted by Diana's neglect, indifference, or unresponsiveness; it shattered Joanne's trust that Diana would protect her from harm. Like Tronick's (2007) still-face research, Joanne internalized a caregiver who did not respond to her natural needs for a parent's response during times when a child expects to receive support, approval, and interaction.

These disrupted relational dynamics as well as the physical abuse and domestic violence had significant impacts on Joanne in several ways. Both Diana and Joanne reported that Joanne was often anxious (hyperaroused) and also experienced sleep problems (night-time anxiety and nightmares). Additionally, Joanne's school counselor observed that she had difficulty with comprehension, focus, and attention and was often impulsive, hitting other children or yelling at her classroom teacher. Joanne's responses to me during our initial sessions mirrored her fear and anger about her primary caregivers. For example, she sometimes demanded my undivided attention when she was engaged in art making, movement, or play and she competed for attention with other child participants when in group activities. On one occasion, she had a violent tantrum when I did not have enough clay on hand for her to complete a project; at another time, she scolded me for being a few minutes late for a session. It was easy to see that Joanne feared abandonment and had a difficult time self-regulating her emotions when confronted with situations she could not completely control or circumstances that felt unsafe.

In Joanne's case, abuse from her father and a sense of abandonment by her mother contributed to her attachment difficulties. Her attachment role also became disorganized because she had to assume the role of the caregiver when Diana's drug addictions prevented her from providing appropriate parenting to her children. During group sessions, Joanne often took on an adult persona, caring for other children and insisting on becoming my "helper" role during sessions. At times, she even gently challenged my role as facilitator, insisting on controlling how art and play materials were shared and making decisions for participants on activities and themes for expressive work. It was clear that even though technically Joanne was a child, she often felt more comfortable in the role of an adult with responsibilities to care for others in ways she possibly wished Diana would care for her.

In brief, Joanne would benefit most from expressive arts that addressed her emotional reactions and stress responses, created a sense of safety, and, to some extent, reinforced attunement to others and social awareness. She also would benefit from experiencing a positive relationship with me through sensory activities that recapitulated early attachment experiences via nonverbal and right-hemisphere interventions. In other words, I hoped our work would help Joanne recover an identity of "being a child" with an adult who responded, rather than abandoned her, in times of stress or need for approval and validation.

Initially, Joanne was able to easily show me through drawings that she felt detached from her abusive father by literally leaving him out of the picture. When working with children like Joanne, I generally start with arts experiences that are neurodevelopmentally related to lower parts of the brain (brainstem, midbrain, and limbic system) and designed to be self-soothing and self-regulating. Although Joanne was 10 years old, I introduced a few activities that I might use with much younger children, such as listening to various soothing rhythms, playing drums and percussion instruments together, and recalling favorite songs from preschool days. I introduced felt markers with different smells of familiar foods for drawing activities and a variety of tactile materials for art making, taking on the role of someone who provides materials for creative self-expression that is accepted with unconditional regard. At other times, I taught Joanne some child-friendly yoga poses, including some that made us laugh because we enjoyed being "silly" together. We practiced breathing together like hibernating bears or buzzing bees, strategies that were also part of child-friendly yoga practices. I taught Joanne several child-appropriate mindfulness activities such as balancing a long peacock feather on the tip of her finger and a colorful, self-created butterfly on the tip of her nose. All of these interventions were selected to support self-soothing experiences (see Chapter 6). Additionally, I was making a "right-brain-to-right-brain" connection with Joanne by communicating with her through hands-on activities rather than words alone (left hemisphere and higher brain) and using creative interventions to build a relationship.

While it took many weeks before Joanne could engage in these initial sessions without angry or anxious feelings, she eventually began to feel safe in our relationship. She began to let me know what activities she enjoyed instead of communicating through tantrums, and she even made suggestions that indicated she felt comfortable collaborating with me (e.g., asking if we could "make cookies together" or use materials "to build a house for a mother bird and her baby birds").

At this point in our relationship, I asked Joanne to share her feelings with me through art expression in more embodied ways. She felt safe enough to show me with colors, lines, and shapes "how your body feels when you worry" and "where in her body she felt worry, fear, and anger" (Chapter 7). I also introduced her to some simple musical instruments (drums, rattles, kazoos, and various percussion instruments) and encouraged her to make sounds to communicate her body's feelings to me without words. Joanne began to use this activity as a way to convey to me how she was feeling at the beginning of each session. With my help, she was also able to begin to recognize situations when she felt these emotions in her body, what types of situations caused her to become distressed and how her body felt when she experienced worry, fear, or anger.

DYADIC EXPRESSIVE ARTS THERAPY

My role as a provider of sensory means of self-expression, with unconditional positive regard for the outcome, became the bridge for Joanne to experience secure attachment with me, reinforcing the idea that an adult could be consistent and co-regulating. While we made a good deal of progress in enhancing our relationship, Joanne was moved to foster care in another town along with her brother, Mark, and we had to suspend expressive arts therapy for the foreseeable future. Joanne's therapy continued for another year with a counselor after my work with her ended. However, before we terminated our sessions together, Diana was allowed to begin to reestablish her parenting role with Joanne and was asked to participate in several mother–child creative arts therapies sessions with us.

In subsequent meetings with Diana and Joanne, I repeated several of the activities I used with Joanne, but with Diana as an active participant. Like many parents who are faced with personal challenges including addictions, Diana herself needed expressive arts strategies for self-regulation. Because she was in a violent relationship with her husband for most of their married life, she understandably needed some self-soothing experiences as well. Because it was likely that Diana had missed out on positive attachment with her parents, I tried to at least give her a few dyad sessions with Joanne that Diana could use to build a more secure relationship with her daughter. In particular, I focused on some simple creative activities that Diana could initiate with Joanne at home, including drawing together to music, creating joint family art pieces, and creating playlists of music for relaxation. More importantly, I was able to introduce some experiences of collaborative, attachment-enhancing activities such as building a dollhouse together from shoeboxes and making puppet families from socks. While I do not know the ultimate outcome of our work together, I do know that Joanne, Mark, and Diana were eventually reunited and that Diana, with the help of addictions counseling, was able to maintain a drug-free existence.

CREATING TOGETHER: REPAIRING RELATIONSHIPS THROUGH COMMUNITY

Dyadic and family expressive arts therapy are two ways to bring together caregivers and children to strengthen positive attachment, repair ruptured relationships, and practice co-regulation through creativity and play-based experiences. But there is another important component that capitalizes on relationship as a reparative factor within a larger and possibly more powerful context: community. Judith Herman (1992) captures the value of community in reparation and recovery from trauma:

> Traumatic events destroy the sustaining bonds between individual and community. Those who have survived learn that their sense of self, of worth, of humanity, depends upon a feeling of connection with others. The solidarity of a group provides the strongest protection against terror and despair, and the strongest antidote to traumatic experience. Trauma isolates; the group re-creates a sense of belonging. Trauma shames and stigmatizes; the group bears witness and affirms. Trauma degrades the victim; the group exalts her. Trauma dehumanizes the victim; the group restores her humanity. . . . Mirrored in the actions of others, the survivor recognizes and reclaims a lost part of herself. At that moment, the survivor begins to rejoin the human commonality. (p. 214)

These words have guided my belief in the reparative possibilities for group and community applications of expressive arts therapy for several decades, creating a basis for intervention with families, neighborhoods, and community—especially in work with those individuals impacted by school shootings and natural or human-made disasters. In fact, the most powerful way to apply expressive arts to capitalize on relationships may actually be through group and community work because the expressive arts naturally lend themselves to interaction between participants. While many individuals may only be able to feel secure with a one-on-one relationship with a therapist, expressive arts experiences that include a sense of meaningful community contain the transformative qualities that Herman so clearly articulates. Macy, Macy, Gross, and Brighton (2003) provide an example contrasting individual versus group music experiences: "When [an individual] moves to music, he experiences connection; the same individual moves to music and experiences peers mirroring that movement, affiliation is experienced; vocalization accompanies the shared movement, integration may begin" (pp. 65–66). When participants are not musicians, playing musical instruments or drumming within a small group of people establishes relationships and congruence; even lack of harmony is recognized, heard, or implicitly felt by participants. Similarly, painting a mural together or acting out a scene together can result in relationships with others that naturally include moments of community and connectedness.

As psychotherapists, we may not always have the opportunity to operate outside traditional clinics and hospitals or our private practice offices to provide services in community settings. However, expressive arts therapy does have a tradition of doing so, since much of it has taken place within groups and communities that are not part of what we define as typical psychotherapeutic care, including programs that take place on neighborhood streets, places of worship, and open studio arts programs. When we begin to reframe trauma-informed practice to include experiences of healing-centered engagement (Chapter 2), how we address trauma reparation and recovery expands beyond clinic and agency walls, making new perspectives possible. In particular, community becomes the central element in supporting the trauma-informed principles of resilience and culture because the intersectionality and uniqueness of the individual are more likely to be addressed. When expressive arts therapy takes place outside of medically oriented settings, the emphasis on the community becomes a source of strength in recovery rather than a way of simply "fixing the trauma symptoms."

While I have been fortunate to have been able to provide expressive arts therapy in a variety of community settings, one experience in particular demonstrated trauma-informed, healing-centered engagement programming. It integrated the role of a neighborhood as a healing factor and participants' use of the arts in their own transformative process toward resilience and well-being.

EXPRESSIVE ARTS AND RESILIENCY PROGRAM WITH AT-RISK ADOLESCENTS

While working within a public school system as a contract therapist, I was invited to establish resiliency-based expressive arts programming with a group of male adolescents who attended an urban middle school. The administrator who contacted me described the group as being composed of boys who had physical and sexual assault in their histories, lived in what was the most violent neighborhood in the city, and were at risk for dropping out of school completely. Because the school administration had predetermined a theme of resilience, it was left up to me and the participants to decide how to develop a weekly expressive arts program to enhance self-efficacy and strengths.

Because I quickly realized that I was not the perfect match for this group, I decided to enlist a male teacher at the school who agreed to co-facilitate and assist in designing the program. The participants' initial presentation during the first group meeting was pretty familiar to me; it was similar to the responses of children from violent homes who experienced multiple assaults and neglect that I described earlier in this chapter. But these participants also brought the history of their neighborhood with them to the group, which included a belief that gun violence on the streets was to be expected and the police were not to be trusted. Recent events within the community easily validated both of these beliefs and explained much of the group's feelings of defeat and lack of trust that the future would improve conditions in their neighborhood. Despite all of these challenges, the boys quickly made it clear to us that they "didn't need any fixing" or "counseling" because many of them had "been there" already without success.

For the first several weeks, we decided to just listen to the boys' stories; for me, it was important to hear and understand the narratives of what life was like in their neighborhood and their school before working toward any specific projects or activities with them. In order to gain some compliance and participation, sharing of stories was rewarded with the option to introduce me to music that communicated the narratives of the streets they went home to every night, streets that were filled with stories of homicides, drug raids, and human trafficking and homes where interpersonal violence and lack of caregiver attention were regular occurrences. Hip-hop, replete with a few explicit lyrics, was the favored musical genre for telling these stories; most participants knew the complex contents of numerous songs verbatim.

During the fourth meeting of the group after listening to numerous stories and music that seemed to emphasize the ever-present chaos and unpredictability of events both on the neighborhood streets and within families, I was moved to ask the participants, "Is there anything that is consistent in your neighborhood?" While I wondered if I would get any type of an answer at all, one boy immediately responded, "Trees." Caught by surprise, I simply asked, "How so?" He was very clear about this answer, saying, "Around here, buildings fall down. Car windows get shot out. People like my cousin, they die from drugs or guns. Some people run away from here. But the trees stay put." I was equally stunned and impressed by the simplicity and wisdom of his answer. After opening the discussion to the larger group, it was not difficult for all participants to come up with personal observations about why "trees stay put," including vivid descriptions of why the trees were strong and resilient, despite the multiple threats and dangers within the neighborhood. It was obvious that what one boy saw as consistency resonated with other participants as a symbol of an entity that could withstand the harshness and challenges they all encountered on a daily basis. We made an agreement at that point to use the concept of "tree" as the starting point for a resiliency-based expressive arts project for the remaining sessions. In brief, we co-created a concept for making small-scale collage trees (Figure 4.3) that expressed "where I come from" on the roots, "who I am now" on the trunk, and "what I can do" on the branches and foliage.

To move this experience into the realm of narrative and dramatic enactment, I asked the boys if they would be willing to "witness" each other's trees and leave words of strength for each creation. Each artist then used the words received from each participant to write a poem or short prose about the images, focusing on resilience. The readings of the narratives (including some that were reminiscent of hip-hop lyrics) created from words given as witness to another's strengths were unequivocally powerful. They also became authoritative statements of hope and self-efficacy that were heard through dramatic readings and given well-deserved applause and praise by the group. The participants were so proud of these initial

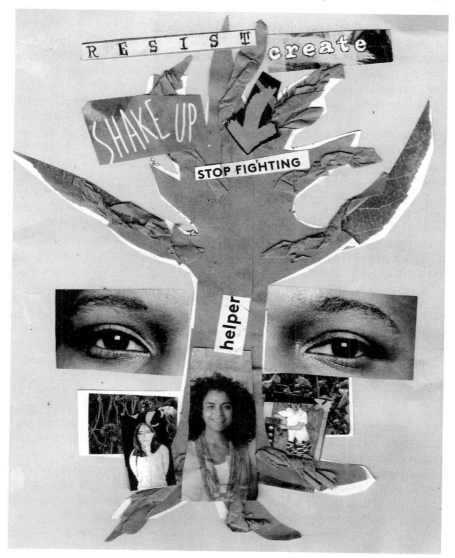

FIGURE 4.3. Collage tree image of "where I come from, who I am now, and what I can do." From the collection of Cathy A. Malchiodi (not to be reproduced without permission from the author).

creations that they asked for one additional iteration—to make life-size painted trees based on the individual collages. It quickly became clear that the trees were not just statements of strength; the participants embraced them as reflections of themselves through initiating an additional process that expanded the original experience.

In many trauma-informed groups located in mental health and health care settings, this may have been the typical ending of a time-limited program. Because this group was situated within a neighborhood in a non-traditional setting, community leaders, including members of the clergy, teachers, and mentors, were involved in the boys' progress and recognized the importance of their accomplishments in the group. As a result, they asked me and the co-facilitator if there was some way to continue the process that had unfolded since it had been so successful. In particular, the leaders wanted to explore ways to make the larger community aware of what these young people were able to achieve in order to recognize the boys' hard work and their expressions of strength and resilience. Although the group had formally ended, we were able to take the participants' creative output one important step further by securing a local artist to work with the boys to produce a large-scale mural of all the trees together in a "forest" on the wall of a building in the center of the neighborhood. At that point, I was only involved as a consultant and occasional supportive "painter" alongside the group members. I was pretty proud, however, to be a small part of this final result that allowed the boys to see their stories unfold in a way that positively impacted their entire community.

This example resonates with all that Herman envisioned when she articulated the healing role of community in reparation from trauma. In most cases, trauma-informed applications of expressive arts therapy continue to take place within settings separated from larger relational networks such as the neighborhood presented in this example. However, despite the limitations of a clinic office or health care facility, the concepts that Herman formulated are essential to fully address the challenges of those exposed to traumatic events because they inevitably include one's community as the "strongest antidote to traumatic experiences" (1992, p. 214).

RELATIONAL QUALITIES OF EXPRESSIVE ARTS THERAPY

While expressive arts therapy integrates psychotherapeutic frameworks within its approaches, certain specific characteristics found in expressive arts therapies come from the arts themselves. Three concepts are particularly relevant to how expressive arts enhance and support relational moments in treatment: (1) recovering the individual's creative life, (2) bridging the space between individual and therapist, and (3) using artistic sensibilities.

Recovering the Creative Life

As discussed previously, the experience of trauma changes interpersonal relationships; it also alters other parts of life, including intrapersonal aspects (relationship with one's mind, body, and spirit). The intrapersonal can include what we sometimes call the "creative spirit," the capacity to enjoy self-expression, exploration, and experimentation with abandon and spontaneity and without self-doubt, both individually and in the company of others. For this reason, imagination and play do not always come naturally or easily to traumatized individuals, despite a prevailing mantra that everyone is "creative."

A key relational piece of expressive arts therapy involves supporting the process of recovering what I call the individual's "creative life," the natural capacity for playfulness believed to be present in all individuals (Panksepp, 2004). Early in my work with abuse and family violence, I was struck by what James (1989) observed about how trauma impacts children's creative lives: "Traumatized children who have not come to terms with what has happened to them may be afraid to play, fantasize or dream, because unbidden memories or thoughts may begin to emerge" (p. 4). Although we believe all children are naturally capable of play, they simply may be too overwhelmed by stress reactions due to complex trauma. For this reason and others, possibilities for recovering a creative life may be temporarily disrupted or, in some cases, the necessary conditions for it to develop may have never been present to begin with. In particular, if primary relationships were interrupted early in life, playfulness may not have been encouraged and in fact, now may feel foreign or even unsafe. If attachment problems are unresolved, children simply may never have had the consistent, prosocial experiences that support the sense of mastery and self-efficacy necessary to play and creativity.

Many children I have worked with are unfamiliar with drawing materials, clay, and paints; have never played with puppets or sandtray miniatures; and never have had the opportunity to use a drum or other simple musical instruments. Often, my very first goal in initial sessions with children is to begin what can be a long process of helping them learn to play and introducing them to various expressive arts media and to rekindle or introduce the experience of "fun" in their lives. A secondary goal is to help them feel safe enough to risk freely engaging with unfamiliar toys, props, and media, conscious of any hyperarousal while they tentatively attempt to explore art media, toys, and props, fearing inevitable repercussions if they spill paint or accidentally break something.

Adults come with similar challenges, including trauma reactions that overtake attention and focus. They often bring additional scenarios and questions about engaging in creative experiences and play at all, wondering if this is the right approach for them and sharing viewpoints that "play is silly," "art is a waste of time," and "self-expression is not serious stuff."

Many soldiers who are referred to my practice because of traumatic stress come to the first session with these beliefs and are only willing to give expressive arts "a shot because other soldiers felt it helped" or because "my clinic doctor recommended it." At the initial appointment, it is not very difficult to pick up on their hesitation. For example, some choose to sit across the room from me, in part because they need to keep a distance until they know more about what was going to happen and what they will be asked to do in this "art thing."

The concept of unconditional positive regard that underscores acceptance of all parts of the individual's process, without judgment or evaluation, plays a central role in helping traumatized individuals recover creative lives. Play therapists often describe this form of regard as "I delight in you," an explicit and implicit communication from the therapist to a child that expresses enthusiasm, appreciation, and unconditional acceptance. It is also an essential stance to reinforce a sense of secure attachment within the therapeutic relationship. If we are fortunate early in life, we experience delight from caregivers, seeing it in their faces and sensing it through gestures and prosody in response to our actions. Badenoch (2008) refers to the concept of delighting as "the sweetness that lets us know we are loved no matter our state" (p. 261). In expressive arts therapy, it can be an authentic response to a particular experience, a spontaneous moment of surprise or novelty or the reflection of multiple interactions.

In her explorations of "what is art for," Dissanayake (1995) emphasizes the interplay of mutual affection, creativity, and interpersonal play in humans found in early attachment relationships and the role of "delight" as follows:

> What mothers convey to infants are not their verbalized observations and opinions about the baby's looks, actions, and digestion—the ostensible content of talk to babies—but rather positive affirmative messages about their intentions and feelings: You interest me, I like you, I am like you, I like to be with you, You please me, You delight me. (p. 91)

In these interactions, the caregiver's voice, facial expressions, and gestures are given spontaneously, authentically, and playfully, conveying a sense of delight in whatever the child is displaying or communicating. The child reciprocates with similar delight through voice, facial expressions, and gestures. Schore (2003) refers to this experience as one of mutual love, "an interpersonal context of right-brain accelerating positive emotional arousal . . . the sources of right-brain intrapsychic creative inspiration" (p. 77).

While there are many moments during an expressive arts therapy session when response is not necessary, it is important to remember that most individuals, particularly those who have experienced developmental or relational trauma, benefit from "delighting" through active responses to their play and creative output. Most children and adults I see have suffered not only from interpersonal violence, but also from experiences of abandonment where nonresponse from significant others or bystanders compounded the impact of traumatic stress. For this reason, my preferred style of interaction is to provide vocal, facial, and gestural encouragement in response to what an individual accomplishes, honoring the energy as well as the courage it takes to engage in self-expression of difficult feelings and sensations through arts-based expression. Making simple, clear statements about the expressive arts process such as "You've got this," "Let's have fun today," "It took a lot of courage to do what you just did," or "It's okay to just play" are necessary messages for individuals who have rarely heard encouraging words from anyone. In brief, recovering the creative life through expressive arts happens through the therapist's responses to help individuals "feel felt," be witnessed, and trust the process. This can only be accomplished if the individual experiences not only your attunement and empathy, but also acknowledgment of verbal and nonverbal communications, including the individual's creative process and output.

Finally, the foundation for helping traumatized individuals recover their creative lives is based in introducing ways to safely and gradually develop an arts-based language through creative expression, imagination, and play. Subsequent chapters describe strategies for how to go about this, emphasizing ways that therapists can help individuals explore and develop this language through art, music making, sound, movement, improvisation, and writing.

Bridging the Space between Us

Winnicott (1971) observes that play provides a space between therapist and child, a space where empathy occurs. I see that space a little differently than Winnicott does when it comes to integrating expressive arts within the psychotherapeutic relationship. While it is a space within which to experience empathy, it is also a space that may feel confusing, uncomfortable, threatening, or even dangerous, depending on the individual's level of traumatic stress and its previous relational origins. Entering into an expressive arts therapy relationship, even when the therapist is perceived as benevolent and safe, still has its challenges for most individuals who lack trust in others due to previous relational or interpersonal trauma. It also may bring up discomfort or unfamiliarity with play and creativity as sources of emotional reparation and well-being because these experiences were absent from the earliest caregiver–child relationship.

In applying any of the approaches in this book, thinking about just how to bridge the space between "us" (individual and therapist) is the first step in supporting a reparative relationship. It is supported by the foundational elements of safety (Chapter 5), self-regulation (Chapter 6), body awareness (Chapter 7), and specific strategies expanded throughout the rest of the book. All of these important foundations are critical in order to establish trust in "us" as well as to strengthen the individual's capacity to transform what has ruptured mind and body into a sense of well-being and resilience.

While bridging the therapeutic space takes many forms and cuts across many stages of treatment, expressive arts therapy differs from talk-based approaches in specific ways. One is the use of props and media to establish ways for individuals to connect with us and enter into a psychotherapeutic relationship in the least threatening ways possible. These ways respect the person's tolerance for arts-based experiences and the body's need for safety and self-regulation, particularly during initial sessions. The following brief example explains the use of props and media to develop a relationship with an individual challenged by interpersonal trauma.

Using Props to Bridge the Space

Tory, a 26-year-old woman who had suffered many sexual assaults, was referred to me for help with her severe hyperactivation due to traumatic stress. As I eventually learned, she not only experienced multiple incidents of sexual assault as a teenager and young adult, she was also sexually harassed at her workplace. As a result, Tory began to experience severe anxiety and panic attacks. She reported that when anyone came closer than a few feet from her, her hyperactivation was uncontrollable and often triggered overpowering feelings of anger that she self-medicated with binge drinking. These episodes were often followed by long periods of feeling immobilized, according to Tory, times during which she would sit staring at the television screen with no sense of how much time passed.

During our initial session, I asked Tory a question I ask all individuals during their initial sessions with me. "Where in the room would you like to sit and where would you like me to sit?" Tory was very clear that she preferred to be as far from any other person as possible, adding: "Nothing personal, Dr. Cathy, but thank you for asking." She also chose to seat herself in a position where she could watch the doorway to the office. This is a position that many of my clients who have experienced interpersonal violence select, even though my office is secure from outside entry.

While we worked with body-based sensations and self-regulatory practices during our first meetings, I was also very conscious of ways to introduce nonthreatening ways through which we could connect and establish a relationship between us. Because Tory indicated that she was essentially experiencing what I guessed were freeze responses, I wanted to get her moving in some way, especially since she was previously active as a long-distance runner and a part-time aerobics instructor. In order to establish connection through movement with individuals who are not comfortable with close proximity to another person, I introduce a variety of props to create a distance, such as stretch fabrics and bands. In this way, Tory could experience pulling against me as well as having a sense of "joining" with me, while still maintaining her space within the dynamic (personal kine-sphere).

In brief, this became a way to safely begin to play with me during the sessions, offering action-oriented possibilities for resistance, with mirror-ing and relating determined by Tory. As Tory started to experiment with moving away, resisting, yielding, moving closer, and feeling more comfort-able with closer proximities to me, it became important for me to help her understand these relational dynamics by verbalizing them as they were occurring. For example, if I noticed her moving away, I simply wondered out loud "how far do you need to move away to feel more comfortable with me?" In this way, we began a series of conversations about the "space between us" as well as how space impacted her body's reactions in relation to other individuals in Tory's life.

Another important component of these prop-enhanced relational interventions with Tory included the use of music as an auditory cue to anchor her in the moment and support the developing connection between us through rhythm and energy. While it is perfectly acceptable to move without music, in most cases I find that individuals can benefit from the addition of music not only to calm and self-regulate, but also to bring vital-ity into the session. While we started out with various instrumental pieces that were relaxing, as our relationship became more playful, I started to get Tory's input on more lively selections we could move to with the stretch bands. Some of Tory's favorite pieces were introduced, including her favor-ites from the 1990s that brought back sensory memories of dancing with friends during less distressing times. While Tory's reactions and trepidation about proximity to others took over a year to resolve through additional expressive arts sessions, her trauma reactions did eventually subside and no longer overtook her daily life. Movement continued to be a regular part of the psychotherapeutic relationship, but eventually we dispensed with props, simply mirroring each other to music as a beginning and ending to sessions.

Out of all the expressive arts therapy approaches, movement is pos-sibly the most effective for addressing, exploring, and establishing rela-tionship, but all art forms can be adapted to support similar relational goals. Communicating through drumming can be a safer replacement for talk for some individuals; dramatic enactment through puppets might be more comfortably performed behind a puppet theater where children can feel anonymous. While building and exploring relationship through dance and movement with Tory was her preferred way of working, in subsequent chapters we present examples of other types of expressive arts props and media that support individuals in similar ways.

Using Artistic Sensibilities

Undoubtedly, clinical education and supervision in trauma-informed prac-tice is a key part of successful relational intervention when it comes to traumatic stress. However, expressive arts therapists, by nature of their backgrounds and training, also bring what I call "artistic sensibilities" to their work because they have experienced the arts through personal experience and time spent in the studio, rehearsal room, or theater. That is, they are generally practitioners who are proficient in various art forms and have made it a priority to engage in dance/movement, music, dramatic enactment, visual arts, and/or creative writing in their own lives. Being a participant in the creative process naturally instills a deeper understanding of the arts as forms of embodied intelligence and nonverbal communication. I know that my training as a visual artist and my experience in theater and improvisation, music, and movement practices have laid an important and unique foundation for my work as a psychologist in how I relate to children, adults, families, and groups. It emphasizes a different type of knowing about how creative experiences serve as ways to establish relational moments with individuals through sensory and body-based activities and within talk therapy. This understanding can be enhanced through education and clinical supervision, but it also is developed through arts-based experiences that support a stance of authenticity when it comes to introducing expressive arts to traumatized individuals.

If you are not an expressive arts therapist, it is certainly possible to apply creative interventions and arts-based relational principles in practice by developing your own "expressive arts sensibilities." Understand that the effectiveness of using expressive arts to establish a relationship with individuals and to repair relational ruptures is not located through simply replicating any specific directive or activity. It is found through integrating some degree of personal knowledge of the arts, creativity, imagination, and play when attending to the individual's moment-to-moment expressive responses. This includes feeling comfortable with assisting clients' creative process when needed; working with the body by using one's own physical presence to instruct and demonstrate, relaxed with improvisation and enactment; and maintaining a sense of play and, most of all, fun to encourage exploration and experimentation.

CONCLUSION

Positive attachment, social engagement, and a sense of belonging are essential experiences in recovering from traumatic events. The relationship between individual and therapist is the fundamental change agent in all psychotherapeutic methods, including expressive arts. Because of their multidimensional nature, expressive arts provide unique ways to support positive, reparative relationships because they go beyond verbal exchanges that capitalize on implicit, sensory-based relational moments. These moments are also key to another critical element in trauma work—establishing an internal sense of safety.

CHAPTER 5

· · · · · · · · · · ·

Safety

THE ESSENTIAL FOUNDATION

I first met Rose, a 29-year-old adult sexually abused throughout childhood and adolescence, when she requested an appointment to explore the possibility of some expressive arts therapy sessions with me. At our first meeting, she brought four sketchbooks filled with crayon and felt marker drawings that she had completed over the past year. Rose explained to me that previously she never had engaged in any type of creative expression except in classroom art projects as a child. She purchased her first sketchbook, felt marking pens, and crayons at the supermarket and started to draw almost every night before going to sleep. When I asked how Rose came to make drawing at bedtime a nightly ritual, she said, "Ever since I was sexually assaulted I haven't been able to fall asleep except with medication. Every night at bedtime I start to feel so afraid that I panic even though I know I am safe now from [name omitted] abusing me or anyone else hurting me. Once I started to doodle and draw, I realized that I could lose myself for a little while. I just don't feel any fear while I am drawing and I can even feel like I am in another place."

Rose discovered on her own that drawing gave her some relief from hyperactivation and a respite (the experience of "silence" described in Chapter 2) from fearful moments related to traumatic memories of the violent assaults she endured for many years. She intuitively sought out a way to distract herself from distress through self-expression each night in order to calm her body's flight reaction to perceived danger. When I first encountered Rose and listened to her story, I was impressed by how clearly she articulated an essential component of trauma-informed practice—the establishment of safety (Herman, 1992). Establishing safety not only includes attention to physical danger and threat to an individual; it also encompasses the person's psychological and somatic internal sense of safety when danger and threat are not present. Multiple and chronic traumatic experiences, like those Rose survived, often diminish the individual's confidence, self-efficacy, and capacity to trust in oneself, relationships with others, and the environment. As a result, an internal sense of safety within body and mind is weakened.

Perry observes, "Because trauma—including that caused by neglect, whether deliberate or inadvertent—causes an overload of the stress response systems, which is marked by a loss of control, treatment must start by creating an atmosphere of safety" (in Perry & Szalavitz, 2017, p. 134). Trauma-informed practice encourages the therapist to recognize this important foundation and to realize that each individual has unique, automatic, and instinctual survival responses to situations perceived as unsafe or threatening responses. Supporting safety, discussed in this chapter, developing reparative relationships (Chapter 4), and providing strategies for self-regulation (Chapter 6) create a comprehensive and necessary foundation for effective applications of expressive arts therapies to address traumatic stress (Malchiodi, 2012c, 2014; Steele & Malchiodi, 2011). For some individuals, this can be accomplished in initial sessions; for others with complex trauma histories, it may be an ongoing goal that requires repeated intervention and creative strategies to support and reinforce. In all cases, addressing safety is essential to successfully applying expressive arts therapy as trauma intervention.

TRAUMA AND FEAR

In subsequent sessions, Rose struggled with repeated fear-related reactions that are common to most individuals who are challenged by psychological trauma and reminders of traumatic events. For many individuals, the fear that takes hold following a trauma can feel as bad or worse than the emotions felt at the time of the events themselves. For Rose, the onslaught of trepidation and anxiety was unpredictable, coming from many sources including environmental cues, fragments of memories, and flashbacks to actual situations she survived. For most people, fear responses decrease over time, but for individuals like Rose who experienced multiple adverse events, fear is unavoidable, paralyzing and difficult to overcome. As van der Kolk (1996) points out, "Fear needs to be tamed in order for people to be able to think and be conscious of their needs" (p. 205).

Although the first goal of expressive arts therapy in ameliorating traumatic stress is to establish a sense of safety, the sensory nature of expressive arts therapy sessions can also vividly reveal how individuals respond to perceived threats from others and the environment. Fear reactions can be stimulated by seemingly benign moments in expressive arts experiences that mimic or trigger trauma memories. While I have encountered many examples of this phenomenon during clinical practice, one instance in particular taught me a great deal about how quickly fear manifests itself in young survivors of interpersonal violence through play and art therapy. During a group session with six school-age children, an accidental spill of a water jar quickly activated a variety of fear-related responses from the participants. The child who knocked over the water jar immediately reacted with a freeze response to what was an anxiety-producing moment for him and intensely watched me for a reaction. While I reached for the paper towels to mop up the spilled water and reassured him that everything was fine, two other children jumped from their seats and ran through the door (flight response); they kept running until they found a hiding place in the changing room adjacent to the indoor swimming pool. Another two children hid beneath the table (flight) and became silent and watchful (freeze). The remaining child disappeared into the restroom and vomited in the sink. In retrospect, I realized that each child reacted to the implicit experiences of the spilled water just as they would as if someone in their own homes had spilled milk at the dinner table. They each felt a risk of physical punishment for what had happened. It is also obvious that none of these children felt completely safe, and the sensory qualities of what happened triggered multiple responses, including hypervigilance, escape routines, and protective strategies because survival was threatened. In brief, their fears reflected a mistrust of adult authority (the therapist), an individual who was perceived to be capable of retaliation in ways similar to an abusive parent or caretaker and was therefore "unsafe." I am also convinced that I might not have learned as much about these children's fear responses through anything but an art and play session where responses to activities mimic real-life situations and tap multiple sensory experiences.

Mass traumas have also taught therapists a great deal about the role of fear in their aftermath. For example, after the terrorist attacks on September 11, 2001, most people who were exposed to the events observed a change in their general outlook, reporting that they were more likely to see the world as a dangerous place in which anything could happen. As a result of their fears, some avoided specific activities such as air travel or situations such as public places or high buildings during the months after the terrorist attacks; others experienced a pervasive feeling of generalized fear and anxiety on a regular basis. Fear was often compounded by televised news that included a constant barrage of images and information about the attacks, reinforcing the level of hyperarousal through repeated exposure to implicit and explicit memories of the original events.

Levine (1997), in *Waking the Tiger*, observes that "the body reacts profoundly in trauma. It tenses in readiness, braces in fear, and freezes and collapses in helpless terror" (p. 6). While fear may involve thoughts and emotions, most of all it brings about terrible discomfort in the body. For many trauma survivors, these physical sensations can be intolerable to the point of doing whatever it takes to eliminate them. Individuals may respond with avoidance, desperately trying not to think about an event, yet replaying the event in their minds despite their best efforts to escape it. For others, fear does not take the shape of distinct memories, but manifests as a nervous system that is on high alert (accelerated heart rate, shallow breathing, gastric upset) and constantly on guard for threats. Individuals (like the children described in the vignette) may feel that danger is always present; they may be fearful of specific environmental or sensory cues, and they may be easily startled by sounds or movement. Others respond to fear with collapse and dissociation to escape the unbearable sensations of terror in the body; drugs, self-cutting, food, and other more destructive strategies may be used in an effort to make the body's response to fear go away.

Because fear is so central to traumatic events, it is a core issue that must be initially addressed to help individuals of all ages begin the process of reparation, post-trauma. Without a sense of safety, it is less likely that any individual will be able to fully engage in expressive arts or trust the therapeutic relationship. Most importantly, people's perceptions of fear do not come from reason or logic, but instead emerge from the body's implicit experience. The neurobiology of responses to danger and threats is one starting place in understanding just how to address fear-related sensations with expressive arts and to support an internalized sense of safety.

THE NEUROBIOLOGY OF SAFETY

Responses to danger are physiological reactions traditionally known as *fight, flight,* and *freeze* (sometimes called collapse) (Cannon, 1932). Trauma experts define these reactions as neurobiological responses to threat. The thinking brain (neocortex) is often automatically dominated by the midbrain (in particular, the amygdala) during moments of fear (Perry, 2009; Rothschild, 2000). This means that the midbrain goes on high alert and signals the sympathetic nervous system to release chemicals to prepare the body for fight or flight. If it is not possible to escape or fight, the limbic system then engages the parasympathetic nervous system to initiate a freeze or collapse response in the body, resulting in immobilization, restricted breathing, and decreased metabolism. In humans, freeze reactions may include psychological dissociation. Threat and danger signals may include real threats such as possible assault or physical harm, but they can also be as simple as humming fluorescent lights, the whir of a fan, or the popping sound coming from a car engine, causing individuals to automatically feel unsafe.

While fight, flight, and freeze are widely accepted as standard reactions to unsafe situations, it is also important to understand the individual's own unique responses to fear-inducing events. For example, Magda, a survivor of a hostage situation, explained to me that because she could not "fight or flee," she felt the need for some sort of action-oriented response. She developed a relationship with her captor over time, using appeasement as a strategy. As it turned out, her strategy was successful in preventing physical assault until she could actually escape (flee) her imprisonment. Other individuals may also feel shame or guilt if they are unable to escape danger or fight off a perpetrator, believing that their collapse (freeze) is a sign of weakness or incompetence. In these cases, it is essential to provide psychoeducation to explain that any response to fear-inducing situations is a normal reaction to an abnormal experience.

While understanding an individual's fight, flight, freeze, and other responses to distress are important to interventions that support safety, several specific neurobiology concepts are relevant when applying expressive arts therapies to trauma-informed intervention. These concepts include (1) safety as an embodied experience, (2) safety and the nervous system response, (3) safety and the continuum of arousal, and (4) safety and private logic.

Safety as an Embodied Experience

Over the past several decades, neurobiology has increasingly informed practitioners' understanding of how the body experiences both threats and safety. Beginning in the 1970s, Levine (1997) studied the effects of stress on animals and humans, leading him to develop a body-based psychotherapy model of trauma intervention. He proposed that while animals are not traumatized by threats to their lives, humans are often overwhelmed by threats, resulting in the body's hyperactivation and dysregulation. In order to ameliorate the impact of trauma events, therapy must address the body's experience of trauma to reduce the sensations of helplessness and paralysis. In a classic example of how the body is central to trauma reparation and self-efficacy, Levine describes an initial session with Nancy, a client who experienced agoraphobia and migraine headaches. Twenty years earlier, she had undergone a traumatic childhood surgery that included being bound and anesthetized with ether. During the session with Levine, Nancy displayed a freeze response and became hyperactivated when reliving the moments before the medical procedure, repeating out loud the expectation that she would certainly die from the surgery. In response, Levine had a vision of a charging tiger and suggested to Nancy that she was indeed being chased by a tiger and that she should run for a nearby tree. Nancy began using her body to imagine escape by kicking her feet as if to run from the impending danger. It was in that moment that Levine first realized that humans need to complete the same self-protective acts as animals when they are threatened with danger. In Levine's view, Nancy finally was able to instinctively use her own body to eventually resolve what had overwhelmed her (agoraphobia and migraines) for two decades. Levine uses this anecdote as an example of the intimate connection between somatic responses and trauma recovery.

Similarly, van der Kolk (1994, 2014) explained that "the body keeps the score," proposing that it is the body, rather than the mind, that controls how individuals respond to trauma and that they are much less impacted by conscious appraisal than nonverbal, implicit memories. He observed that once people get close to re-experiencing their traumatic experiences, they become too upset to speak in many cases. He notes that when people feel threatened, they first reach out for help, support, and comfort from those around them. If no help is found or if danger is imminent, then the body reverts to the next level (fight or flight) to survive by either escaping to a safe place or fighting off the threat or attacker. If unable to escape, the body's tries to survive by literally shutting down (freeze or collapse) and dissociating from the present. According to van der Kolk, this is the "ultimate emergency system" (p. 83). For example, children who have no escape from an abusive caregiver often become physically immobilized in response to the situation. Freeze/collapse is a common reaction of chronically traumatized individuals whose safety has been repeatedly threatened, whereas acute trauma may result in fight-or-flight responses.

In brief, talk alone may not be enough for real change to occur, and a way to physiologically calm the body is necessary to help the traumatized individual tolerate threats stimulated by trauma memories. As a result of his work in the aftermath of a large-scale natural disaster, van der Kolk realized that physical movement has a positive impact on the body's ability to cope with psychological trauma when confronted with danger. More importantly, if individuals cannot reestablish their sense of efficacy after a trauma and create a sense of safety, they may develop post-traumatic stress responses. What most individuals really need is the practitioner's focus on helping them safely explore their felt experience, physical sensations, and somatic reactions.

When integrating expressive arts into sessions, the embodied experience of trauma is possibly the most relevant neurobiology principle related to safety. As highlighted in earlier chapters, the action-oriented qualities of expressive arts therapies are relevant to the body's need to literally get moving and become active when confronted with threat. Creative endeavors can distract attention from internal sensations of worry and fear; Rose is a good example of someone who found a way to momentarily escape fear, worry, and hyperactivation through refocusing herself on drawing in her sketchbook. For her, engagement in expressive arts also approximated some of the self-protective acts Levine noted as reparative and the self-efficacy inherent to physical movement, mastery, and action cited by van der Kolk. She was literally "quieting her mind and body" through the repetitive actions of drawing within the confined space of a sketchbook to prevent self-harm and other adverse outcomes.

Expressive arts and their relationship to embodied experiences are described in more detail in Chapter 7 as approaches that capitalize on the somatic experience of trauma and how each individual specifically encodes distressful events. In particular, the role of movement and various forms of body scans as subjective maps of feelings and sensations are explained as key approaches to help traumatized children and adults identify dominant reactions.

Safety and the Nervous System Response

Stephen Porges's (2012) polyvagal theory provides all therapists with a clear account of how the nervous system can guide us in applying expressive arts therapy. As explained in Chapter 4, the *social engagement system* refers to a type of nervous system response that Porges explains as a mixture of activation and calming that operates out of a unique nerve influence. Essentially, it helps us navigate relationships, become more flexible mutually with others, and gain a sense of belonging. The social engagement system is a key concept in establishing a reparative expressive arts psychotherapeutic relationship between the individual and the therapist.

With specific reference to safety, Porges explains the perception of safety through the autonomic nervous system (ANS), which is usually understood as a two-part system including the sympathetic branch (accelerate) and the parasympathetic branch (brake). He notes that the ANS actually has three branches that hierarchically increase the perceptions of danger; the additional branch is the ventral vagal parasympathetic or "social engagement system" that allows individuals to feel secure in relationships with others. One branch sequentially takes over another as a means of protection and survival. Thus, at the perception of danger, the sympathetic branch takes over from the ventral vagal nerve. If the fight-or-flight possibility is blocked, the parasympathetic takes over from the sympathetic.

As described previously in Chapter 4, neuroception (Porges, 2004, 2012) is an unconscious process that helps individuals distinguish between what is safe and what is not safe. This distinction happens automatically, before conscious recognition of safety or danger within the environment takes place. When the individual perceives safety, the social engagement system is enhanced. The neuroception of safety is apparent in flexible interactions with others, including eye contact and reaching out for help. Ogden and colleagues (2006) note that neuroception of safety is also manifested in autoregulatory actions through body-based responses such as grounding, deep breathing, and an aligned posture.

The social engagement system decreases the fight, flight, or freeze response, changes the heart rate, and reduces the release of the stress hormone cortisol. According to Porges (2012), many traumatized individuals develop faulty neuroception, "an inability to detect accurately whether the environment is safe or another person is trustworthy" (p. 17). For example, when individuals feel unable to protect themselves from danger, their ability to regulate arousal fluctuates from hyperalertness to hypoactivity (dissociation) and the social engagement system is compromised. This model suggests that all individuals need substantive experiences of safety, especially in the earliest years of life, to develop a healthy social engagement system. The social engagement system, in turn, supports positive attachment and successful interpersonal relationships.

Because expressive arts emphasize gesture, intonation, rhythm, visual, tactile, and proprioceptive experiences, they have the potential to help individuals both "sense" safety and "feel" more secure with others and their environments. For this reason, polyvagal theory is key to applications of expressive arts therapy in several ways because of similar characteristics that support a sense of safety. For example, the vagal nerve influences many forms of communication (listening, facial expression, and vocal patterning and tonality) and if a communication is perceived as safe. In brief, understanding this principle helps us quickly understand how to create vocalizations, facial expressions, and gestures that soothe the individual during hyperaroused states. One simple variation of a vagal response I have used for many years is called the "Lassie Twist" (Etcherling, 2017), so-called because it mimics this famous beloved dog's slight turn of the head when engaging eye-to-eye with an individual, along with a relaxing vocal cadence. The combination of these sensory-based communications not only is soothing, but also conveys interest and attentiveness.

Porges's own experiences with music informed resulted in an important discovery about the vagus nerve with regard to breathing. As a young person, Porges was a clarinet player and recalled the effect of his breathing patterns required to play the instrument. Based on this understanding, he observes that extending exhales for a longer period of time activates the parasympathetic nervous system. In working with Rose, I became aware of how teaching her to extend her exhales helped her step out of her stress responses and move closer to experiencing a sense of safety in her own body. In contrast, using typical breathwork, such as equal inhales and exhales for a count of 4 or 5 seconds, quickly accelerated Rose's fear reactions. While some simple movements like running in place could dissipate her hyperarousal, simply extending exhales when she felt stressed became a practice that she could easily apply outside of our sessions.

Safety and the Continuum of Arousal

The perception of danger is not a static experience; that is, each individual possesses various thresholds ranging from attentive to threatened to terrorized. Perry (2009) explains this through a continuum of five states of increasing arousal in the following order: calm, aroused attention, alarm, fear, and terror. Perry states that when an individual is in each of these states of arousal, a different region of the brain is more dominant. For example, when an individual is calmly attentive, executive functioning is possible and the person can make decisions, problem-solve, and reason. However, when the individual is in a state of alarm, the limbic part of the brain takes hold and limits cortical functioning; this makes thinking and reasoning less possible. If terrorized, the brainstem/lower brain is activated and the person may feel distracted, overwhelmed, and chaotic. Perry notes that in cases of chronic interpersonal trauma during the early years of life, children may experience long periods of hyperarousal that may in turn increase an overall sense of alarm and eventually fear and terror. As a result, these children exhibit alarm and fear when they encounter certain sensory cues such as sounds, smells, or facial expressions. In other words, a fear or terror response occurs in the lower brain that compromises the limbic and higher brain, and individuals of any age may have no conscious awareness or understanding of their automatic reactions to hyperarousal or dissociation, to various sensory cues. In a sense, almost everything is perceived as a threat, including even the most innocuous interactions with therapists.

Tanya (described in Chapter 2) demonstrated various responses that mirror Perry's continuum of increasing dysregulation. When I first met with her at residential treatment, she was often fearful of me and with good reason as it turns out. Adults who were supposed to be caregivers had physically and sexually violated her in the past, and in Tanya's experience, her mother and grandmother also failed to protect her. Tanya understandably began to display alarm and terror when she learned that the individual who sexually abused her in the past was returning to her neighborhood and had visited her home. In order for me to be able to help her resolve previous traumatic experiences, addressing Tanya's sense of safety became essential so that she could not only reduce her level of hyperarousal, but also begin to feel safe within the residential treatment environment and with me. Similarly, Rose responded to various environmental and relational cues with extreme terror, often dissociating in an effort to temporarily escape overwhelming hyperactivation. In those moments, creativity, imagination, and play were temporarily inaccessible for her, including drawing in her sketchbooks. In brief, in order to fully engage individuals in any arts-based expression, it is important to identify where the person is on the continuum of arousal in order to address any feelings and body-based sensations of alarm, fear, or terror.

Safety and Private Logic

Although many types of traumatic events can alter one's internal sense of safety, interpersonal violence challenges it emotionally, socially, cognitively, and even somatically. When asked if she had a safe place to go to when her mother and boyfriend got into a fight, Emma, a 13-year-old survivor of multiple abuse and a witness to chronic violence in her home, reported:

"The social worker asked me about safety when we saw her last year for play therapy. I have never had safety. I told her that I did not know what it is. I feel safe with my mom sometimes. But other times I am afraid because she was not able to protect me from her boyfriends. I have tried taking the breaths that the social worker taught me. But if one of my uncles (mother's boyfriends) starts to touch me, I know that is not safety. I know the sound of his footsteps outside my bedroom is not safety. Even at this place [residential foster care] when I hear foot-steps outside my room I freeze up. I don't hug or touch anyone because it could lead to something bad. Sometimes just thinking about being touched gives me a pain in my stomach and my head. I can never stay calm because if I do I might not be ready for what can happen next. I don't know when there will be a fight at home or if my mother will be crying. If you ask me what my safe place is I will tell you 'I don't know.'"

Emma's responses are common to many children and adults who have witnessed or experienced multiple situations of interpersonal violence and abuse. On the continuum of arousal, she stays between alarm and terror in order to feel in control of her survival. She has also clearly developed what Adler (2002) calls *private logic*, an internalized story and pattern of reactions. Adlerian therapists emphasize that individuals often have their own private logic based on unique perceptions of the self, others, and the environment. These are convictions that are not part of cognitive awareness and are usually automatic; they reinforce a person's thinking, feelings, and actions in a consistent way. In order to address these responses, therapists generally try to have individuals explore their beliefs and definitions of self and worldviews. The practitioner also assumes that the individual's behaviors are adaptive coping strategies; in other words, these strategies comprise the person's private logic. This logic replaces what we often call "common sense" or objective reasoning.

Natural and human-made disasters often induce short-term private logic in even resilient individuals. As previously mentioned, events like the terrorist attacks in the United States on September 11, 2001, changed how millions of people responded to perceived threats in the days and weeks after the disaster because their previous beliefs about safety and national security were temporarily altered. Similarly, experiences of interpersonal violence, abuse, or neglect over time can permanently alter how individuals perceive verbal and nonverbal communications from others, including therapists. These individuals develop a private logic to help them negotiate relationships and situations, adapting to circumstances to survive what is perceived as danger or threat.

Narratives about private logic and personal safety are often clearly expressed in art expressions created by children and adults who have survived interpersonal violence and chronic trauma. For example, survivors

including isolation, abandonment, coercion, or even threats of death. Arts-based expressions through drawings, movement, or enactment may communicate a worldview that complying with assault (danger) may be what is required for acceptance and protection—that is, a sense of emotional, social and/or financial security, despite a violent relationship. This is a dynamic commonly experienced by individuals who are caught in the cycle of domestic violence and are unable to leave the violent relationship for various reasons. Private logic can occur not only in the form of trauma narratives, but also through behavioral reactions stimulated by tactile, visual, proprioceptive, auditory, and other sensory-based experiences common to expressive arts and play therapy groups. The vignette presented earlier in this chapter describing children's reactions to spilled water during a group session is another good example of the variety of private logic in response to a single event.

ESTABLISHING SAFETY IN INITIAL EXPRESSIVE ARTS SESSIONS: OVERALL CONSIDERATIONS

In strategizing how to introduce expressive arts, I always assume that the most uncomfortable sensation a child or adult may be experiencing in initial sessions is that one's own body does not feel safe. For this reason, I expect that the individual's body may respond in what seems like unpredictable ways with anything from hyperarousal and avoidance to dissociation, lethargy, and withdrawal. While the neurobiology of safety provides a helpful framework for understanding and addressing these responses, expressive arts interventions are also guided by three basic dynamics in treatment: (1) safety with others, (2) safety within the environment, and (3) safety within oneself. The first two areas are influenced by internal and external perceptions of "who one is safe to be with" and "where it is safe to be." The third dynamic—safety within oneself—is related not only to the ability to self-regulate, but also to a sense of personal empowerment. This is the level of internal confidence that one has an actual influence on one's life, mind, and body. These three dynamics translate into two trauma-informed practices key to supporting safety through expressive arts: *presenting oneself as safe* and *presenting the process as safe*.

Presenting Oneself as Safe

When working with individuals who may easily become anxious or distressed, therapists must often first present themselves as "safe" before any other effective intervention can begin. When I began working at a busy medical clinic, I immediately noticed how many individuals were often anxiously sitting in a large reception area waiting for their appointments. I actually thought about how I often felt when I was scheduled to see a new doctor or therapist: I would become agitated or uncomfortable in meeting that individual for the first time in an examination room. So I began to wonder just how I might be able to help new psychotherapy clients feel safe with me before we even began our initial session together. Rather than have the reception staff call their names or lead them to my office to meet me for the first time, I purposefully walk into the waiting area and start an informal conversation with the receptionist. It is a form of enactment on my part to give any new clients a chance to see and experience me and begin to attune to our relationship. During this bit of theater in the waiting area, they learn the cadence of my voice, hear my friendly laughter, notice my gestures and body language, and see what I look like well before going through to the second reception area where we will formally meet before going into my office. They get a preview of "coming attractions" before they actually enter what will be an unfamiliar environment to meet their psychotherapist. While this is a very helpful approach to use with children, adults and families appreciate it too. During subsequent sessions, individuals begin to recognize the sound of my voice as I am coming into the entrance of the waiting area. In working with trauma survivors, this simple procedure can be reassuring, demonstrating positive regard for individuals and setting the precedent for the ritual of meeting and greeting that builds trust and positive relationships.

When working with children or adults, giving them a tour of the expressive arts therapy or play therapy room helps them acclimate not only to the helping professional, but also to the environment where the therapy takes place. While an expressive arts environment can be perceived as inviting and positive, first encounters with it may feel just the opposite for some individuals. Marcos, a muscular, 6-foot-tall, 27-year-old military veteran who was referred to me for counseling and expressive arts therapy to help with his hyperactivation and traumatic brain injury, looked very hesitant as he first entered the room. After we talked for a few minutes about his challenges and personal goals, I asked him if he had heard of expressive arts as a treatment and, if so, what he thought about it. Marcos responded, "M'am, I am not so sure about this, to tell the truth. I have heard that other soldiers think it has helped them. But I am not so sure about painting pictures. I think it might be easier for me to talk than do art. But if I survived battle, I guess I can survive this." Then he added with a wink, "M'am, I'm a soldier, I take orders seriously. Dr. W sent me to you, so I will follow your orders." Despite his humor and willingness to try art therapy, Marcos's hesitation about being in a novel environment and being asked to make art or music and engage in movement or imagination reflects what many individuals unfamiliar with expressive arts therapy may feel.

An important way to support safety during an initial expressive arts therapy session involves asking several basic safety-related questions in order to give individuals a sense of control over the immediate environment. As previously explained when developing trust in the psychotherapeutic relationship, I asked all individuals these questions: "Where do you want to sit in this room?" "How would you like to arrange the chairs?" or "Where would you like me to sit?" These are key questions that respect individuals' level of comfort as well as empower participation. Marcos was quick to reply that he wanted his chair to face the door so that he could see the entry to the therapy room. As a military veteran, being able to observe one's environment for possible threats or changes is a key part of a soldier's training. Some individuals may become anxious if they are seated in the middle of a room away from walls, preferring to lean their chairs or their backs against a wall, while others want to be seated in a place where they can see a door or window in order to be able to monitor them.

Presenting oneself as safe is also predicated on establishing the reparative, empathetic relationship (Chapter 4). Kossak (2015) underscores this as a core principle in expressive arts therapy, noting, "Without safety there will never be any kind of relational trust built, and in turn there will never be any kind of attunement" (p. 73). Crenshaw (2008) adds that children do not verbally share or symbolically express their experiences, stories, or memories unless they feel that an empathetic individual is present. He notes:

> If the child does not have a trusting relationship with an adult perceived to be caring and capable of responding to their pain in an empathetic way they will not feel safe and nothing therapeutic will happen. This process cannot be rushed, pressured or forced. It has to evolve in a natural way as a result of the child or family gradually coming to view the healer as committed to their well-being. (pp. 94–95)

Crenshaw's words are equally true for adults whose traumatic experiences have left them feeling insecure and responding to the world as an unsafe place. The critical difference between social support and empathy is that empathy communicates to individuals that they are truly heard and seen by the helping professional.

Finally, as emphasized in Chapter 4, how helping professionals respond to creative expressions is key to supporting a sense of safety in expressive arts experiences. Overall, a nonjudgmental atmosphere is important because creative expression is part of each session; ensuring that all communications, including nonverbal creative ones, are accepted is essential. Sometimes therapists believe it is important to be able to interpret the meaning of artwork or other creative expressions to their clients. While meanings may clearly be present, responding with brain-wise and body-relevant questions, supportive observations and calming intonations of voice, gesture, and body language are much more important than any interpretation. These types of actions reinforce an implicit sense of safety, instilling trust and building an empathetic relationship between therapist and individual.

Presenting the Process as Safe

Applying expressive arts approaches adds new dimensions to treatment that are not always found in other methods. Safety is supported not only by what is verbally communicated, but also by the therapist's presentation of opportunities for play, imagination, and creative self-expression. These opportunities include but are not limited to the following: (1) providing choice and pacing exposure, (2) establishing structure and predictability, (3) identifying the window of tolerance, (4) finding a sensory comfort level, and (5) supporting mastery.

Providing Choice and Pacing Exposure

First and foremost, it is important that practitioners clearly convey that individuals have the right to decide their level of participation in expressive arts and what is comfortable to explore. Verbal disclosure of traumatic memories, the body's sensations, and experiences is an initial safety-related issue for most individuals, and as Rothschild (2011) notes, "There is no reason to revisit your past if you do not want to or if you do not see a value in doing so" (p. 49). Many practitioners still ask individuals to "draw what happened" or specifically explore details of traumatic memories through arts-based experiences. These approaches can be counterproductive and even harmful if the person feels pressured to recapitulate painful memories and experiences. Like Rothschild, I believe there certainly may be situations where reparation and recovery do not necessarily result from revisiting past traumatic memories with words or through arts-based expression of specific trauma narratives.

What is important is the individual's own pacing and control of creative expression. The value of expressive arts is the possibility it offers for nonverbal communication of feelings and perceptions related to painful or distressing experiences, providing both a relatively safe way to "tell without talking" (Malchiodi, 2008) and a form of "breaking the silence" (Malchiodi, 1990, 1997). In particular, children exposed to violence or abuse convey trauma through nonverbal behavior; they benefit from being in control of when and what they express as they begin to establish a sense of safety and trust. Their anxieties are generally diminished once they realize that they are not expected to verbalize or draw anything about what they witnessed or their own experiences of abuse and neglect. While I always indicate that I am there to help them with their feelings about "what happened," I also add these options: "You can always choose to tell me as much or as little as you want to while you are here with me"; "Some children who come here like to tell stories through drawing, painting, or clay, and others like to make up stories using the toys and games that are in this room"; "Some people who come here like to use the musical instruments to speak by making up songs or sounds."

Similarly, adults need to clearly know that they are free to communicate as much or as little as they wish to through creative self-expression or language and that when something is too difficult or overwhelming, they can leave it and return to it when they feel ready. Statements that support safe participation are key, including "Remember, you can stop participating at any time an activity feels too activating"; "If I am asking something too uncomfortable, please let me know to stop by raising your hand"; "You are the best expert as to what is helping and what is hurting during our sessions together." These statements reinforce the important point that creative expression is an *invitation* rather than a demand to disclose distressing feelings or memories when appropriate and according to the pace of the individual.

While expressive arts- and play-based approaches offer relatively safe ways to communicate nonverbally, they also may be novel or unfamiliar experiences for many people and potentially agitating rather than self-regulating, even with structure and pacing monitored. Despite what we know about the impact of traumatic stress on the senses, many arts and play therapists still repeat a mantra that expressive arts are "always" a safe way to communicate. This well-worn generalization does not always hold true. The degree of perceived safety in engaging in expressive arts therapy may change over time with the support of the therapist, but initially it is dependent on the individual's perceptions, previous experiences with creative expression, and capacity to imagine and play.

Establishing Structure and Predictability

When I was a graduate student working in an outpatient mental health clinic, I ham-handedly facilitated a group art process that demonstrates how lack of structure and predictability influences individuals and groups. Each participant was given a piece of potter's clay with which they could "make anything you want to." My professors suggested that "free expression" was always a good approach because it provides unrestricted choice and thus promotes spontaneous communication and creative freedom. While that theory may hold some truth, in practice this approach can also produce surprising responses that are not necessarily therapeutic or trauma-informed. Within a few minutes of working with clay, one of the participants began to pound his clay loudly and erratically (a response on the sensory/kinesthetic level of the ETC); it was not long until the entire group responded by pounding their clay, too. While this moment could be reframed as somewhat cathartic, it was counterproductive in the short term, causing many group members to become extremely agitated and anxious. I was becoming agitated too, and I quickly decided that the only response I could make was to meet the group exactly where they were in their own process. I began to pound a piece of clay, first to the beat of the group, and then I slowly altered the rhythm of the pounding, moving the group rhythm to a more organized and relaxed beat. After a few very tense minutes (possibly more tension-producing for me than for the group), I was able to alter the tempo and the sound level of the pounding, returning the group to a more relaxing and productive art process.

Most therapists clearly understand the importance of structure in their work and its value as a key component of trauma-informed intervention. Introducing expressive arts adds a sensory dimension that can stimulate chaotic and sometimes unpredictable responses. Structure can be as straightforward as the boundaries defined by the edges of a piece of paper or space within which to move one's body; the rhythm of music or sound; a limited number of toys or props; or co-created warm-ups or rituals to begin each session. It can also be in the form of simple directions, such as "Just use one color and just make marks with the chalk on the paper. Don't worry about making an image or what your drawing will look like." Or "Take a rattle, tambourine or drum, follow my rhythm, and we'll start slowly, counting one, two, three."

Identifying the Window of Tolerance

The "window of tolerance" (Siegel, 2010) is the area of arousal within which an individual can comfortably participate in expressive arts therapy. Sensitivity to this continuum is key to supporting safety. This window is bounded by two common trauma responses: hyperarousal (overactivation) and hypoarousal (withdrawal or dissociation). When individuals respond in either way, they are experiencing something intolerable and possibly something sensed as unsafe. While many individuals have the ability to return to their tolerance zone, many individuals challenged by traumatic stress may not have the same capacity. In these cases, it is important to understand not only what can be tolerated in terms of creative expression, but also how to appropriately pace expressive arts in a way that maintains that individual's comfort zone.

Lamott (1994), in her memoir *Bird by Bird: Some Instructions on Writing and Life,* provides a story that I often share with older children, teenagers, and adults to help them identify their window of tolerance for expressive arts intervention. Lamott's brother, age 10 years, had to write a report on birds, due the next day. Although he had been given 3 months to write it, he left the project until the last minute and understandably became overwhelmed by the magnitude of the assignment. Lamott's father put his arm around his son's shoulder and simply said, "Bird by bird, buddy. Just take it bird by bird" (pp. 18–19). This short story not only explains how overwhelming the process of recovery can be, but also explains the window of tolerance we will be working within and how we will be taking small arts-based steps that can be safely tolerated rather than stretching one's limits, only to feel worse as a result.

Certain verbal approaches are particularly helpful in supporting an individual's window of tolerance when speaking about arts-based expression. In other words, direct disclosure of trauma memories and experiences can accelerate arousal (alarm, fear, terror) in some individuals, causing distress or dissociation. While expressive arts may naturally bypass the discomfort of disclosure, for some individuals a "shift in perspective" is needed. Milton Erickson used a process called *refraction,* a form of parallel communication as a way to shift the course of conversation without direct confrontation (Marvasti, 1997). In play therapy, for example, it is essentially a way of using a prop or puppet to indirectly communicate a story. Similarly, in drama therapy, stories and enactment are strategically introduced to convey parallel experiences and to create what is called "aesthetic distance." In brief, both refraction and aesthetic distance allow individuals to maintain enough distance to feel safe and infer meaning when ready.

Projection is another way to support the window of tolerance. It is basically a shift in perspective from a first-person to a third-person narrative in communication, in contrast to the historical definition of projection as a form of defensive behavior in response to threat. In a trauma-informed practice, projection allows a child or adult to communicate uncomfortable memories or feelings in a safe manner through an expressive art form or through talking about the arts expression in a third-person narrative. For example, if I ask a child to show me a "fear" through a drawing, clay sculpture, or puppet play, I then ask, "If that fear could talk, what would that fear say?" I am not requesting a first-person disclosure, but instead am allowing the child to establish a safe distance from the experience being conveyed. Similarly, I may ask an adult to write down five words that come to mind (a top-down cognitive approach) after completing a drawing or a movement experience. The five words can be used to create a story or poem to verbalize an experience or perception from a third-person stance. The goal is to allow individuals to establish a distance between themselves and distressing reactions so that they can authentically express uncomfortable feelings, perceptions, and thoughts (for more detailed information, see Chapter 8 on trauma narratives).

The concept of post-traumatic play (Gil, 2010; Terr, 1990) is a good example of the window of tolerance in children and guides therapists as to whether to invite nondirected play or to intervene to adjust experiences to help children reach their optimal tolerance zone. Gil (2010, 2016) notes that there are two types of post-traumatic play behaviors: one that brings resolution (optimal tolerance) and one that does not (hyperarousal or hypoarousal). Gil further defines these types of post-traumatic play as either more *dynamic* or more *stagnant.* In dynamic post-traumatic play, children generally exhibit identifiable affect and variable interactions with the therapist and experiment with adaptive responses through creative expression. Over time, these children often find release and relief as the result of play activity.

In contrast, children who are stagnant in their post-traumatic play may have restricted affect and limited interactions with the therapist; themes remain constant and repetitive, and children may seem tense or frustrated by their interactions with props and toys. The window of tolerance is being noticeably stressed by stagnant play activity rather than comforted by it. According to Gil, the play itself may become "stuck" because it does not have the proper distance (optimal tolerance) from the individual. These concepts are particularly relevant to pacing both play therapy and expressive arts therapy sessions. For example, an individual who is able to use media and props with an increasing sense of mastery and self-direction has an optimal window of tolerance compared to the individual who frequently becomes distressed by making choices, using media creatively, and experimenting with play activities.

Finding a Sensory Comfort Level

In my experience, many traumatized individuals come to sessions with their own unique set of sensory reactions that can impact the window of tolerance. For example, Alexa, a 33-year-old woman whose history of exposure to multiple sexual assaults caused her to seek treatment for traumatic stress, sat before me at her first appointment with tapping fingers and sometimes a shaking leg. With rapid speech, she explained that she keeps her apartment very cold so that she can wear a 15-pound weighted blanket to bed because it helps her feel calm and "held." If she does not use the blanket, she feels so agitated that she cannot sleep at all. Certain kinds of music put her on edge, and she can only listen to ambient sounds; bright lights make her uncomfortable, and to avoid getting a headache, she sometimes wears sunglasses indoors. During most sessions, Alexa had to wrap the weighted blanket around her in order to participate in art making because otherwise she felt too anxious to continue, despite learning some simple ways to relax through ambient music and breathwork. Other individuals may need me to adjust lighting or play white noise, specific sounds, or music on my iPad to keep them feeling grounded. The same sensory qualities of expressive arts that have the potential to soothe and self-regulate can also feel overstimulating or uncomfortable for some children and adults. In other words, the senses of traumatized individuals may be on the "defense." In these cases, it is crucial to establish a sensory comfort level in order to successfully introduce expressive arts into sessions.

Early in my psychotherapy training I became fascinated with the concept of sensory integration (Ayres, 1976), which is a foundation of occupational therapy. Jean Ayres, occupational therapist (OT) and psychologist, developed a theoretical framework for sensory integration that describes how the neurological process of processing and integrating sensory information from the body and the environment helps affect regulation, learning, and behavior. At the time I first read Ayres's book, I was working with adolescents in classrooms who were labeled "learning disabled." They seemed to have a poor sense of balance (vestibular reactions), lack of perception of their bodies in space (proprioception), an inability to stay focused, various auditory distractions, and complained about lights being either too dim or too bright. After working with these adolescents for several weeks, I also realized how many of them seemed to have a good deal of trauma in their backgrounds. I decided to refer myself as a "patient" to a local OT in order to learn at firsthand about sensory integration and how an OT addressed individual problems. This learning experience turned out to be invaluable for my later work involving the connection between sensory input and traumatic stress in traumatized individuals.

During decades of work with abused and neglected children, I have regularly encountered young clients who seem to have many of the same sensory responses as the adolescents I saw in classrooms. These children are agitated by certain sounds and musical rhythms and have sensitivities to tactile qualities of paints or other media. Some children can only tentatively touch clay when wearing gloves. Others repeatedly fall out of their chairs, regularly trip over toys and props, and easily lose their balance when I introduce simple movement activities. It is important to monitor these sensory responses and others because they influence the individual's window of tolerance and inform what adjustments to arts-based experiences are needed, especially in initial sessions when focus on safety is crucial.

Of all the forms of sensory comfort found in the expressive arts, music is possibly the most relevant to supporting the body's sense of safety. While individuals may have specific musical preferences, there are some basic characteristics of music that can guide choices that support a feeling of "being held," similar to the weighted blanket Alexa found comforting. Music that has the tempo of a resting heartbeat, slower rhythms, low pitch, and no lyrics is generally relaxing for most individuals and modulates arousal levels. When introducing movement into sessions, I often use background music to help anchor the individual in the moment or simply to reinforce a calming sense of being held through soothing rhythms and tones.

Singing also has a powerful impact on most individuals because it is an experience that can be simultaneously calming and energizing. I introduce singing more often than breathwork because individuals will naturally learn to breathe more deeply through singing while gaining the soothing benefits it produces. Some studies (Collingwood, 2018; Thoma et al., 2013) demonstrate that singing releases endorphins and oxytocin, which helps relieve stress; this is a cumulative outcome, reducing levels of cortisol and thus measurably lowering stress over time. Singing becomes even more powerful when it is performed with the therapist or with a group; it deepens trust and attachment between individuals and becomes a form of co-regulation (Chapter 6).

Supporting Mastery

The experience of mastery is central to trauma reparation and enhancing a sense of resilience (Chapter 9). Mastery is also at the core of feeling safe within oneself and within one's environment. In work with children and adults who were hospitalized because of cancer or other life-threatening medical conditions, I learned how essential an internalized sense of efficacy can be in their recovery and perceptions of wellness. Serious illness threatens previously held beliefs about life because individuals often find themselves losing control and feeling fearful, powerless, and confused (Malchiodi, 2013). Fortunately, creative expression can help medical patients to regain some measure of control in their lives, leading to a sense of efficacy. The active processes found in expressive arts involve numerous opportunities for mastery, including freedom to choose and master materials and media. These experiences can contribute to feelings of autonomy and dignity when other aspects of life seem out of control. Ultimately, this translates to a sense of safety in one's own body for individuals whose lives are threatened by illness.

Similarly, traumatic events can also rob people of an internal locus of control, particularly when one's mind and body reactions are overwhelming and unpredictable. In other words, resolution of trauma begins with reestablishing "lost resources" (Ogden et al., 2006) through action-oriented mastery that supports self-efficacy and a perception of safety. When applying expressive arts, the previously mentioned concept of post-traumatic play explains how individuals make sense not only of traumatic events, but also attempts to master them through action. Children and adults may also engage in "post-traumatic art" (Malchiodi, 2014a), which is similar to post-traumatic play, repeating a particular narrative through imagery in an attempt to gain control over it. To some extent, Rose felt that she was intuitively attracted to drawing and collage-making for the very purpose of mastering something distressing that had happened to her during childhood through repetitive images and symbols. While these self-directed activities provided short-term experiences of self-regulation, Rose shared that her drawings also "helped me to survive" during moments when her hyperarousal became overwhelming and she desperately needed to feel safe within her own mind and body.

While expressive arts therapy generally emphasizes process over achievement of a final product, many individuals benefit from mastering self-regulation through arts-based experiences (Chapter 6) throughout trauma recovery. In other words, opportunities for creativity and play are not only a way to redirect focus away from hyperactivation, but also can simply become learning processes, in and of themselves, resulting in a sense of competence and confidence.

SPECIFIC APPROACHES TO ESTABLISHING SAFETY IN INITIAL EXPRESSIVE ARTS THERAPY SESSIONS

Many ways to support safety are well known to most therapists who work with traumatized individuals. For example, some approaches may help individuals identify external resources, including interpersonal support (family, friends, pets, communities) and activities (hobbies, physical exercise, self-care routines) that contribute to a sense of safety to some extent. A conversation that revolves around personal safety for those in danger of assault and describes how to appraise threats to self and what to do if one is at risk for physical or emotional harm is essential. For many individuals who have experienced traumatic events such as natural disasters or interpersonal violence, there are also necessary external resources that are part of physical safety. These resources include medical evaluation, identification of future threats, and development of plans to manage any ongoing crisis. There are also internal resources such as spiritual beliefs and personal strengths that contribute to a sense of purpose as well as memories of past experiences that provide a sense of security and control.

There are unique possibilities that support a sense of safety through expressive arts. The following section explains several relatively simple approaches that can be adapted for work with children and adults. They focus on four safety practices that are particularly important in early sessions: (1) using playful psychoeducation, (2) reviving imagination, (3) practicing the felt sense, and (4) developing creative rituals.

Using Playful Psychoeducation

In trauma-informed practice, psychoeducation is a primary concern in early sessions. It often focuses on helping individuals learn about the impact of trauma on the mind and body, as well as self-regulatory skills that support an internal sense of safety. The overall purpose is to reduce the stigma, confusion, and shame that individuals may experience as a result of traumatizing events or diagnoses such as post-traumatic stress.

There are many approaches to psychoeducation, but since I am an expressive arts therapist, I lean toward trying to make any learning fun, especially when one is addressing trauma and the brain. I generally use art expression to do this, offering individuals either a simple, hand-drawn image of a brain or a visual, preprinted outline of the three parts of the brain and the two hemispheres (see Appendices 2 and 3); I may even playfully use an outline to help the individual understand "what might be going on in my

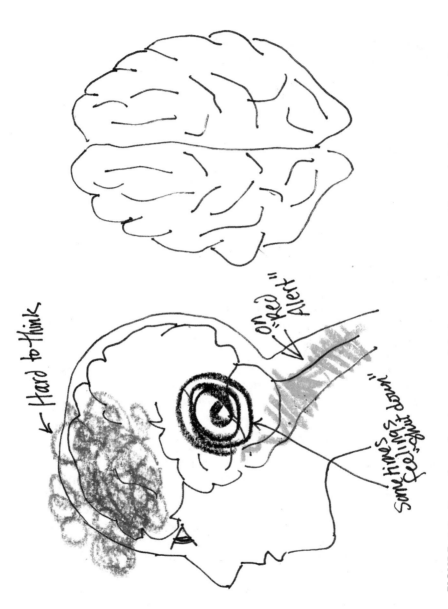

FIGURE 5.3. One of my drawings created during a session to provide psychoeducation on the brain and trauma. Reprinted with permission From the collection of Cathy A. Malchiodi (not to be reproduced without permission from the author).

brain" (Figure 5.3). Using an outline of the brain was especially effective with Marcos, the military veteran described earlier in this chapter, because his diagnosis of traumatic brain injury in addition to post-traumatic stress caused him to become interested in just how "my brain is handling this TBI [traumatic brain injury] and PTSD thing." His initial concerns about his medical treatment and expressive arts therapy sessions focused on perceptions of being "defective" because of his inability to control his hyperalertness and recurrent and intrusive memories. While Marcos understood how trauma can result in these reactions, seeing it in a visual form helped him to more easily understand that he was experiencing normal reactions to abnormal experiences. It also stimulated his interest in learning more about

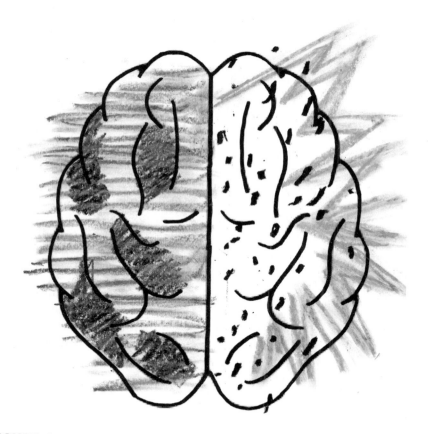

FIGURE 5.4. Marcos's drawing of how his "brain was doing." On the left side, he depicted his "loss of words" due to combat trauma; on the right side, he created lines and shapes to show "how everything has gotten way, way out of control." From the collection of Cathy A. Malchiodi (not to be reproduced without permission from the author).

how trauma impacts mind and body and in taking a risk to create his own visual images. When I explained that some experts believed that traumatic events impact the right and left hemisphere in different ways, he produced his own drawing of how he perceived what his "brain was doing" using the two-hemisphere brain outline (Figure 5.4). On the left side, he depicted his "loss of words" due to combat trauma, and on the right side, he created lines and shapes to show "how everything has gotten way, way out of control." While psychoeducation was an effective first step for Marcos, it also introduced him a little to the expressive arts, helping him to develop some visual language to continue to communicate what he was experiencing as a returning soldier who had survived multiple events.

Adults are not the only ones who take to this playful approach to psychoeducation; with some adjustments, children enjoy it too. One prop I use quite frequently is a colorful three-dimensional model of the brain that I keep on my desk. If a child seems interested, I often mention that "sometimes our brains actually change when we worry or experience bad events." At that point, I might make a drawing similar to the one I created for Marcos, asking children "What do you feel is going on in your brain lately?" This may lead to a dead zone in our conversation, but usually it results in a response ("It's kind of crazy in my head sometimes" or "My head hurts a lot") or the children may add to my drawing or create one of their own (Figure 5.5). If all of this goes according to plan, I can introduce the idea that it is possible to "change our brains" by remembering or imagining happy, fun, or calm times. The latter, of course, is part of a longer process of transforming trauma stories into new, reparative narratives. But in initial sessions, playful psychoeducation reinforcing the idea that change is possible is a first step in supporting belief in the expressive arts process.

Reviving Imagination

As discussed in an earlier chapter, imagination is a compelling part of expressive arts approaches in trauma reparation; the ability to imagine new possibilities is a key factor in eventual reparation and recovery (Chapter 10). But it is also a challenge because imagination may not always be easily accessed by all individuals because of traumatic stress and its impact on mind and body. The presence of fear is a particular barrier to imagining new narratives, especially for individuals with a history of chronic trauma or interpersonal violence. In other words, asking a traumatized person to go to a place of the imagination can be a frightening or at the very least, an overwhelming experience. Despite these challenges, imagination is an essential foundation for not only overcoming trauma, but also for harnessing the potentials of expressive arts to support reparation. The goal is to gradually begin to revive and use imagination to alter the body's sense of traumatic stress.

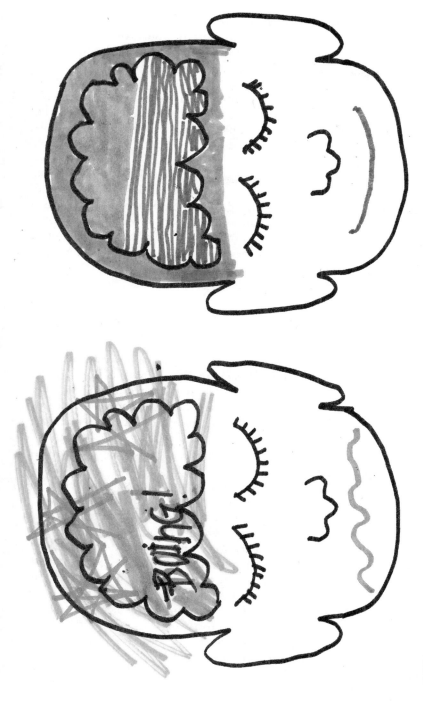

FIGURE 5.5. Child's drawing in response to the question, "What's going on in your brain lately?" On the outline he depicts the idea that "it's kind of crazy in my head sometimes" (left image). After practicing self-regulation during the session, he was able to show "when my brain is not going BOING" (right image). From the collection of Cathy A. Malchiodi (not to be reproduced without permission from the author).

One commonly used directive to tap the imagination about safety involves asking individuals to "draw a picture of your safe place" or to "make a collage of your safe place." These directives are often accompanied by guided imagery or breathwork to calm and relax the person. I generally do not use this arts-based strategy for several reasons. First, this question has exactly the opposite effect on many individuals because it stimulates all kinds of memories of their inability to find a place to be safe. It also can be a reminder of how an individual could not escape a perpetrator or a dangerous situation to get to a safe place, resulting in feelings and sensations related to guilt and shame.

Guided imagery, though helpful for some individuals, may cause some children and adults to relinquish adaptive coping strategies such as aroused attention or heightened alertness, strategies that have helped them to survive perceived dangers in the past. For example, for individuals like Rose, vigilance is a means to gain safety and with good reason. Rose, as noted earlier, came to treatment with a history of complex trauma with multiple instances of physical and sexual abuse that occurred over 12 years of her childhood. Rose felt that she was a failure because she had been unable to defend herself from her perpetrators. When I asked her about her sense of failure in fighting or fleeing, Rose sighed, "I just couldn't run fast enough, I couldn't get help and I couldn't scream loudly enough." While she knew these thoughts were irrational, Rose said that she now saw everyone as a possible adversary, worrying that she might also alienate me because of her mistrust and level of fear. When working with individuals like Rose, giving the impression that one is being asked to "let one's guard down" before a foundation for safety has actually been established is not only counterproductive, it threatens any survival skills the individual has painstakingly developed.

Francine Shapiro (2018), the originator of eye movement desensitization and reprocessing (EMDR), provides some helpful guidelines for accessing the imagination when the therapist is attempting to support safety in individuals like Rose who bring complex trauma histories to treatment. Shapiro cautions that any suggestion of imagery may inadvertently come with negative associations: "Some clients will say, 'Well, my safe place used to be in my closet with my teddy bear. Every time mom and dad argued, I would go there.' . . . Or, 'Oh, the beach is a wonderful place except for the time I got raped there'" (2012, p. 54). In my experience, prompts such as "the day you adopted your dog," or "Can you recall a comforting phone call or visit you received from a friend?" are sometimes necessary when traumatized individuals cannot easily call forth a positive memory.

Shapiro also underscores a key principle in accessing any memories or imagined images or providing any prompts—noticing the sensory experiences that come up in the body and being able to identify sensations that feel positive. This principle can be combined with helping the individual to notice changes in breathing when a positive sensory experience is present by placing one hand on the part of the body (stomach or chest) where the breathing begins. In this way, when the image and sensory characteristics of safety are accessed at other times, the individual can also identify the breathing pattern associated with a safe place.

One expressive arts approach I frequently use with both children and adults goes beyond the limited sensory experience of "draw a safe place." When asking an individual to explore and make tangible a positive resource for survival and self-soothing, it is important to involve multiple senses that are novel, pleasurable, and stimulating in positive ways. But because many traumatized individuals do find personal safety to be a difficult topic, I combine expressive arts with the "shift in perspective" that I previously described. I also introduce a prop that is generally perceived to be "fun"— in most cases, a rubber duck. I have used this prop not only with traumatized children but also with adults, who find they have many personal associations to the duck. Rather than consider what makes oneself feel safe, I invite clients to "take care of the duck" and provide an environment where the duck feels safe, thus shifting the perspective from the person to another

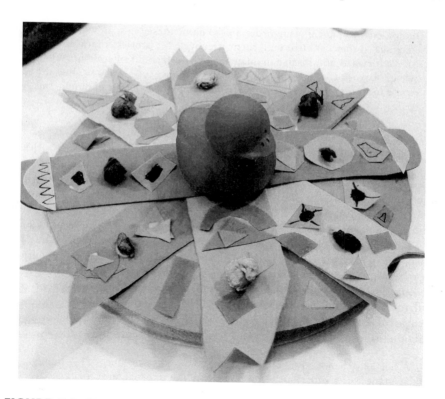

FIGURE 5.6. Keeping the rubber duck safe. From the collection of Cathy A. Malchiodi (not to be reproduced without permission from the author).

entity to be protected. Providing evocative materials such brightly colored tissue paper, feathers, glitter, yarns, and embellishments makes the experience not only more novel and fun, but also much more sensory and inviting than drawing, which tends to be more oriented to cognition and narrative (Figure 5.6). This simple shift in perspective of caretaking another entity outside oneself can be applied in many different ways in arts- and play-based approaches to safety. Just a small change in viewpoint often helps those individuals who have no real or imagined "safe place" to experience positive sensations by "pretending" it is happening to someone other than themselves.

Practicing the Felt Sense

When explaining the technique of "name it to tame it," Siegel (2011) advocates beginning with the higher brain as an effective strategy to address safety:

> What kids often need, especially when they experience strong emotions, is to have someone help them use their left brain to make sense of what's going on—to put things in order and to name these big scary right-brain feelings so they can deal with them effectively . . . stories empower us to move forward and master moments when we feel out of control. When we give words to our frightening painful experiences—when we literally come to terms with them—they often become much less frightening and painful. (p. 32)

Here Siegel is observing that by helping a child name the behavior, the storytelling capabilities of the left hemisphere can help calm the emotional responses of the right hemisphere. This strategy can be effective for individuals of any age who are capable of higher-level functioning and decision making (the cognitive/symbolic level of the ETC). However, executive functioning is not always available to individuals who are struggling with trauma reactions, making it difficult to get them to start with language.

Levine (1997) provides another way to go about this through the "felt sense." It is a concept that is more resonant with expressive arts therapy approaches to safety that begin at the sensory/kinesthetic and perceptual/affective levels of the ETC to address implicit (sensory) that may eventually lead to explicit (declarative) narratives. Eugene Gendlin (1982), credited with formulating the original concept of the felt sense, describes it as an individual's internal body awareness. He conceptualizes it as follows:

> A felt sense is not a mental experience, but a physical one. . . . A bodily awareness of a situation, person, or event. An internal aura that encompasses everything you feel and know about the given subject at a given time—encompasses it and communicates it to you all at once rather than

detail by detail. Think of it as a taste, if you like, or a great musical chord. (p. 32)

According to Gendlin, the role of the therapist is to help individuals become aware of internal sensations and how they transform. As people shift their focus from the felt sense of distress to one of well-being, emotions and perceptions change from vulnerability to self-efficacy.

Similarly, Levine (2015) and others who practice from a somatic perspective use the term *felt sense* to describe various body-based experiences related to trauma reactions. Even when individuals become more aware of their body's sensations, they still often need a process to access the felt sense. Levine offers several ways to gradually enhance the capacity to heighten awareness; these approaches are particularly useful in early sessions with traumatized individuals to support safety through learning to utilize one's own felt sense. The first approach involves simply obtaining a book, illustrated calendar, or magazine (nature or travel) with a lot of photo images. In my office, I keep a bin of photo images of various scenes and situations, pre-cut from magazines or printed from the Internet. It is essential to begin the process by guiding the individual through a gentle examination of current physical sensations, including how the body is making contact with the floor or chair; the tactile qualities of clothing; and feelings of tightness, temperature, hunger, thirst, or sleepiness. The individual can return to these sensations at any time during the process, along with the breath.

Next, the individual begins to look at one photo image, noticing any responses to it. Levine (1997) suggests responses such as "Is it beautiful, calming, strange, mysterious, haunting, joyful, sad, artistic, or something else? Whatever your response is, just notice it" (p. 75). Given that most people hardly ever have a single response to anything they encounter, it is not unusual to have several reactions to an image, so multiple impressions are normal. The felt sense is cultivated through identifying body-related sensations that come up when viewing an image. In other words, does a sensation arise in a certain part of the body? If so, what does that sensation feel like? Is it loose, tense, heavy, light, cool, warm, energizing, or something else? I may have individuals use "mark-making" or "colors, lines, and shapes" to show me those sensations on a body outline, as described in Chapter 3. Simply looking at several images, experiencing what sensations are evoked, and naming these sensations are enough to begin to access and learn to use the felt sense in the early stages. As part of this process, it is important to identify images that embody the felt sense positive and soothing sensations; the individual can return to these images, which serve as "resources" for safety when they are needed to reduce arousal. As the individual's level of safety in engaging the felt sense expands, more evocative images related to family, people, or events can be used to gradually and safely explore the body's sensations that may contribute to traumatic stress.

The felt sense that Levine refers to is a bit different from the practices that Gendlin (1996) proposed as "focusing-oriented therapy." Also, the idea of a felt sense is not new to expressive arts therapy and has been applied via expressive arts for many decades to help people communicate the body's experiences and perceptions of trauma and loss (Malchiodi, 2006). For example, Rhyne (1973) describes using "your body's senses to get in touch" by drawing "feeling states" as part of the Gestalt art therapy approach, which includes movement, sound, and visual arts. Rapaport (2009) provides a detailed framework for all the expressive arts as ways to identify and communicate Gendlin's felt sense concept through simple drawing, movement, sound/music, or any number of sensory-based expressions. She notes that in order to establish safety in applying focusing-oriented expressive arts therapy, therapists also assist individuals in the practice of "being friendly, accepting and welcoming" (p. 92) toward the felt sense. This is known as the "focusing attitude" and is essentially the experience of compassion and loving-kindness toward the self, similar to mindfulness. As Thich Nhat Hanh (2011), explains: "I have learned that the most important thing to transmit . . . is our way of being. So our presence, calmness, gentleness, and peace are the most important things we can transmit" (p. 37). In order for the individual to learn a focusing attitude, the therapist, too, must transmit the felt sense of welcoming and unconditionally accepting the client's felt sense experiences.

Rose's experience with learning the focusing attitude toward the felt sense is a good example of how it can become a pivotal piece in supporting safety. Once she mastered the basic skills needed to access the felt sense through gradual exposure to various photo images, I explained some basic mindfulness practices and the idea of "being friendly, accepting, and welcoming" toward all felt senses, even those that were uncomfortable or distressful. While Rose indicated that she was not quite ready to be "friendly to a lot of hurt in my life," she did want to accept and welcome the various felt senses in her body that helped her survive numerous years of abuse. At that point, we decided to co-create a simple "guardian figure" (an image chosen by Rose based on her spiritual beliefs) that included not only Rose's acceptance and welcoming of these felt sense experiences, but also my own focusing attitude of compassion and loving kindness toward Rose for all that she survived. Her images focused on "love," "nurturing," and "reliable." With her permission, I added "brave" because my felt sense of Rose was that she was undoubtedly courageous throughout her life and because she decided to commit to treatment.

This process of transforming the focusing attitude into a tangible art expression extended over several sessions not only as a way to support safety, but also to encourage Rose to practice self-regulatory skills and gradually begin to acknowledge and "welcome" more uncomfortable sensations related to traumatic stress. Co-creating the figure also allowed Rose to welcome and accept my positive regard for her ability to be creative, experimental, and successful in taking risks. For adult survivors of childhood physical and sexual abuse, arts-based interventions that might work well with children often provide similar opportunities for adults to revisit the sensory, implicit experiences necessary to the early development of internalized safety and trust. Through co-constructing the guardian image, Rose had the experience of being witnessed and appreciated for completing a creative task similar to what one might engage in during childhood. While this simple figure did not immediately resolve her overwhelming fears and hyperactivation, it visually captured a benevolent entity and a nonjudgmental, accepting observer that provided an implicit representation of Rose's own internal courage that she could revisit as needed. I encouraged Rose to speak through it at some of our early sessions not only to provide a safe way to communicate difficult narratives, but also to serve as a tangible reminder of her own inner strengths. In this sense, Rose was gradually practicing positive felt sense states in a manner similar to Levine's (2015) concept of "resourcing" (Chapter 6), using this particular image as a focus when distressed.

Developing Creative Rituals

Rituals are commonly used to reinforce consistency and structure within many forms of counseling and psychotherapy. Most individuals who have experienced repeated or chronic trauma throughout the lifespan benefit from culturally based rituals that soothe and reinforce a sense of safety. Common rituals include greetings (handshakes or other interactions agreed upon by the individual) and closure (saying goodbye, celebrating endings, and observing routines at the close of a session). These experiences can be even more meaningful if they are accompanied by sensory experiences such as specific arts-based activities, including movement, familiar songs, or stories.

As Perry (2009) notes, repetition not only is the foundation of self-regulatory processes, but also instills a sense of safety within oneself and the environment. The type of repetition Perry refers to is currently being integrated into programs that support safety through expressive arts. For example, the Israel Center for the Treatment of Psychotrauma (2014) developed the building resilience intervention (BRI) model, which encourages the development of resilience in children and parents in its ongoing trauma intervention programs with survivors of terrorism and war. It is a model protocol that can be adapted to any stressful situation. In the BRI model, children are encouraged to focus on their strengths while expressing their experiences of bombings and life-threatening circumstances. They practice safety rituals that are integrated within songs and movement not only to help them recall what to do when threatened, but also to pair positive sensory elements, especially physical action, with self-efficacy when in danger. In another example of their arts-based resilience-building activities, children are directed to invent a device to deal with rocket bombings; children create depictions of imaginative devices that vacuum up missiles and send them out into space, or they invent safe places that can escape the missiles' detection. The goal is to enhance the sensory experience of personal empowerment through active, hands-on participation.

A ritual I find particularly helpful involves "clearing the space with the arts," which is part of the focusing-oriented art therapy approach (Rappaport, 2009). It is a sensory and perceptual means for individuals to take a meaningful inventory of what is in the way of "feeling all fine," which for traumatized individuals translates to the body's sense of safety. In brief, the individual is asked to identify several things that are currently hindering a sense of safety or well-being in the present moment. The therapist guides the individual in sensing and perceiving these stressors and asks the individual to use one or more of the expressive arts (images, sounds, music, movement) to place these stressors at a distance from the body as follows:

> Take a few deep breaths . . . being friendly and accepting to whatever is happening within right now. Imagine yourself in a peaceful place. When you are ready, ask, "What's between me and feeling 'all fine' right now?" As each concern comes up, just notice it without going into it. Imagine a way to set the issues at a distance from you outside the body—such as wrapping each concern up and setting it at a distance from you; placing it on a park bench nearby, or any imagery that come[s] to you. As you put each issue aside, sense how it feels inside. Check again; except for all of that, am I "all fine?" and see if anything else comes up. See if there is an image that matches your inner felt sense of the "all fine place." When you are ready, express your experience through the arts. Some people prefer to only create the "all fine place" while others like to include the stressors they are setting aside and the "all fine place." Trust what is right for you. (Rappaport, 2015, p. 200)

The addition of expressive arts increases the felt sense experience for most individuals. First, it helps individuals to more clearly express implicit experiences of "what is getting in the way" (what threatens safety) and "what is the all fine place" (safe place) in ways that the therapist can actually witness. When "clearing the space with arts" is initially practiced through an expressive arts activity, individuals can then later more easily imagine "clearing" when concerns or stressors arise outside the session.

Distancing is an additional practice that can be added to the experience. For example, creating visual symbols for "what is getting in the way" and then placing them in a paper bag and then determining how far the bag needs to be from oneself in order to make one feel comfortable and safe. While many individuals find just sealing up the bag and placing it a short distance from them feels right, there are a wide range of responses. Some clients ask me to carry the bag outside to the waiting room, and they even have a specific area in mind for me to place the bag. One client made her decision about distance with both levity and pragmatism. She knew exactly where she wanted her bag of "what's getting in the way" to go—out into the clinic parking lot in the trash collection bin for eventual removal to the county recycling station.

As an adult survivor of numerous incidents of physical and sexual abuse, Rose had some initial challenges in "clearing the space." But she was willing to practice it numerous times to begin to put aside traumatic memories and body sensations that overwhelmed her. In her case, I initially started with a "top-down" strategy, asking her to simply write words, use mark-making or symbols with felt pens on paper, or choose magazine images representing "what was getting in the way of feeling safe" in the moment. In other words, I was actually calling on her higher brain (cognitive/symbolic) to name "what is getting in the way" because it helped Rose to feel more in control and to verbally name what was getting in the way; expressing emotion (affect) and body sensations were simply too overpowering for her and only escalated her hyperactivation. She specifically asked that the colorful paper gift bag containing her words and symbols stay with me in the therapy room. We brought it out during most sessions so that Rose could add anything new to the container. In brief, the point of using expressive arts in this manner is to give traumatized individuals a means to at least temporarily put aside fears that get in the way of feeling safe.

CONCLUSION

For Rose, Tanya, and others who have experienced traumatic events, it is essential to address fear-related responses in early sessions for several reasons. First, they result in uncomfortable physical sensations that keep the body in a state of alarm, trepidation, and uneasiness. Relief from a repeated internal perception of threat not only is welcome, but also increases one's sense of self-efficacy and empowerment to meet other challenges associated with traumatic events. Mediating fear through supporting safety also involves introduction of self-regulatory strategies to reduce hyperactivation, dissociation, and other counterproductive coping reactions. This, the subject of the next chapter, is a key foundation in any expressive arts approach designed to reduce the body's sensations of fear and assist individuals in discovering specific and novel ways that will decrease their stress and help them feel safe.

CHAPTER 6

● ● ● ● ● ● ● ● ● ● ●

Self-Regulation

FUNDAMENTALS OF STABILIZATION

Helping professionals who work with traumatized children or adults know that one of their first challenges is helping individuals address trauma reactions activated by seemingly benign events. As discussed in Chapter 5, an unstoppable, automatic physiological cascade often brings on distressful sensations of alarm, fear, dissociation, or other responses. A teenage client summarized the terrifying nature of this cascade in her description of a simple trip to a grocery store to pick up some bread and milk for her mother. "I was just trying to find the bread my mom likes. Then I saw a man who looked like my grandfather, and I panicked. I almost threw up in the store. I had to leave without the food and I ran all the way home." The adolescent had been sexually and physically abused by her grandfather when she was a young child. Although the grandfather had been dead for more than 7 years, the experience of interpersonal violence was still very real to her. Just seeing a person who reminded her of the perpetrator had a powerful effect on her body to the point of nausea and extreme terror. Similarly, an adult client explained the startle response she had when she saw someone simply lift a hand to wave at her. It immediately caused her to recoil because it mirrored the same motion her husband made right before he started to physically assault her. Although these reactions may have helped these individuals avoid or escape harm in the past, they now have become automatic dysregulated responses to environmental cues that are unpleasant and disruptive.

As a result of repeated exposure to traumatic events, individuals may be highly reactive, avoid situations that activate fear and anxiety, and lack control over emotional and physiological responses to stress. Those who

164

have experienced early developmental trauma or attachment problems have similar reactions, yet they do not know or understand why they may be in a constant state of hypervigilance (sympathetic nervous system) or be dissociative, emotionally detached, frozen, or in state of collapse (parasympathetic nervous system). Because implicit memories can be so powerful, the brain and body respond instantaneously as if what happened in the past is happening in the here and now, even when the person knows the source of the memory.

Assisting individuals in addressing the intense physiological responses caused by trauma is essential to initial work with any child, adolescent, adult, group, or community in distress. People who have experienced interpersonal violence (physical abuse, sexual assault, or witness to violence events), war, or natural disasters are particularly in need of strategies for self-regulation leading them to eventually feel calm enough to relax, repair, and recover. Before exploring the details of painful memories, it is important to introduce therapeutic experiences that support an internal sense of stabilization and begin to help individuals find sources of self-regulation. Expressive arts therapy is an action-oriented method designed to help children and adults develop these sources. This chapter provides examples of various arts-based approaches that can be adapted to support stabilization with individuals, groups, and communities.

SELF-REGULATION AS A CRITICAL COMPETENCY

Along with supporting an internal sense of safety, *self-regulation* is an initial critical competency that forms the basis of any future successful intervention. The term *self-regulation* is used to describe the capacity not only to control one's impulses, but also to be able to soothe and calm the body's reactions to stress. It is the ability to modulate affective, sensory, and somatic responses that impact all functioning, including emotions, somatic responses, and cognition. Additionally, it refers to the brain's executive function, which can delay actions or initiate them if necessary. In other words, individuals who are self-regulated can delay gratification and suppress reactions in order to become mindful of consequences or alternative, appropriate responses. The term *affect regulation* is also used to describe healthy ways to manage and release stress, including how we cope with sadness, joy, challenges, anger, worries, and fear. For the purpose of this chapter, I use the term *self-regulation* because it encompasses all forms of regulation, particularly how one responds to the body's sensory reactions to distress.

Dysregulation occurs when individuals are unable to feel or identify emotions and body-based sensations and when feelings and physiological responses overwhelm them. Because these responses remain unresolved in many traumatized individuals, they often make unhealthy attempts at self-regulation in the form of substance abuse, smoking, self-mutilation, overeating, or overworking; or anxiety, panic, depression, disrupted sleep; or compulsive behaviors. Extreme arousal can result in dissociation and alexithymia—the inability to put feelings into words (see Chapter 8).

Perry (2009) defines self-regulation as a core strength that is critical to the healthy development of one's capacity to respond to stress. As described in Chapter 5, he explains safety through a continuum of five states of increasing arousal (calm, aroused attention, alarm, fear, and terror), emphasizing that self-regulation becomes more difficult as arousal increases. Goleman's (2012) concept of an "emotional hijack" is somewhat similar to Perry's concept. According to Goleman, the amygdala takes the mind on somewhat of an emotional rollercoaster in response to stressful circumstances. These responses are immediate, overwhelming, and at times inappropriate given the nature of a perceived threat; that is, these responses are faster than the thinking brain (executive functioning). Goldman's concept also seems to be a "physiological hijack" because not only anxiety and other powerful emotions are activated in traumatized individuals, but also somatic responses such as increased respiration and heart rate, muscle tension, nausea, and other body-based reactions. Additionally, a "cognitive hijack" takes place because traumatic stress disrupts executive functioning and impacts thought in a variety of ways. For example, when an individual is preoccupied with hypervigilance, worry, and fear reactions, it is difficult to use higher functions to pay attention, comprehend, or retain information easily.

Tanya demonstrated various responses reflecting Goleman's concept. A series of emotional hijacks brought her to residential treatment, including defacing buildings with graffiti and brief, violent outbursts that she later regretted being unable to control. In order to help Tanya resolve previous traumatic experiences, I knew that she first needed to develop some self-regulatory skills that would help her reduce her high level of arousal (fear of sexual assault). Marian, also discussed in previous chapters, observed that she often experienced an uncontrollable sense of alarm when confronted with situations that triggered the possibility of panic occurring; she was emotionally and physiologically hijacked by fear of being unable to continue to drive her car if sensations became overwhelming. Marian could easily describe in detail the feeling of terror that occurred with occasional nightmares she had about the bus accident she survived. In the initial sessions, the goals for both Tanya and Marian were to help them achieve calm and relaxed alertness (alert attention) and a state where the threat of "hijack" was decreased and problem solving and reasoning were possible.

For Tanya, Marian, and many other traumatized individuals, the experience of trauma "does not tell time" and dysregulation can occur at any moment when environmental or relational cues replicate aspects of the original traumatic events. In other words, the sensory qualities of the original distressing events spontaneously stimulate a cascade of hyper-arousal, avoidance, dissociation, or other responses when actual danger is not present. LeDoux (2015) observed that in order to begin the process of transformation, we have to notice these inner experiences of distress. According to LeDoux, van der Kolk (2014), and others, internal (intero-ceptive) experiences and implicit memories of the original events dominate the executive functions that recognize external (exteroceptive) cues in the environment. The way to begin to identify interoceptive experiences and implicit sensations is through self-awareness and conscious notice of emo-tion and sensations in the body, rather than the avoidance that comes with constant focus on others and the environment.

For this reason, introducing ways to self-regulate through expressive arts is an initial and essential foundation for gradually redirecting focus toward implicit (interoceptive) experiences. Once individuals have adopted several creative strategies to address the body's uncomfortable sensations, they also begin to feel empowered to take charge of how they respond to the internal perceptions triggering these reactions. They then can begin to become effective self-regulators who can sustain calm and restful alertness when they are anxious or fearful and can more quickly adapt, with an enhanced capacity to meet distressing situations successfully.

EXPRESSIVE ARTS: USING THE SENSES FOR SELF-REGULATION

Over 100 years ago, Freud (1920) observed a behavioral response that underscores why we should use "action" rather than words alone to address dysregulation stemming from traumatic stress. He called this response "the compulsion to repeat," noting that individuals who do not remember dis-tressful events are likely to repeat those experiences both in treatment and in life. In other words, these repressed memories are repeated in the here-and-now rather than allowing the experiences to live in the past where they originated.

While my psychotherapeutic stance is not psychoanalytic, Freud's concept does highlight an important characteristic of all forms of expres-sive arts therapy— they are action-oriented processes that may help trau-matized individuals "repeat" the memories Freud cited, but in a different form. Traumatized individuals are, in fact, action-oriented in the sense that they instinctively use various unhealthy responses to address self-regulation, as mentioned at the beginning of this chapter. They also simply may not have the appropriate language (speechless terror or alexithymia) to express their feelings and body-based sensations, they may dissociate, lack-ing the ability to articulate their emotions; and their somatic responses may have become dysregulated. The kinesthetic/sensory qualities of rhythm, movement, enactment, visual imagery, touch, and sound found in expressive arts naturally involve active participation rather than talk-only. Also, verbally analyzing and interpreting dysregulation, along with a focus on "what's wrong," do not necessarily support self-regulation. According to some practitioners, these strategies may actually increase dysregulation (Heller & LaPierre, 2012).

In addition to being action-oriented, specific applications of expressive arts therapy have many unique dimensions that can enhance self-regulation. In particular, they support the following areas either as a primary strategy or as an adjunct to other effective approaches: (1) *grounding and anchoring,* (2) *sensory-based co-regulation and shared regulation,* (3) *mirroring and entrainment,* (4) *bilateral movement,* (5) *relaxation and mindfulness practices,* and (6) *affect regulation.*

Grounding and Anchoring

The concepts of grounding and anchoring are commonly used as forms of self-regulation practices within many therapeutic approaches. *Grounding* techniques generally refer to ways for people to focus on some aspect of external reality and often involve using the senses to reinforce being in the here-and-now. It is a strategy often introduced in early sessions to help individuals stop or at least slow down stress responses and emotional or physiological dysregulation. For individuals whose distress responses are overwhelming and easily activated by implicit memories, grounding can be effective because it involves sensory-based experiences designed to interrupt anxiety, panic, dissociation, or attention lapses. The goal is generally to help the person return to the here and now rather than remain stuck in a reaction to something in the past or that might happen in the future.

Many of the grounding techniques I use have more to do with sensory-based experiences than with arts-based approaches. For example, various rhythmic breathing techniques or the introduction of aromatherapy (strong smell such as eucalyptus) or gustatory experience (pungent taste of ginger candy) are fairly straightforward grounding experiences. If effective, they simply create a shift in attention to external senses, such as identifying things that one can see, hear, or smell in the present. A conventional strategy used by many therapists asks the individual to scan the immediate environment and describe that environment in detail using all of one's senses. For example, "the walls are light green, there are three brown folding chairs, there is a cinnamon smell coming from the next room, there are sounds of cars passing by outside." Other grounding techniques include various repetitive protocols, such as counting, using a specific grounding phrase ("I'm safe in this room"), bringing one's senses to a specific part of the environment, stamping one's feet, and employing imagery (imagining ocean waves going in and out). While these techniques can effectively support grounding, introducing a strong sensory element in the moment (tasting a pungent candy or holding a tactile object) adds an essential component to the process. Additionally, in applying any grounding technique, it is important to have the individuals rate their experience before and after in order to understand whether or not the experience is perceived as effective. Simple 0-to-10 Likert scales, or a template with faces showing "happiest" to "saddest" for children, are common qualitative instruments.

Anchoring is another term that is sometimes used to describe the process of using specific cues or experiences to bring one's attention to the present moment or to shift sensations from anxious to calm. It is similar to grounding, but in expressive arts therapy it usually involves some sort of arts-based sensory cue (sound or music) or creating an object (specific art expression). It is also something that the individual can return to for self-regulation. Goleman (2012) describes a powerful example of anchoring used as part of "Breathing Buddies" in the New York City public school system. It is part of the Inner Resilience Program, a curriculum established after the World Trade Center attacks on September 11, 2001. The program includes both specific grounding and anchoring practices, including a sound (a bell's chime), as well as holding stuffed animals and deep belly breathing as a method of anchoring with children. While a variation of mindfulness breathing is involved, the bell and special toy provide children with sensory-based anchors. The goal is self-regulation, which, when achieved, supports students' success in classroom learning by increasing attention, comprehension, and problem solving.

The advantage of using expressive arts is that they can be both sensory-based and creative ones tailored to developmental, cultural, and personal preferences and relevance. Many grounding and anchoring practices ask clients to simply imagine a grounding image, but this can be an impossible request for a highly stressed individual. In contrast, expressive arts require active participation while taking advantage of various senses to help increase focus on something other than distressing implicit reactions or memories, or they can serve as an immediate distraction if necessary.

Grounding and Anchoring with Children

When individuals do not have an identifiable and healthy way to self-soothe when stressed, I often invite them to create something that can be used for anchoring in the present and for use outside the therapy session. For children, this can involve making a tactile object such as a stuffed toy, a painted rock, or other special object. Sometimes, too, even a simple art expression can be helpful if it is relevant and meaningful to the child. For example, Katy, an 8-year-old girl who survived a recreation vehicle accident, had to be hospitalized for several operations and difficult medical procedures. Early in the course of her treatment, she developed fear reactions, insomnia, and claustrophobia during X-ray procedures. Because Katy could carry very little with her to the medical treatments, we decided to create a pocket-size "thumbprint friend" who could accompany her during her multiple stays in the hospital. The first iteration of this friend was created by Katy's thumbprint on an index card; she added various features to the thumbprint to give it a face and personality (Figure 6.1, top). On the back of the index card we drew a five-pointed star (Figure 6.1, bottom), which was part of a simple breathing exercise that proved specifically effective for Katy. Katy carried her thumbprint friend with her to all her doctor visits and radiology appointments, proudly showing it to the technicians and telling stories about how it was created with her own thumb and drawing skills. This form of grounding (breathing) and anchoring (image) worked for Katy, and during another session we decided to create a more tactile, three-dimensional version by making a small doll out of pipe cleaners (chenille stems), wrapping it with colorful yarn, and adding various embellishments and a thumbprint face similar to the original one. Because this version was bendable, it also became another way that Katy could communicate her feelings about her accident and medical interventions, using dramatic enactment and storytelling (from sensory to narrative) stimulated by the doll.

Integrating Yoga with Expressive Arts for Grounding and Anchoring

An expressive arts colleague and a trained yoga practitioner, Emily Johnson Welsh (personal communication, 2017), introduced me to a grounding and anchoring practice that integrates both a relatively simple yoga pose and an arts-based experience. The pose, Tadasana or "mountain pose," is one that most people can easily practice and master in a short amount of time. One caution that needs to be observed when introducing any yoga poses within sessions is to ensure that the individual is not experiencing any blood pressure issues, dizziness, or lightheadedness. I work in settings where most individuals have their doctors' permission to participate in simple physical activities; if you do not have this permission, it is important that the individual engage only in yoga that is within the range of their limits and abilities. Since I am not a trained yoga practitioner, when I work with groups, I prefer to have a yoga practitioner lead this part of the experience. However, this pose is relatively simple, and most therapists can learn it with supervision from an experienced yoga teacher.

The Tadasana pose basically requires the person to take a standing position and place weight evenly across the balls and arches of the feet, breathing rhythmically and focusing on the present moment. It is best done with bare feet because, in order to perform it correctly, one must lift one's toes and spread them apart. If there is a problem with balance, be sure to ask the person to stand with feet at least 6 inches apart or at a comfortable distance (feet positioned directly under hips). I find that practicing this pose against a wall for proper alignment is a good variation for many

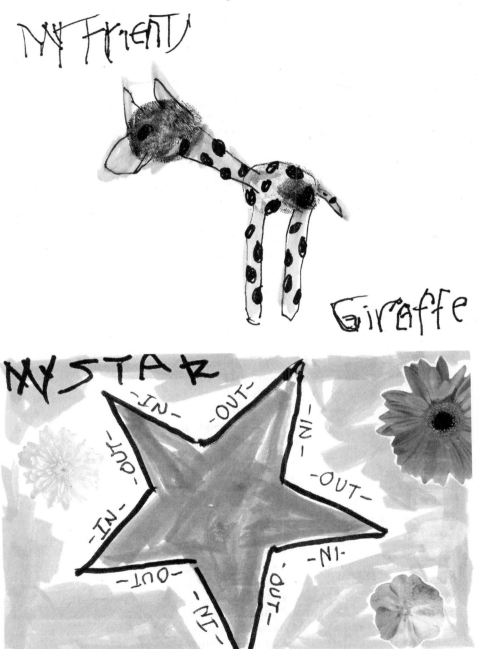

FIGURE 6.1. Child's "thumbprint giraffe friend" and star breathing practice on index cards. From the collection of Cathy A. Malchiodi (not to be reproduced without permission from the author).

individuals. The Tadasana pose with eyes closed is more of a challenge to the window of tolerance (i.e., one's sense of safety and ability to balance), but it will help the individual begin to put additional focus on body-based sensations. For complete instructions on this pose, see Appendix 6.1 at the end of the chapter.

The Buddha reportedly said, "The foot feels the foot when it feels the ground." The Tadasana pose is an experience of grounding as well as a conscious awareness of how the "feet feel the feet when they touch the ground." An anchor can be created through taking the perception of that grounding experience and translating it into a simple art expression. The point is to try to capture at least some of what it is like to sense feeling where the body is in contact with the floor and how that helps the individual to feel stable and supported. Ultimately, the eventual goal is to help the person sense this stability and connectedness in life. The process is simple—tracing one or both feet (with the person's permission, the therapist might be called upon to do the actual tracing) on paper or large cardstock. At this point, with some prompting and third-hand assistance, I ask the individual to use mark-making, lines, shapes, and colors, choose magazine photos, and/or write words if needed to illustrate the felt sense of Tadasana within the outline of the foot. If it seems appropriate, the space outside the foot outline may also need imagery and/or words because the felt sense of support may be perceived beyond the physical boundaries of the experience. To move the experience through the ETC, asking for a narrative about the experience facilitates the process of articulating the self-awareness that LeDoux (2015) and van der Kolk (2014) observed as a necessary step in interoception. Here is a brief example from an individual who suffered from severe panic attacks triggered by stress responses to open spaces and crowded social situations:

> "The mountain pose was much harder than I thought it would be. After all, it ought to be easy to just stand in one place. But the more I tried to stay in one place, the more I felt unbalanced. Cathy helped me to find a way to feel stable by slowly suggesting different positions for my feet and letting me lean against a wall until I felt okay to stand on my own. I never realized that by just focusing on how my feet were touching the ground and how spreading my toes as far as I could made such a difference. My whole body changed. I felt just a little better sense of control over my breathing and my feelings in that moment. The fear in my chest actually got smaller. It's not gone yet, but feeling the strength of being a mountain surprised me because I have felt so afraid for so many years now because of my panic attacks. Moving from the yoga posture to art making was a very revealing experience for me. It really helps me to look at that image I made and remember the experience of being supported by my own feet and my body."

While the grounding (Tadasana) is the key component, the additional arts-based experience and narrative not only capitalize on the bottom-up approach, they also create the necessary anchors that can serve as additional tangible resources for the individual in the future.

Sensory-Based Co-Regulation and Shared Regulation

In Chapter 4, the importance of attunement was highlighted as an essential part of the expressive arts psychotherapeutic relationship. It is the therapist's capacity to respond with both insight (knowing what one feels) and empathy (knowing what others feel) to the explicit and implicit communications of clients. Attunement is not only perceiving what individuals say, but also attending to eye signals, facial gestures, tone of voice, posture, and even breathing rate. It is also an embodied response because, as therapists, we actually feel a connection to our clients and their expressive work through our own physiological responses to individuals in order to support self-regulation. Attunement operates from the "bottom up" because we perceive feelings in others in the more ancient parts of the brain—the amygdala, hypocampus, and structures underlying the cortex. Therapeutic relationships that resonate these responses between therapists and clients enhance clients' overall functioning and help individuals develop adaptive responses to stress (Badenoch, 2008; Siegel, 2012).

Co-regulation is defined as responsive interactions that provide support, coaching, and modeling and is a variation of attunement. In order to achieve co-regulation, therapists are required to pay close attention to the individual's cues with consistency and sensitivity; it is also dependent on the changing social interactions between therapist and individual over time. Like an internalized sense of safety, it is well documented that a healthy connection early in life between caregiver and infant is essential in shaping an individual's ability to self-regulate throughout life. Numerous studies over decades show that the ability to derive affect regulation from the presence of another individual is a more powerful predictor of whether individuals improve over time than the actual trauma history. A caregiver who is depressed, anxious, angry, or dissociated does not have self-regulatory abilities and cannot pass along this capacity to the child; this compromises the child's abilities to self-regulate and may result in increased vulnerability to stress and trauma. A history of developmental trauma in particular can result in a pervasive pattern of dysregulation (van der Kolk, 1996, 2014).

While the term co-regulation began as a way to describe caregivers' support for infants, it is now used to describe regulatory support that occurs within the context of caring relationships across the lifespan. In one sense, all regulatory dynamics are forms of co-regulation because regulation is best learned through another individual who provides the necessary sensory cues and responses, such as a caregiver or significant other. In expressive arts therapy, arts-based co-regulatory interactions are central to how therapists begin to help client address stress. In general, this form of co-regulation is less dependent on words and is sensory-specific to the characteristics of each expressive art form. For example, arts- and play-based experiences emphasize interaction mostly through tactile, visual, and kinesthetic senses. Music includes sound, prosody, vocalization, and rhythm-based experiences that can be co-regulatory experiences; it also involves social engagement when collaboration or playing instruments is involved. Psychodrama, improvisation, and enactment offer multisensory ways to establish co-regulation through role play, modeling, mirroring, and enactment.

In the field of art therapy, one common approach to co-regulation is called the *third hand*. Kramer (1986) is credited with coining this term and demonstrated its applications with children who were challenged by traumatic events. The third hand refers to the therapist's use of suggestion, metaphors, or other techniques to enhance the individual's progress in therapy and self-expression without being intrusive or imposing values. It also involves the strategic use of the therapist's own active participation through supporting creative expression by mirroring and modeling and occasionally even redirecting the individual's creative process. I have found that the third hand includes being a focused witness to an individual's efforts to engage in art expression and, more importantly, assisting the individual in those efforts. These actions mimic a healthy co-regulatory relationship between a caring adult and child and reinforce the self-regulatory skills the child will need to cope with distressful events throughout life. Third-hand arts and play interventions also echo the concept of the "good-enough parent" (Winnicott, 1971) who supports the individual's efficacy experiences during creative exploration and experimentation.

Shared regulation, a form of mutual regulation, is found in group expressive arts experiences. The synchrony of moving within a group, singing together, and participating in an improvisation troupe or dramatic enactment with others are all social experiences that stimulate shared regulatory moments. Music in particular stimulates an experience of shared regulation among both listeners and participants. The neural networks found in the areas of the brain associated with social cognition and music production are highly activated when the participants are playing their instruments and when ability to connect with each other while playing music is exceptionally strong (Sanger, Müller, & Lindenberger, 2012). While there are many ways to use expressive arts to create moments of shared regulation, having participants engage in line and gesture drawings on large sheets of paper while listening to various types of music is a very simple strategy. In my experience, participants naturally pick up on each other's rhythms and begin to synchronize their movements even when drawing to music within a group setting.

Mirroring and Entrainment

In contrast to talk-only, expressive arts experiences have a distinct advantage as a form of co-regulation and shared regulation because rhythm and synchrony are central to arts-based approaches. *Mirroring* and *entrainment* are two essential techniques that support regulation on a sensory and kinesthetic level.

Mirroring

Mirroring is a commonly used approach to establish and enhance the relationship between the individual and the helping professional. Within the expressive arts therapy, it is generally described as the embodiment or reflection of an individual's movement or nonverbal communications. The goal of mirroring is not only imitation of postures, facial expressions, and gestures, but also includes attunement between the individual and practitioner. The brain's mirror neuron system is believed to be at least one part of these experiences of attunement, empathy (Goleman, 2012), and mirroring (Gallese, Eagle, & Migone, 2007). These neurons refer to a special type of cell that fires not only when a person performs an action, but also when the person observes someone else make the same movement. For example, when you see someone stub a toe on a concrete curb, you might immediately flinch or shudder with sympathy, sensing what the person's pain or distress is actually like. This is an example of the ability to instinctively understand and respond to what another person is experiencing. Research on mirror neurons and related aspects of neurobiology have also informed the larger domain of interpersonal neurobiology. While the mechanisms behind these specific brain cells are not completely understood, they have implications for helping professionals in terms of both mirroring and attuned relationships.

Mirroring is common to almost all expressive arts approaches, but it is particularly relevant to dance/movement because of the kinesthetic level of expression and interpersonal aspects involved. For example, expressive arts therapy group sessions, including those for trauma survivors, often begin with a movement sequence or simple stretches in which everyone reaches up to the sky and down to the earth in a rhythmic manner. Participants are simply asked to pay attention to their breathing and their bodily experiences and to do as much or as little as they feel comfortable with in terms of movement. For individuals who are not yet comfortable with moving their bodies or those who find moving in a group overwhelming, I often keep things simple by just inviting participants to "mirror me," allowing everyone to feel at ease in just following along rather than inventing their own movements. In facilitating this process, I am observing the energy of the group and individuals; for example, is the energy level high, calm, lethargic, or neutral? Depending on the nature of the group, participants may eventually be invited to demonstrate their own stretches, with other participants repeating the movements. The goal is to get group members to move in self-regulating ways and eventually become attuned to each other through movement. Trauma-sensitive yoga is another option (Chapter 7) that involves specific movements; breathing and relational dynamics between practitioner and participants emphasizes attunement as a self-regulatory experience. The overall goal of mirroring in the form of movement is to help individuals experience their bodies in a safe way as the basis for any additional self-regulating experiences.

One of the first things that I demonstrate to parent–child dyads working on attachment and co-regulation is mirroring through the simple kinesthetic/sensory activity involving joint scribble drawings. Both parent and child choose a felt marker or crayon, and each has the opportunity to be the leader in scribbling on a large piece of paper. In other words, the child may be the leader of the first drawing, and while he or she scribbles with a pen on the paper, the parent follows the child's lines at the same time with his or her pen. Sometimes we reverse roles and the parent becomes the leader of the scribble, with the child following or, in some situations, the therapist may be the leader or follower. While there may be interpersonal goals within this activity, it is also a way for the participants to mirror each other in a nonverbal way, to attune to the other's behavior and sensory, nonverbal cues, and to encourage a parent to develop ways to respond to the child. In coaching a parent to engage in this experience with a child, it is important to help the parent prepare the child for the activity. I often suggest to a mother, for example, that she make eye contact with her child, use a calming prosody and vocal cadence, and tell the child that they will be playing a game together with crayons on paper. I also may suggest that the mother make some sort physical contact with her child, such as giving a light touch on an arm or upper back and placing their chairs as close together as is comfortable for them at the table. I may model the activity with either the parent or child as co-scribbler, asking one of them to be the leader of the scribble drawing while I follow, or vice versa. A brief example follows.

CASE EXAMPLE. LEE ANN

Lee Ann, a 22-year-old mother, and her 6-year-old son, Jared, were survivors of years of interpersonal violence; Lee Ann experienced physical abuse from her family of origin and from other partners before she married Jared's father. Initially, Lee Ann was enthusiastic about mirroring Jared's scribbling across the paper, but she quickly became frustrated and angry when Jared was not able to follow her scribble and drew over her lines. She felt that Jared did this on purpose and that he was being "oppositional and defiant" (descriptors she learned from a school psychologist who previously evaluated Jared) in response to what she believed were the rules of the activity. In this case, I reframed the experience to help Lee Ann understand that Jared's marks were not necessarily marks of aggression toward her, but simply reflected the limited developmental motor skills of a young child who was also challenged by traumatic stress. I redirected the moment to a more trauma-informed perspective and suggested that perhaps Jared's marks were, in part, a positive action of "making contact with her mark-making during the scribble chase." I remarked that Lee Ann could say to Jared, "I feel really happy when our lines touch. My lines are happy when your lines touched mine in the picture."

The overall goal in this simple arts-based conversation on paper is not only to reinforce a positive relationship through tactile, visual, and kines-thetic senses, but also to enhance the parents' or caregivers' ability to initi-ate co-regulating responses with their children through mirroring as well as attunement. As a young mother who had experienced physical abuse and years of distress, Lee Ann understandably became upset when Jared responded in ways that reminded her of the violence and chaos she expe-rienced in her family of origin. In this case, both parent and child could benefit from sensory-based activities that involve mirroring and support positive attachment as forms of co-regulation that contribute to a founda-tion of self-regulation throughout the lifespan.

A similar approach that capitalizes on mirroring via simple arts-based activity is to introduce a "two-way conversation on paper." This two-way conversation can be presented in several ways, but most commonly two people are asked to simultaneously respond to each other's mark-making on paper nonverbally through drawing. This can involve mirroring each other's marks or simply drawing together on the same sheet of paper. I often introduce this approach to parents and children as well as couples who work in dyads on "conversations." As with the joint scribble drawings, be prepared to provide some additional coaching and third-hand interven-tion.

Entrainment

Entrainment, also called *rhythmic synchronization,* is another expressive arts approach that can support self-regulation, co-regulation, and shared regulation. Entrainment occurs when the rhythm of one experience syn-chronizes with the rhythm of another. For example, babies hear their first rhythm in utero listening to their mothers' heartbeats; the natural way to calm infants is to sway, rock, or pat them to the rhythm of a resting heart rate. In expressive arts therapy, heartbeat, motor activity, and brain activ-ity can fall into synchronous rhythms through the therapist's voice and through sensory experiences that match a resting heart rate (60 to 80 beats a minute), slow it down, or speed it up and energize individuals.

Perry (in Perry & Szalavitz, 2006) highlights the extraordinary impor-tance of rhythm in our lives, emphasizing that if our bodies cannot generate the most fundamental rhythm of life—the heartbeat—we cannot survive. He notes, "Our heart rate must increase to power fight or flight, for example, and it must maintain its rhythmic pulse despite varying demands placed on it. Regulating heart rate during stress and controlling stress hormones are two critical tasks that require that the brain keep proper time" (p. 142). Any variations in this essential rhythm impacts not only emotions and physical responses; they also effect relationships with others, putting stress on developing and maintaining positive attachment because entrainment is inevitably disrupted.

The previously described group movement experience involving mirroring has elements of entrainment; the facilitator can lead group members in synchronizing their movements for the purpose of self-regulation. While other arts-based approaches include aspects of entrainment, music and sound are most often used because rhythm is at the core. Musical entrainment is defined as a process of providing a musical rhythm at a different tempo from the personal tempo of the individual (Shultis & Gallagher, 2016). The person's rhythm, whether in the form of respiration or heartbeat, adjusts to the music automatically and unconsciously. There are also specific approaches such as music-assisted relaxation (MAR) to enhance physiological and psychological relaxation (Gardstrom & Sorel, 2016), which emphasizes that certain music experiences have a measurable calming effect that decreases agitation. In the field of music therapy, MAR is often combined with progressive muscle relaxation (tensing and releasing muscles throughout the body) or autonomic relaxation (passive focus on heart rate, breathing, or body temperature). Additionally, Moore (2013) observed that music listening and singing not only entrain, but actually help individuals shift away from activating memories. Similarly, a therapist's voice can be utilized to promote entrainment via tempo and rhythm, thus promoting self-regulation.

Music can be used as entrainment through its role as an auditory cue to enhance experiences of calm or of energy. Hyperactivation and dissociation impact how individuals "keep the beat" internally; one way to address this is to co-create playlists of music for a smartphone or other device, depending on individual needs. For example, Tanya tended toward dissociation and withdrawal, so we created playlists of music that would not only help to ground her when she "spaced out," but also entrain her to feel energized and positive. In contrast, Marian, who experienced panic reactions, benefited from a playlist that included gentle instrumental music with rhythms at the beat of a resting heart rate. In the case of both Tanya and Marian, it was also important to understand their personal and cultural experiences with music because of all the expressive arts, music is the one that most quickly stimulates emotional responses and past memories. Because each individual has had specific experiences with music, it is best to approach entrainment by finding out more about preferences, memories of music, and even what sound volume is soothing rather than agitating or unproductive.

Bilateral Movement

An arts-based approach that I use regularly with individuals of all ages involves various forms of bilateral movement. Simply put, it means using both sides of the body for dance/movement or drawing/painting. The sensory integration concepts I discussed with reference to safety (Chapter 5) are often associated with bilateral movements and are techniques found in occupational therapy to assist individuals in organizing specific sensations. In the process of reparation from psychological trauma, various forms of bilateral stimulation or movement are effective in engaging cross-hemisphere activity in the brain, and there is a growing body of research on EMDR (Shapiro, 2018) and similar methods. While there is no hard evidence for bilateral expressive arts approaches, I speculated that it may be effective for some of the same reasons (Malchiodi, 2003, 2012a) and may be complementary or "value-added" to approaches like EMDR (Urhausen, 2015).

I have used bilateral drawing for several decades as part of my expressive arts therapy sessions; I actually learned it during art courses as a way of "loosening up" before beginning to draw or paint. Florence Cane (1951) is one of many early artists and educators who observed an important connection between the free-form, kinesthetic qualities of gestural drawing on paper and the embodied qualities of the experience. In her work with children and adults in the mid-20th century, Cane hypothesized that it is important to engage individuals through movements that go beyond use of the hands to engage the whole body in natural rhythms. She referred to these experiences as "liberating exercises" and as necessary preparation for image making. In particular, she observed that the large swinging gestures that come from the shoulder, elbow, or wrist had a restorative capacity that supported healthy rhythms in the body and mind. Cane would encourage individuals to practice these rhythmic movements in the air and then later transfer them to paper with drawing materials. Bilateral drawing methods (McNamee, 2003, 2004) have also been used as forms of self-regulation in trauma-focused intervention and in combination with EMDR, although no standardized protocols or evidence-based research exists at this time.

Elbrecht (2018) has explored applications of bilateral drawing extensively for the last several decades, defining it as a *sensorimotor art therapy* approach to addressing trauma and as *guided drawing* (Figure 6.2). It was taught to Elbrecht by Mary Hippius, a psychologist and Jungian depth analyst. Elbrecht has brought the method into the 21st century by integrating concepts from Peter Levine's (2015) Somatic Experiencing®, Bessel van der Kolk's (2014) body-based approaches and Pat Ogden's (Ogden & Fisher,

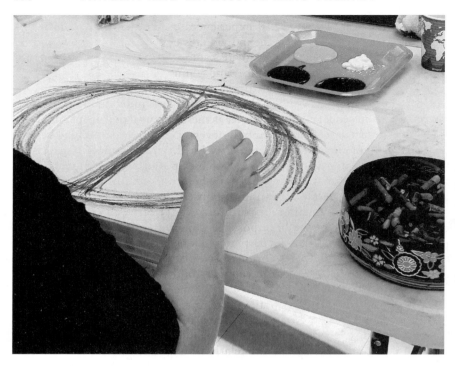

FIGURE 6.2. Participant engaged in guided drawing. From the collection of Cathy A. Malchiodi (not to be reproduced without permission from the author).

2015) Sensorimotor Psychotherapy. She underscores that this approach incorporates sensory awareness and concepts found in mindfulness practices. Because this method is helpful when focusing on the body's sensory-based experiences and its relevance to Somatic Experiencing (Levine, 2015) and Sensorimotor Psychotherapy (Ogden & Fisher, 2015), it is also discussed in more detail in the next chapter.

Bilateral drawing is particularly useful as a grounding technique because it is an active and generally nonthreatening experience for most individuals. In work with trauma reactions, it is particularly useful with those who are easily hyperactivated or susceptible to freeze responses. These individuals often need experiences that involve movement in order to reduce their anxiety and decrease sensations of feeling trapped, withdrawn, or dissociated. Making marks or gestures on paper with both hands can shift attention away from the distressing sensations in the body to a different, action-oriented, and self-empowered focus. It capitalizes on large muscle movements, body-based experiences observed by Cane to be self-soothing, and begins to alter the individual's own internal rhythms.

Elbrecht (2018), however, provides some insight into the complexities of using bilateral movements with some traumatized individuals who may need to initially build internal supports from the top-down (cognitive to sensory) and to develop trust in the psychotherapeutic relationship. According to Elbrecht, it sometimes is better if these individuals begin by creating "images of biographical or symbolic events; they may assemble collages or sculpt figures. This is more in line with their experiences of a session, and it is often necessary to build resources" (p. xxi). For example, I began with a top-down approach with Tanya before introducing bilateral work due to her frequent dissociation in response to environmental triggers and alternating hyperarousal in the form of severe anxiety. In particular, her need to remain hyperalert for possible danger made it impossible to get her to move much at all in our first sessions. I spent most of our initial sessions working on co-regulation through engaging her in some of the activities I was providing to the younger children at the facility—enjoying sandplay with miniatures; learning to trust me through my third-hand support during art-making activities; listening to me read from storybooks with gentle prosody; and engaging them in singing familiar rhymes and songs. In brief, Tanya and I needed to spend some time together to develop a predictable routine and a secure relationship before we proceeded to more action-oriented experiences.

When I was finally able to introduce the idea of bilateral movement, I simply asked Tanya to make gestures in the air and to pretend she was drawing on a large invisible piece of paper. I then invited her to transfer those marks and gestures onto a large paper with chalk and oil pastels (Figure 6.3). Plain brown wrapping paper is especially good not only because of its size and durability, but also because individuals can use white or light-colored chalk pastels. This simple art activity became a relaxing and self-regulating experience for Tanya at the beginning of each session. We experimented with several variations of the method, including using a "favorite color" and an "unfavorite color" to have a visual conversation with each other on large paper. In other sessions, I introduced playful suggestions such as draw "energized," "angry," "sad," "calm," and other mind–body states, asking Tanya to choose colored chalks in both hands to quickly sketch her sense of each emotion. If she felt stuck, she could simply draw in the air, moving her hands, wrists, shoulders, and then her entire body. I mirrored and moved with her, sometimes using music as an anchor for our mutual gestures. While this example reflects how I structured bilateral work with Tanya, I often begin most sessions with some sort of bilateral movement either in the form of drawing in the air and/or on paper in order to help individuals "loosen up" for other creative expression, including art making, movement, musical engagement, play, or dramatic enactment.

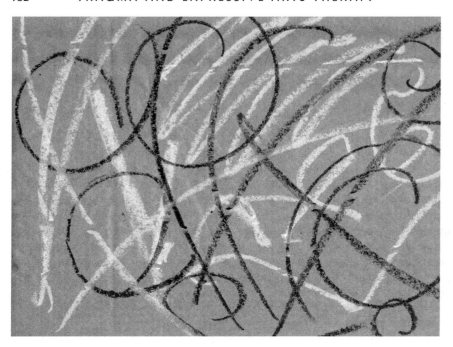

FIGURE 6.3. Transferring gestures and movements to brown paper. From the collection of Cathy A. Malchiodi (not to be reproduced without permission from the author).

In the residential setting where I met with Tanya, I did not have one important prop for bilateral drawing that I have in my clinic office—a long table painted with black chalkboard paint, which has a surface for drawing with colored chalks or pastels. My colleague, Elizabeth Warson, an EMDR practitioner and art therapist, introduced me to this idea, which she uses as a central part of her work with adolescents and adults (personal communication, November 2, 2017). This table is an inviting place to simply doodle on without the worry of making permanent marks because anything expressed on it can be easily erased with a chalkboard eraser or wiped away with a cloth. To encourage individuals like Tanya to engage in bilateral drawing, I can stand at one end of the table and demonstrate specific movements with chalk on the surface that the individual can mirror while watching me. This can also be a form of entrainment because I change the tempo and variety of lines I create in response to the individual's pace and capacity. The table legs can be folded inward, allowing the table to be placed against a wall for drawing while one is in a standing position. This stance is similar to what Cane originally envisioned as "liberating" for bilateral movement.

Relaxation and Mindfulness Practices

Relaxation

Relaxation protocols are popular strategies used to support self-regulation with individuals of all ages, particularly with those who experience post-trauma hyperactivation. There are numerous effective relaxation protocols such as progressive muscle relaxation and stress inoculation (Meichenbaum, 2004). Trauma experts have also developed various specific strategies that help people to decrease uncomfortable physiological reactions. For example, Levine (2015) proposes a series of simple postures to help one's body literally "slow down" when anxious or fearful. These postures involve various placements of hands on the head, heart, and stomach, along with rhythmic breathing.

The "four B's" (brake, breathe, brain, and body) are fairly common techniques that I learned from occupational therapists who use these practices to address sensory integration by inducing relaxation in some way. These systematic calming methods can be used to help both children and adults to self-regulate and regain a sense of self-control. These techniques are largely movement-based and body-oriented. In conjunction with these approaches, I also often ask individuals to "show me through colors, lines, shapes, or mark-making" what the felt (body) sense of the experience is for them. The drawing then serves as a visual anchor that can be used as an additional reminder of each practice and as a resource. Each exercise is designed to help individuals begin to sense what is going on in their bodies, redirect attention, and facilitate a relationship toward the self that is caring, gentle, and nurturing. It is also important to capitalize on attunement, mirroring, and entrainment by modeling and doing these exercises with individuals.

1. *Brake.* When an individual feels out of control, anxious, fearful, or even terrorized, it is important to learn ways to "brake" as one would do to slow down an automobile. Rothschild (2000) uses the term *putting on the brakes* to describe an important practice that helps to keep the hyperarousal at a manageable level. From a sensory integration perspective, "putting the brakes on" decreases excess energy and helps release muscle tension. To accomplish this, a simple movement of pressing the palms of the hands together in front of the chest for 5–10 seconds is often effective. Many individuals need to repeat this movement several times to really engage the muscles in the arms and shoulders.

2. *Breathe.* Similar to mindfulness practices (discussed in the next section in more detail), learning to breathe properly helps a person to regain a sense of body awareness and restore a sense of calm and helps to stabilize and ground the body. Most individuals can begin to learn proper breathing by placing both hands on the abdomen or one hand on the abdomen and

one over the heart. Another common prompt that sometimes helps is to follow a breathing chart with one's finger while breathing; this orients the individual to breathing in and out through tracing the sides of a drawing of a five-pointed star, a figure eight, or a square (four sides) (see Appendix 4). For those individuals who are extremely anxious, the chart is a visual anchor for the breath.

3. *Brain.* To create a sense of both alertness and calm, I ask individuals to place their hands on top of their heads and press with a light pressure. This not only calms the body, but also activates the brain. It is particularly useful for individuals who dissociate or withdraw during a session by gently bringing them back into the here and now.

4. *Body.* Because self-regulation and a sense of safety are so closely related, a self-hug (crossing arms in front of the body) with gentle pressure may help some individuals. The sensation of squeezing pressure on the arms and shoulders not only increases body awareness, it also increases a sense of security, calm, and focus (this is effective for both hyperarousal and dissociation). With children, including a soft toy as part of the hug experience is also helpful. Levine (2015) uses a similar approach, explaining it as tapping the sense of being "contained" because the body is essentially the container of all sensations and feelings. In other words, once people can actually feel the container (their bodies), any hyperactivation does not feel as overwhelming. An additional variation that many people find self-soothing and deactivating involves placing the left hand on the head and the right hand on the heart area, focusing on any sensations of energy and temperature change, and observing any energy flow between the hands (Levine, 2010).

Mindfulness

Mindfulness is now a well-known practice that has a long tradition within many cultures; it generally involves the experience of silence described in the four-part model in Chapter 2. Historically, it is rooted in spiritual meditation that is quite different from the current secular psychotherapeutic applications of mindfulness. In contrast, neuroscience and psychology view mindfulness as a method that can self-regulate the brain and body; increase self-management physically, emotionally, and cognitively; evoke the relaxation response; and decrease stress responses (Kabat-Zinn, 2013). Its wide-ranging benefits include lowered blood pressure, reduced inflammation, slower breathing rate and respiration, and greater immune system response. It has also been shown to increase the brain's gray matter, which is involved in memory, attention, emotional regulation, and other functions (Hölzel et al., 2011). Rothschild (2010) recommends mindfulness as one possible strategy for trauma recovery because it helps some individuals become more aware of somatic sensations, feelings, and thoughts as sources that both cause stress and create calm. It is also increasingly combined with expressive arts therapy approaches (Rappaport, 2015) to focus awareness on the present moment, while acknowledging and nonjudgmentally accepting feelings, thoughts, and body sensations.

Although applications of mindfulness are pervasive among various forms of psychotherapy, there are challenges in introducing it to many traumatized individuals (Treleaven, 2018). While the "here-and-now" is relevant, reducing hyperactivation triggered by thinking about the past or worrying about the future, some forms of mindfulness can create increased arousal. Many years ago, I had a personal experience of dysregulation during a mindfulness activity presented in a social work course on complementary and alternative approaches to stress reduction. The instructor introduced a standard protocol, asking participants to close their eyes, keep both feet on the floor, and maintain good posture. This seemed innocuous enough to me, and so I complied. However, when he asked us to begin taking deep and regular breaths and empty our minds, I immediately started to feel an uncomfortable change in my chest. A sense of panic swiftly followed, my eyes bolted open, and I lurched forward in my chair. The instructor noticed my response but did not halt the protocol; nor did he address my obvious discomfort. I stubbornly continued with the activity under duress; as soon the break came, I ran out of the classroom to escape whatever was causing severe dysregulation and wondered why I had not achieved the peace and calm that was promised as a result of being mindful.

Because my reaction was so dramatic, I followed up on the experience, engaging in several sessions with a psychotherapist to see if I could learn more about the origin of my panic and what triggered it. From what we could tell, during the deep breathing I was flooded with imagery from a particularly difficult session with a client who disclosed how he was held hostage as a child and repeatedly beaten by a family member. That story also reminded me of an event I never quite recovered from during my childhood—hearing a cousin being beaten with a belt by my uncle while I was forced to sit and remain silent in the room next door. Those two memories (the client's disclosure and my inability to prevent my cousin's beating) somehow became connected; my memory of my cousin's abuse was unresolved and apparently resurfaced during the process of mindful breathing. Once I became aware of this connection and addressed my traumatic memory, I was able to engage in the form of mindfulness the instructor presented without panic or distressful images. I also realized that asking traumatized clients to suddenly become mindful without some additional supports could leave them extremely agitated or even cause a relapse into an intensely traumatized state.

Within her framework for dialectical behavior therapy (DBT), Linehan (2014) explained the need for an anchor when introducing mindfulness practices to individuals who do not respond well to following their breath or other body-based sensations that arise when focusing inward. Some forms of breathing do include an identifiable anchor (following the rise and fall of the abdomen or the sensation of breathing in the throat or chest), but they are still far from a neutral experience for many traumatized individuals and do not provide the necessary grounding that Linehan cites. To address this problem and enhance mindfulness as a self-regulatory practice, integrating an anchor within the experience supports the nervous system while decreasing dysregulation. Some individuals may only need to focus on feeling their feet on the floor or holding a weighted stuffed animal or object to feel grounded and anchored. But by making the anchor more sensory and tangible, it is easier for many individuals to return to it when they are distracted.

"Drawing the breath" is a common exercise that combines mindfulness practice with art making for the purpose of awareness, self-regulation, and grounding. Initially, I often invite individuals to try a short period of rhythmic breathing and relaxation (with eyes open or closed) and ask them to observe their breathing with friendly, nonjudgmental awareness, noticing how slow, deep breaths move in and out of the body. Those who find this short exercise difficult have the option of moving to the next part, which involves using drawing as a sensory-based anchor. On a large sheet of paper, I then invite people to use drawing materials (chalk or soft oil pastels) to simply "make marks" that represent the movements of the breath as it goes in and out of the body (Figure 6.4). For some individuals, suggesting specific rhythmic shapes is helpful (clockwise circles and counterclockwise circles or a bow shape). This can involve bilateral mark-making similar to the bilateral drawing described in the previous section. Another variation does not involve drawing at all but rather simply repetitive arm movements, slowly swinging one or both arms up and down, right to left, and in broad circles clockwise and counterclockwise. Whatever sensory experience is used as an anchor for breathing, the goal is to help the individual inhabit their bodies in a neutral or positive way, while breathing rhythmically in order to support self-regulation.

While most of the literature and research on mindfulness has focused on adults, there is a growing body of knowledge that supports its application to children and adolescents for self-regulation and decreased stress responses as well as an overall sense of psychological wellness (Huppert & Johnson, 2010). With some adaptation and inclusion of anchors to support safety, mindfulness can be an important part of self-regulation for traumatized children. Visual metaphors and symbols embedded within any mindfulness practice are one key strategy. For example, while learning deep breathing strategies to relax the body, children can be asked to imagine "breathing a cloud." Willard (2010) offers this adaptation for relaxation, imagination, and mindful awareness: "Pick out a cloud; you may want to start with a small one. Focus on that cloud and just breathe into that cloud. With each breath, watch and see that cloud change shape or start to get

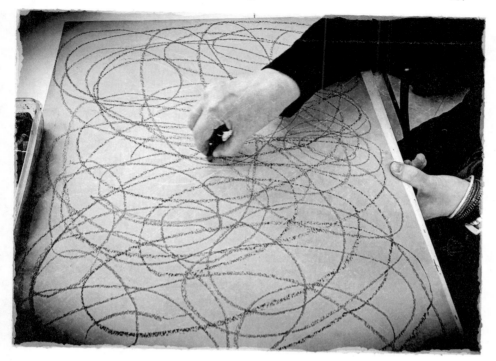

FIGURE 6.4. Drawing "breath."

smaller or larger. If your mind wanders, just try to bring your attention back to the cloud. Just remain focused on the cloud, watching and breathing until it gradually fades away" (p. 36).

Willard's suggested imagery is often effective, but introducing a sensory-based, tangible experience can be much more effective for some children. When using the metaphor of the cloud as the anchor, I invite children to create their own tactile clouds with cotton, soft wool, or fake fur adhered to a small piece of cardstock. Before we do any breathing exercises or visualizations, we spend some time noticing what these "clouds" feel like and describe these sensations and where we feel them in our bodies. One other effective strategy involves creating a "mindfulness jar," a glass jar filled with water and glitter in it that a child and I co-create. When the jar is shaken, it shows the child (or adult for that matter) what an agitated mind might look like (glue the lid to the jar to prevent any of the contents of an "agitated mind" from accidentally leaking). Taking deep breaths while watching the jar's contents settle slows down the mind and body. Children learn that as the glittery contents of the mindfulness jar eventually settle, they too will feel less agitated. In brief, the mindfulness jar provides not only an anchoring object, but also a visual form of entrainment in addition to providing an easily understood example of both agitation and eventual calm.

Affect Regulation

I use many of the same methods in this chapter to release my own stress, provide self-regulatory experiences, and soothe my own brain and body. But in particular, I have used these approaches to support affect regulation and, in particular, to produce a more positive mood. I have some very simple ways to "feel better" and less distressed through implicit memories. For example, in my office I have a favorite coffee mug from Café Du Monde, a famous New Orleans landmark that serves delicious coffee and beignets—deep-fried pastries with powdered sugar on top. Every time I have a cup of coffee in that mug I almost immediately recall the spring-like weather, a pleasant light rain, the smell of the beignets, and the good friends who were there at the café on that morning. In my mind, I see the shops in the French Quarter, the open market, and the horse-drawn carriages making their way down the street; my body immediately feels relaxed and joyful. Despite any challenges I am facing in the moment, it is one of many sensory memories I can call upon to change my mood to positive. It is one experience that I can rely on to increase a feeling of joy throughout my body, both by seeing or imagining the coffee mug and the sights, sounds, smells, and tastes associated with it. In other words, it is a resource that can help one redirect focus to more pleasurable sensations when distressed or activated.

While it is easy for some individuals to recall a positive sensory memory that can self-soothe and calm them in the moment, it is not so straightforward for most traumatized individuals. Trauma inhabits the body in ways that not only dysregulate, but also often strip people of the ability to recall a pleasurable event or to access the necessary imagination to experience enjoyment. During decades of work with children who experienced developmental trauma, I saw how repeated traumatic stress, internalized shame and guilt, and disrupted attachment with caregivers robbed these children of the ability to feel joy and pleasure. Helping individuals regain their body's memories of positivity is a key part of all self-regulation, but for those who have experienced multiple traumatic events, developmental trauma, or repeated exposure to interpersonal violence, this can be a pretty challenging, though not an impossible outcome. This is where talk therapy and even many of the body-based approaches that reduce the impact of traumatic stress are limited in comparison to expressive arts. As described in Chapter 1, the expressive arts may elevate mood because of their tendency to help us experience the subjective feeling of "aliveness." The sensation that one is living life with vitality, joy, and connectedness are key factors that support our internal sense of positivity.

Neuroscience provides some emerging explanations for why engaging in the arts increases a sense of positivity and improves mood. For example, neuroscience researcher Kelly Lambert (2010), by simply creating meaningful objects with one's hands, can alter mood because handwork actually mediates anxiety and depression. Lambert specifically looked at the "accumbens–striatal–cortical network," a system in the brain that connects movement, emotion, and thinking and could be an underlying source of symptoms associated with mood disorders. These areas account for slow responses (accumbens), perceived loss of pleasure (striatum), and negative feelings (limbic system) and form what Lambert defines as the "effort-driven rewards system." A well-engaged effort-driven rewards circuit, however, seems to help individuals meet emotional challenges, thus ameliorating depression and anxiety to some extent. Lambert specifically cites repetitive activities such as knitting and tending a garden as effort-driven reward-giving activities, but "making things" of any kind that involve a hands-on investment in creating objects that give pleasure may have a similar impact.

The expressive arts may also mediate depression and anxiety as a result of the experience of creative "flow" (Csikszentmihalyi, 2014) that results from engagement in activities that are absorbing and somewhat challenging. Common terms for flow are being "in the zone" or "in the groove." This sense of flow is achieved when completely absorbed or immersed in an activity. Similarly, flow naturally decreases the perception of hyperactivation or stress. Flow is often referred to as a natural form of mindfulness, but it is actually a different state of being. But like mindfulness, it is often an experience of inner quiet that induces a sense of well-being.

There is a growing body of data on various expressive arts approaches that under certain conditions increase a sense of positivity and general well-being. Music therapy has a long history of applications of music and sound to support positive mood and regulate affect (Ghetti & Whitehead-Pleaux, 2015; Pelletier, 2004; Schafer, Sedlmeier, Städtler, & Huron, 2013). Dance/movement therapy also is successfully applied to support self-regulation and reduce stress (Brauninger, 2012), as do many body-based, movement-oriented approaches, including yoga (Woodyard, 2011). Similarly, specific art-making directives indicate that at least short-term "mood repair" is possible. Dalebroux, Goldstein, and Winner (2008) conducted a study to evaluate art expression as a form of short-term mood repair. After viewing a film that induced a negative mood, participants engaged in one of three tasks: (1) creating a drawing expressing their current mood (venting), (2) creating a drawing depicting something happy (positive emotion), or (3) scanning a sheet for specific symbols (distraction control). The greatest improvement occurred after creating a drawing depicting something happy, possibly because it redirected feelings or served as a form of catharsis. Similarly, Drake and Hodge (2015) compared drawing and writing activities, finding that drawing is more effective in "mood repair" than writing, although both activities improve mood through distraction more than by venting about feelings. Finally, Diliberto-Macaluso and Stubblefield (2015) conducted a study that concluded that painting a theme that the art maker defined as "happy" following an angry mood resulted in a positive impact on one's emotional state. The results indicate that art making may help mediate mood through sensitively redirecting creative expression toward positive rather than negative mind states.

Journaling is a fairly simple practice that therapists can introduce to trauma survivors of all ages to support positive mood. A visual journal (also called an artist's journal or art journaling) is a book of unlined pages used to regularly record images (drawings or collages) and written text in any combination. There is anecdotal support for visual journaling as a form of emotional release and insight, but the emerging research indicates that it may have physiological results, including stress reduction and self-regulation. Mercer, Warson, and Zhao (2010) demonstrate a decrease in anxiety levels and negative affect. Other studies with adults support physiological results from regular visual journaling, particularly in the areas of immune function and cortisol reduction (Warson, 2013; Warson & Lorance, 2013).

Writing, even if consisting of only a few words, phrases, or sentences, can also be an important part of the process, for expressive writing is a way to decrease stress and increase a sense of well-being. Pennebaker and Chung (2011) observe that, while not all studies of expressive writing support an increase in positive mood, overall writing about emotional topics is associated with significant reductions in distress. They note that a comparison of a group of students who used bodily movement to express a traumatic expressive and another group who used movement followed by writing about a traumatic experience showed that the latter group had significant improvement in physical health and grade point average. In this case, it seems that kinesthetic/sensory expression (movement) of trauma is not sufficient and that cognitive (language) expression is required to show improvement. While regular visual expression through journaling may increase positive mood and decrease stress in the short term, it is also possible that adding writing to the activity has additional, long-term benefits.

APPLYING EXPRESSIVE ARTS AS REGULATORY PRACTICES

Two case examples illustrate some of the many self-regulatory expressive arts applications and strategies. The first brief example describes a child and parent who have experienced an acute trauma and discusses the role of both individual and dyadic regulatory strategies. The second example underscores how self-regulation can be introduced within a group setting involving disaster relief.

Applying Expressive Arts as Regulation in Acute Trauma with a Child and Parent

In my work in hospitals and clinics, I generally see pediatric patients who have experienced accidents and, as a result, have short-term traumatic stress reactions. I also see their parents who are dysregulated because of what has happened to their child and who are often in need of some self-regulatory skills. In most cases, both caregiver and child can benefit from learning co-regulatory approaches that they can practice after leaving the hospital or outpatient clinic. The following example emphasizes not only how a child and parent can benefit from some simple self-regulation, but also why it is beneficial to do some psychoeducation on arts and play activities so the parent can continue to enhance co-regulation at home.

Case Example. Caroline and Marie

Eight-year-old Caroline and her mother, Marie, survived an acute trauma as a result of a car accident during which Caroline sustained injuries, putting her in the hospital for several weeks for fractures and abrasions. Marie, who was driving the car, only suffered minor abrasions that were treated in the emergency room. The accident occurred as the result of another driver looking away from the road while sending a cell phone text message. Because the accident occurred in a rural area, the nearest hospital was 10 miles away, making the experience of getting medical help frightening for both mother and child.

I first met with Caroline and Marie at the hospital while Caroline was an inpatient. Because of the nature of her injuries and her medical treatment, Caroline had to remain in a stationary position, propped up by pillows and partially restrained in a halo (a device used to hold the head in a certain position). At our first meeting, she was obviously uncomfortable because of the restraints and her inability to move freely. Caroline was also understandably fearful of the many medical procedures she was subjected to, even though she understood that the doctors and nurses were trying to help her recover. In my first meeting with Caroline at the hospital, I quickly realized that multiple medical procedures and the restraints were compounding her distress. Caroline responded to her situation by remaining quiet and noticeably withdrawn rather than complaining or asking for assistance. Marie reported that before the accident and hospitalization her daughter tended to be "shy" and withdrawn and did not seek out support or help from other adults, including Marie. I respected Caroline's choice not to talk as her strategy for coping with an abnormal and frightening situation. I allowed her to use toys and props to externalize her thoughts and feelings rather than to communicate directly about her feelings and experiences. When I asked Marie how Caroline expressed her feelings when distressed, she reported that Caroline often perseverated, retreating to her room and ruminating without relief rather than speaking about her feelings to her mother.

During the first week of Caroline's hospitalization, I had the opportunity to meet with Marie separately on two occasions. She was visibly anxious and disclosed that she often felt panicked, did not sleep well since the incident, and cried almost every day. In part, she was upset by Caroline's hospitalization, but she also confided that she felt somewhat responsible for what happened. She repeatedly observed, "If I had only been watching more carefully I would have been able to avoid that car. Caroline could have been killed." Marie was clearly having repetitive negative thoughts in response to the stress of the incident, reinforcing her own hyperarousal. She also explained to me that she had divorced Caroline's father several years earlier, and being the only parent was difficult because she had sole responsibility for Caroline's care and because of the financial worries that had arisen since she could not work during her daughter's recovery.

A primary goal of expressive arts therapy with hospitalized children like Caroline is to provide ways to help them decrease their distress and frustration and to increase their sense of calm and control (Malchiodi, 2015a). While many issues were involved in addressing Caroline's psychosocial needs, Marie herself was also obviously in need of some support to self-soothe and reduce stress. I also wanted to help Caroline and Marie learn (self-efficacy) regulation strategies that they could practice together (co-regulation) at home after the inpatient stay ended.

Since Caroline was the identified patient, I initially taught her some child-friendly ways to use breathing to calm herself when she felt upset. We practiced mindful breathing "like a sleeping bear," "hissing like a snake," and "roaring like a lion" from *Yoga Pretzels* (Guber, 2005), a colorful set of cards with yoga and mindfulness strategies for children. On other occasions, we simply blew soap bubbles and self-created a pinwheel that she could move with extended exhales (Porges, 2010). Because Caroline tended to withdraw (freeze) when stressed, I also devised ways to get her moving as much as she could within the restrictions of her bed. She had just seen the movie *The Wizard of Oz,* and so I used the characters as a way to help her practice progressive muscle relaxation by "holding your muscles tight, tight, tight like the Tin Man," and "letting your muscles relax like the Scarecrow." If possible, it is helpful to learn what books or media children are familiar with; not only can they become potential sources for breathing, movement, or creative relaxation strategies, but also they are more meaningful to young patients.

When I was able to spend time with Marie, I explained each of the activities I presented to Caroline, and as I do for the parents of most patients, I invited her to join the sessions. Marie was sincerely interested in learning more about what I was doing with Caroline and why. I therefore explained a little bit about co-regulation and why it would be helpful for Marie to be able to continue what Caroline was practicing with me when she left the hospital. Of course, I was also thinking that Marie could benefit from some self-soothing and regulation herself.

Because Caroline was still limited to her bed for much of the time, listening to music and drawing were some of the only options at this stage. I suggested that Caroline and Marie co-create a playlist of songs that they found self-soothing. Such a playlist is not always possible, but fortunately, this hospital provided digital tablets to each child in the pediatric unit. The playlist of songs that Marie and Caroline co-created with my help became the musical anchor used to support a sense of calm and focus while engaging parent and child in expressive arts and play experiences. I also introduced an easy drawing activity that I frequently use with parent–child dyads. It involves using felt marking pens to create an overlapping tracing of the parent's and child's hands on one sheet of paper and filling in the lines and shapes in any way they enjoy (Figure 6.5). To make this activity less stressful, I provide a "cheat sheet" of various types of doodle designs that the child and parent can use for ideas. My goal in this simple activity is not only to provide a co-regulatory experience through relaxing doodling, but also to create what is a symbolic gesture of connectedness in overlapping hands. During the process, I also had time to educate Marie on the drawing media that I use in expressive arts therapy with children at bedside so that she could feel confident in using them with Caroline between sessions.

To help Marie with her intrusive thoughts and to reduce Caroline's hyperarousal, I introduced an expressive arts variation of the concept of "thought catching" (Seligman, 2007). I adapted this process for Caroline and her mother by using a gingerbread figure (Figure 6.6), asking them to imagine reaching to "catch their worry thoughts" and to show me through mark-making and colors, shapes, and/or lines "where the worry you caught is in your body and what it looks like." It was fairly easy to help Marie identify thoughts that led to negative feelings and stress reactions, and she immediately made the connection between negative thinking and how it affected her sense of well-being. While this activity can be used for other objectives, it is one way to not only "catch" negative thinking before it causes stress, but also help individuals begin to understand where they feel stress in their bodies (Chapter 7). Because it was important for Caroline to learn how to communicate her feelings to Marie, Marie began to use this strategy to "check in" with Caroline when the hospitalization ended. Marie also used the strategy to continue her own process of identifying dysregulating sensations and thoughts, understanding that her own self-regulation was important to supporting healthy co-regulation with Caroline.

Post-Disaster Self-Regulation with Families

Working with survivors of natural and human-made disasters is challenging in many ways. Because each situation is different in terms of events and contexts, reactions are complicated and diverse owing to the unique

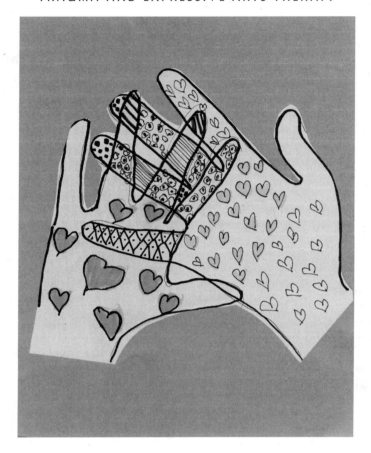

FIGURE 6.5. Overlapping hands by Caroline and Marie. From the collection of Cathy A. Malchiodi (not to be reproduced without permission from the author).

events involved in any mass disaster. For example, helping professionals who responded to the shooting of elementary school children and school personnel in 2013 in Newtown, Connecticut, involved a uniquely tragic situation (Loumeau-May et al., 2015). In cases of natural disasters, such as tornadoes, hurricanes, tsunamis, floods, or earthquakes, survivors have lost property and belongings as well as entire communities and their resources (hospitals, schools, businesses, and places of worship or congregation). They are confronted with the long-term process of rebuilding and reestablishing life in communities where they may have lived since childhood.

As a result of the terrorist attacks of September 11, 2001, in the United States, we have learned a good deal about providing disaster relief. In

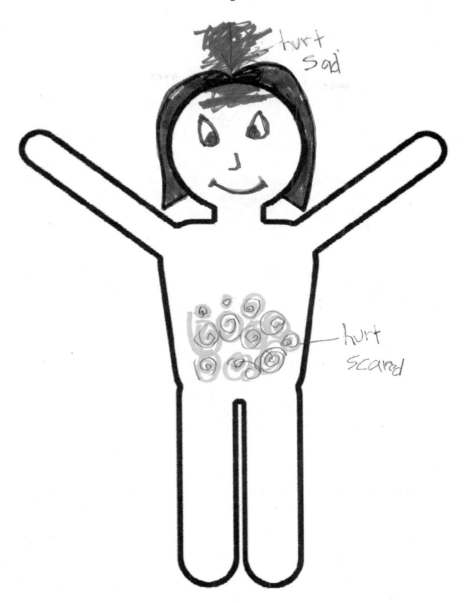

FIGURE 6.6. Catching thoughts on a gingerbread figure. From the collection of Cathy A. Malchiodi(not to be reproduced without permission from the artist).

particular, involving those impacted in their own relief efforts is now rec- ognized as a source of recovery as well as resilience.

Counseling and psychotherapy are generally not part of psychological first aid efforts in the immediate aftermath of disaster. However, children, adults, and families need self-regulatory, co-regulatory, and particularly shared regulatory experiences in most cases. In brief, many individuals are continually retraumatized in the days and weeks after the event by media reports and disrupted by prolonged evacuation, having abandoned what was once home without clothing or money.

During my many years of being sent by various relief organizations to address the needs of those who survived a natural or human-made disaster, I have found the following principles helpful. They capitalize on sensory- based experiences to soothe body and mind after a large-scale traumatic event (Malchiodi, 2012d) and, if appropriate, they can be adapted to expressive arts strategies.

1. *Attunement.* Attunement is an important practice used in the aftermath of a traumatic event. It is much more effective to establish attunement than to delve into feelings. This practice includes simple ges- tures of assistance ("Can I help you find your family?" "May I stay with you in case you need something?"), maintaining good eye contact, and providing undivided attention and affirmation (nodding and other physi- cal cues). If touch is involved, the safest place to invite it is through a handshake or a light touch on the lower arm; these are the areas of the body that are least prone to alarm when touched by another individual. In all cases, even if the individual or group does not seem to be respond- ing to your gestures, your responses will be perceived, remembered, and appreciated later on.

2. *Sensory safety.* Psychological trauma produces a "felt sense" of fear, confusion, and worry in many survivors and is a somatic sensation rather than a strictly cognitive experience. Comfort food, a cuddly toy or blanket, and even a glass of water helps to slow down the body's hyperac- tivation of rapid breathing or heart rate through soothing sensory-based experiences. For this reason, therapy dogs are now commonplace as post- disaster first responders, along with trained animal-assisted therapy profes- sionals, because their presence and interaction with survivors can quickly decrease stress responses.

3. *Here-and-now focus.* Although survivors feel frightened, angry, or anxious about what has happened, it is important to reinforce that they are safe right now in this moment. Even if there is still the possibility of additional distress, helping individuals to "be here now" begins to reduce hyperarousal. For example, helping professionals can ask, "What can you do to give your mind and body a rest right now?"

4. *Connection.* Survivors' connection with others within a community impacted by disaster is important. This connection may include social support given and received by others or for some individuals, becoming active in comforting others. In other words, providing opportunities for survivors to become connected to others in ways that reinforce self-efficacy can reduce distress and enhance self-regulation. Supporting the concept of healing-centered engagement (Chapter 2) is crucial, emphasizing that assistance takes place within the community through the enlistment of community members in actual relief efforts.

5. *Cultural sensitivity.* Trauma-informed practice emphasizes that intervention is not a one-size-fits-all operation. It includes identifying and honoring cultural preferences for assistance. This is particularly important in disaster relief because communities often have specific healing practices, including arts-based practices, that are soothing and reparative in times of trauma and loss.

Shared Regulation after Disaster

A few years ago, a deadly tornado occurred over a large area of the southern United States and resulted in over 40 tornado-related fatalities. The storms began in the morning and continued throughout the day, creating damaging winds and tornadoes that destroyed hundreds of homes in its path. Several rural towns were among those most impacted, with numerous deaths due to intermittent tornado touchdowns and extensive damage to numerous houses, businesses, and mobile homes (trailers with no foundations or basements). As the storm approached these towns, property was swept miles away; some personal property, still largely intact, was recovered by individuals living over 100 miles away. At the time of the event, a school was in the process of dismissing students; many of the students could not leave the school and stayed there as it was destroyed around them. Fortunately, all survived without major injury. However, many other residents of the area were not so lucky; they sustained multiple injuries in addition to loss of personal property and, in some cases, loss of family members and friends.

As with most disaster relief assignments, I usually am asked to meet with families or small groups of individuals in shelter settings, generally within the first 2 or 3 weeks of the event. In this case, I met with several families who were referred for crisis intervention at a local community center in the midst of the areas most affected by the storms. Because 2 weeks had passed since the event, initial shock over what had happened had dissipated, but both children and parents complained of anxiety and sleeplessness and expressed generalized fears about both the disaster and what the future held for them. They had to rebuild their lives, having lost almost everything during the storm. But despite their losses, they were all quick to point out that they were the lucky ones because they knew the families who lost loved ones or sustained serious injuries.

In addition to asking questions that focus on basic needs and ways to practice self-care, I also specifically wanted to learn what types of "healing arts" individuals and families had used in the past to help them through crisis, grief, and loss. As explained in Chapter 2, these healing arts might include songs or music, prayers or chanting, storytelling, movement, or other ways of self-soothing. Because this particular group attended the same Christian-based church, they were easily able to identify prayers and songs that comforted them in the past. Both prayers and songs are not only meaning-making experiences within specific cultures and communities, they are also activities that have the potential to self-regulate participants. Prayer, for example, is often based on rhythmic repetition of words and phrases that reinforce comforting, recognized beliefs. Some prayers—such as the Lord's Prayer, which is well known to all participants—are also self-soothing in cadence and inflection. When I do not know a particular prayer or chant that a community uses, I ask everyone to teach me (self-efficacy), and we all say it together, giving me the opportunity to become attuned to the group as well as reinforcing connection among the individuals present. The families knew several songs, most of which were church-related, that we sang together. Singing familiar songs together not only is important in establishing connection and mutual support; singing has the natural benefit of helping people breathe more deeply and fully. It is a simple, yet culturally resonant, way to introduce self-regulation into a session.

In a subsequent session, I introduced an expressive arts activity that I often use with families and groups for the purpose of self-regulation and connection. I call it the "Group Tangle Doodle" and it requires minimal skill from participants. "Tangle doodle" is another name for patterns and designs created on paper with felt pens or markers, such as the easily available Sharpies®. Families particularly enjoy it because everyone, including children, can contribute to the process. Each group uses a large piece of white drawing paper (18" × 24") on which one or several members draw a simple scribble with black felt pen. They then cut the paper into pieces, one piece for each member of the family. Next, I ask everyone to trace their hand on their section of the paper; children can trace more than one hand on the paper to fill up the space. The families are then asked to "tangle doodle" with felt pens in various colors in the spaces created by the scribbled lines on their sections (Figure 6.7); I provide doodle examples (readily available as clip art on the Internet), so that everyone can try different patterns or devise their own. Because survivors of disasters are often overwhelmed or distracted, I also offer support as needed and serve as a "third hand" in showing simple ways to use the materials, motivating participation when needed, and commenting on progress.

With some groups, it can be helpful to play instrumental music at a low volume; music at around 70 beats per minute is a good rhythm, mimicking

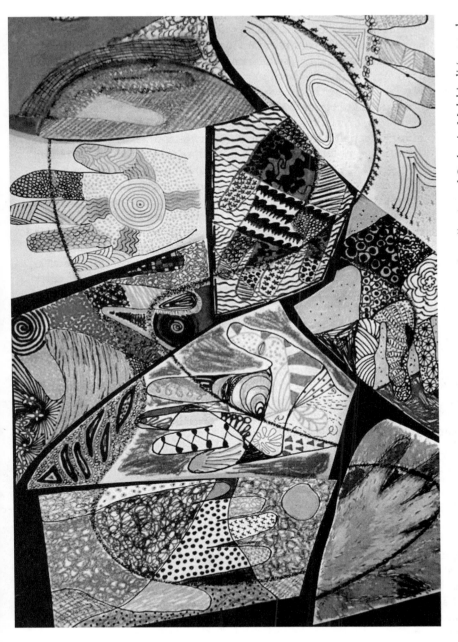

FIGURE 6.7. Group mural created from "tangle doodling." From the collection of Cathy A. Malchiodi (not to be reproduced without permission from the author).

a resting heart rate. Depending on the group, I may play some soothing percussion on what is called a "chakra drum," a small metal instrument that is used for meditation and relaxation because of the sounds it generates. With this particular group, I used my iPad connected to a stereo speaker and played one of many short, soothing playlists I use with groups that lasts approximately 20 minutes, the amount of time needed for most people to begin to relax, breathe more slowly, and decrease their heart rate. I also may ask the groups to try drawing without talking to each and to just focus on their doodling or mark-making. The overall goal is to create a relaxing, self-soothing experience of doodling in order to help participants reach a state of creative flow and engagement in the process. When the doodling part of the activity has ended, the puzzle parts are put back together to assemble a visual representation of connection. The families in this particular group enjoyed taking a "gallery walk" around the room to see other families' drawings and share impressions of each other's creative work.

Because this group was limited to only a few sessions, the focus remained on self-regulation and stabilization. The families learned several self-regulating practices they could use on their own, including self-soothing rituals they already knew (prayer and familiar songs). Two years later I was fortunate to again meet parents from two different families from the group at a local outpatient clinic. When asked, "What did you remember most from the meetings we had after the tornado?," they quickly agreed that it was "singing hymns together" and "that big doodle we did." The singing not only helped anchor them in the moment, but also supported a meaningful sense of connecting with a "higher power" and in doing so, gave them hope. The "big doodle" helped the families remember that they still could have fun together, despite what happened and the losses they endured. While "drawing those doodles," they at least momentarily escaped the stress of the events during that time.

CONCLUSION

Self-regulation is an ability that is optimally learned early in life and is built on a foundation of interactive regulation. For various reasons, traumatized individuals lose the capacity to regulate. In cases of early trauma and disrupted attachment, they may never have adequately developed it, nor have they experienced the social engagement necessary to co-regulate with others. Expressive arts provide a set of uniquely multilayered approaches to enhancing self-regulatory abilities through the sensory-based nature and relational qualities of arts-based experiences. Along with supporting safety, helping individuals develop creative regulatory practices is an essential foundation for conducting deeper work with trauma. These two components are key in introducing the next area essential to trauma reparation—the body's memory and reactions to distress, the subject of the next chapter.

APPENDIX 6.1. Instructions for Tadasana Pose

1. Stand with your feet together and your arms at your sides. Press your weight evenly across the balls and arches of your feet. Breathe steadily and rhythmically. Draw your awareness inward. Focus on the present moment, letting all worries and concerns fade away.

2. Press your big toes together (separate your heels if you need to). Lift your toes and spread them apart. Then, place them back down on the mat, one at a time.

3. If you have trouble balancing, stand with your feet 6 inches apart (or wider).

4. Draw down through your heels and straighten your legs. Ground your feet firmly into the earth, pressing evenly across all four corners of both feet.

5. Then, lift your ankles and the arches of your feet. Squeeze your outer shins toward each other.

6. Draw the top of your thighs up and back, engaging the quadriceps. Rotate your thighs slightly inward, widening your sit bones.

7. Tuck in your tailbone slightly, but don't round your lower back. Lift the back of your thighs, but release your buttocks. Keep your hips even with the center line of your body.

8. Bring your pelvis to its neutral position. Do not let your front hip bones point down or up; instead, point them straight forward. Draw your belly in slightly.

9. As you inhale, elongate through your torso. Exhale and release your shoulder blades away from your head, toward the back of your waist.

10. Broaden across your collarbones, keeping your shoulders in line with the sides of your body.

11. Press your shoulder blades toward the back ribs, but don't squeeze them together. Keep your arms straight, fingers extended, and triceps firm. Allow your inner arms to rotate slightly outward.

12. Elongate your neck. Your ears, shoulders, hips, and ankles should all be in one line.

13. Keep your breathing smooth and even. With each exhalation, feel your spine elongating. Softly gaze forward toward the horizon line. Hold the pose for up to one minute.

CHAPTER 7

• • • • • • • • • •

Working with
the Body's Sense of Trauma

When *The Body Keeps the Score: Memory and the Evolving Psychobi-ology of Posttraumatic Stress* (van der Kolk, 1994) was published, it was perceived as controversial and was dismissed by many practitioners as well as scientists. As a result, body-based treatments for trauma remained generally unrecognized for many years. Fortunately, there is now general agreement that traumatic memory is also a somatic experience, one held in not only the brain and mind, but also expressed by the body. van der Kolk and others have altered the prevailing belief in words as a primary approach and allowed integration of strategies not strictly language-dependent. Non-talk body-based treatments have emerged and are gaining research sup-port, including sensorimotor processing, Somatic Experiencing®, EMDR, trauma-sensitive yoga, and various forms of neurofeedback.

This validation was a veritable monsoon on the desert of talk ther-apy for practitioners who intuitively recognized the connection between expressive arts therapy and the body. The early contributions of Bessel van der Kolk (1994, 1996) and Peter Levine (1997) helped me to clarify the role of the body in applying expressive arts to trauma reparation and recovery (Malchiodi, 2019). Their vision and insight also made it possible for those of us who use expressive arts to recognize the essential role of embodiment in psychotherapeutic work. As discussed in Chapter 1, embodiment is a form of intelligence that informs us about how we perceive and experience the world, but not one that is widely cultivated or taught in Western cul-ture. It is often in direct contrast with the prevailing notions that focus on cognition as the main source of intelligence.

Trauma-informed expressive arts therapy emphasizes the centrality of the body as a source of trauma memory through nonverbal, embodied communication. Unlike talk therapy, all applications of the expressive arts support the need to literally "do something," which can be an important strategy for individuals seeking relief from trauma reactions. This action-oriented characteristic found within expressive arts interventions not only forms the foundation for reparation, but also makes it possible for individuals to actively change their relationship to the body's memories of traumatic events.

As emphasized in previous chapters, trauma is an experience that often disrupts one's internal sense of safety and the pleasure in being within one's body. Accordingly, the goal of any psychotherapy is to sensitively help individuals develop their ability to pay attention to and identify sensations and perceptions within the body in the present moment. While Chapter 6 on self-regulation addressed the impact of trauma on the body and ways to reduce its impact, the following sections focus on the role of embodied communication in trauma-informed intervention and approaches that address body-centered concepts. These include strategies not only to help individuals identify the body's sense of trauma, but also how trauma-informed expressive arts methods can be creative methods for using the body as a resource (Levine, 1997, 2015). The overall goal is to help individuals transform the body's sense of trauma to somatic states that lead to reparation and resolution of distress.

THE BODY'S SENSE OF TRAUMA

In Chapter 1, I described 9-year-old Sally who witnessed repeated violence in her home. While Sally was very responsive and talkative during our sessions, her art expressions seemed to convey a very different story and were unlike anything I had seen in art expressions by children Sally's age. At the time, I wondered if the unusual idiosyncratic characteristics of her paintings could be related to the impact of repetitive stress in her body; I later learned that she had a painful duodenal ulcer. Sally's paintings were pivotal in my thinking about each child I subsequently saw who had endured interpersonal violence and particularly in my thinking about how the body's sense of trauma is communicated. Art expressions and play, as well as expressive arts therapy sessions, can tell us something about the body's sense of trauma that is not always communicated with words. They are powerful windows into the somatic impact of distress, as explained in the following example:

Case Example. Tesha

Tesha came to a domestic violence shelter program at the age of 10 with her mother and two younger brothers. While her physically abusive and violent father repeatedly terrorized Tesha and her family, she consistently managed to maintain an outwardly positive attitude about what had happened. Like Sally in Chapter 1, Tesha assumed the role of caretaker within her family, and at her young age, she endured an enormous amount of stress and took on numerous adult responsibilities to help her siblings and mother. Also, like Sally, her dark and heavily black drawings seemed to tell a different story (see Figure 7.1). In Tesha's case, I also was struck by her repetitive images of what appeared to be physical pain, although I just was making my best intuitive guess. Tesha had no explanation for her images, but gradually I began to wonder if there was something she might not be able to talk about or was afraid to say. In fact, Tesha was in a great deal of discomfort. After she was given a complete medical examination, my colleagues and I eventually learned that she had cluster headaches and severe muscle spasms across her chest. While it is not verifiable that Tesha's images solely represented her physical pain due to these conditions, medical staff agreed that her body was likely responding to the stress of chronic exposure to violence.

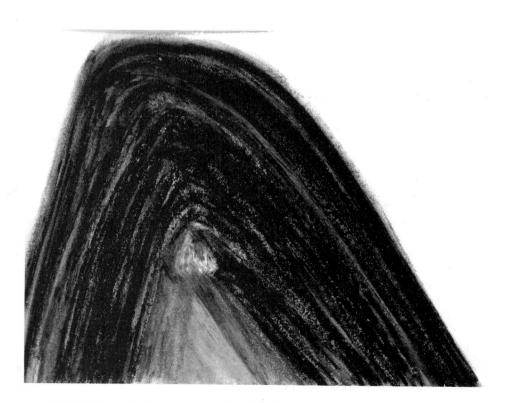

FIGURE 7.1. "Rainbow," one of Tesha's repetitive dark images. From the collection of Cathy A. Malchiodi (not to be reproduced without permission from the author).

In contrast, Tesha's younger brother, Todd, had a different set of somatic responses to the physical assaults he endured. Similar to the way some animals react to danger or threat, Todd frequently displayed a freeze or collapse response, becoming visibly immobile in the art and play therapy room. From a neurobiology perspective, this is the sort of response that an animal uses to protect itself from harm. Immobility helps the animal become invisible since predators tend to notice motion or may avoid it, perceiving that it is dead. But unlike animals in the wild who can exit from immobility (Levine, 1997), Todd often remained frozen for extended periods of time. Eventually, I had to invite and often coax Todd to "get moving" in some way through games, beating drums, or pounding clay to bring him out of his freeze response.

While expressive arts and play can be sources of self-regulation, they also can provide a unique window into the body's response to stimuli because of their sensory-based qualities. Todd initially perceived the art and play therapy room as a dangerous place, full of unknowns and experiences that provoked both freeze and flight reactions. For example, while playing with toy miniatures in the sandtray, Todd happened to lean against the table in such a way that several miniatures fell onto the floor. Before I could reassure him that nothing bad had happened, he was under the table in a state of collapse, possibly seeking to avoid any punishment or reprisal from me. When the perceived danger had passed, Todd responded by running out of the room to find another hiding place. Even the most benign interactions with me or other staff members consistently set off freeze or escape reactions. Like the responses of Tesha and others who have survived intense or dangerous situations such as physical abuse, Todd's body posture and movements to protect himself communicated the memory of past traumas, even though those events were not occurring in the present.

Play therapist Violet Oaklander (2015) observed that "children who are emotionally disturbed due to some trauma tend to cut themselves off in some way; they will anesthetize their senses, restrict the body, block emotions and close down their minds" (p. 6). If their trauma is not addressed early, children like Tesha or Todd carry the body's memories of these powerful events into adulthood, resulting in a body sense or a "gut feeling" that things are not quite right. Whereas Tesha conveyed her distress through drawing, Todd literally acted out his through immobilization and then flight to escape his sense of impending danger.

Many decades before we fully realized the importance of the body in trauma-informed practice, Freud (1920) said, "What the mind has forgotten, the body has not, thankfully." For most traumatized individuals, the fact that the body has not forgotten "what happened" is an important source of information for understanding how their bodies react when experiencing intrusive memories or avoidance. In all cases, the body holds an implicit narrative for how the individual has adapted to what is perceived as dangerous. This narrative is not only communicated by the body, but also potentially through various forms of expressive arts and play.

Three individuals in particular (Peter Levine, Pat Ogden, and Bessel van der Kolk) have underscored the critical need to address the body as central to intervention. Each is key to applying expressive arts therapy within trauma-informed practice. Levine (1997, 2015) clarified the neurobiological impact of trauma on the body, showing that when an individual is threatened, the body mobilizes large amounts of energy in order to defend itself. If the body's energy is discharged effectively, the autonomic nervous system is reset and balance is restored. Because some individuals do not release this energy, causing it to literally become "stuck" in their bodies, a variety of behavioral and physiological symptoms may emerge. In other words, while the body wants to defend itself from threats and distress, it sometimes cannot complete the process that would result in a sense of self-efficacy and safety. According to Levine, when individuals are overwhelmed to the point that this energy is stuck in the body or "scared stiff," the energy needed to overcome a traumatic event is literally locked in the muscles and nervous system. In brief, the goal is to help the person not only release this "stuck energy," but also redirect that energy into an active response, giving children and adults a sense of power to reclaim their own bodies.

Levine (2015) also emphasizes the importance of understanding the body's procedural memory—the impulses, movements, and internal body sensations that effectively guide most people through daily life. These include learned motor responses (bicycling, skating, dancing) that are skill-based and practiced; emergency actions (fighting, fleeing, freezing) that are used to address threat or danger; and fundamental responses involving approach, avoidance, attraction, or repulsion. The fundamental responses are senses that are more basic and instinctually tell us when to avoid people or places or when to reach out and move toward something or someone.

Similarly, Pat Ogden's sensorimotor psychotherapy (Ogden & Fisher, 2015) guides individuals in transforming overwhelming somatic experiences and body-based trauma reactions by working with the body's natural actions. For example, engaging trauma survivors in simple physical responses such as standing up, reaching out, or moving away is central to completing body responses that may have been halted by past traumatic events. Ogden explains what she calls the "somatic sense of boundaries"—the body's ways of signaling who one is safe to be close to and who is not, similar to Porges's social engagement concept. For example, when a boundary is threatened, the individual reacts with tightening muscles, moving away or leaning back. In expressive arts therapy, this is particularly important in noticing the movement, gesture, and body language of individuals who have been assaulted or have been unable to defend themselves from harm or danger.

Finally, van der Kolk (1994, 1996, 2014) has had the most extensive impact on understanding the role of the body in trauma reparation and recovery. To my knowledge, he was the first to identify trauma memories as "somatosensory," nondeclarative communications (van der Kolk, 1994), an idea that has changed the way we view traumatized individuals. The idea that trauma is not just a brain-based experience, but also one that extensively impacts the body became the foundation for the emergence of "bottom-up" approaches to treatment, including applications of expressive arts.

Possibly the most significant contribution to expressive arts is van der Kolk's (2014) observation about culturally relevant, body-based resources that have proven effective in the resolution of trauma for thousands of years. He explains:

> Mainstream Western psychiatric and psychological healing traditions have paid scant attention to self-management. In contrast to Western reliance on drugs and verbal therapies, other traditions from around the world rely on mindfulness, movement, rhythms, and actions. Yoga in India, taiji and qigong in China, and rhythmical drumming throughout Africa are just a few examples. The cultures in Japan and the Korean peninsula have spawned martial arts, which focus on the cultivation of purposeful movement and being centered in the present, abilities that are damaged in traumatized individuals. Aikido, judo, tae kwon do, kendo, and jujitsu, as well as capoeira from Brazil, are examples. These techniques all involve physical movement, breathing and meditation. (p. 207)

Along with my interest in cultural anthropology, the idea that these "self-management" strategies have existed throughout human history formed the foundation for identifying the four major healing practices in Chapter 2.

The arts have been "the voice of life experience far longer than medicine or psychology and have served people and communities as a means to process suffering, pain, celebration, and healing eons" (Gray, 2015, pp. 170–171). Expressive arts therapy emerged as a field from these ancient healing traditions to become more formalized psychotherapeutic practices, including movement-based approaches. This set of practices also reflects the concept of healing-centered engagement (Chapter 2) and the essential role of self-management in trauma reparation and recovery. In applying any form of expressive arts to address the body, it is essential to understand and identify individuals' traditions and rituals that are already part of their worldviews of healing. These traditions form the basis for culturally relevant interventions, particularly when it comes to addressing the body's experience of trauma.

THE BODY, MOVEMENT, AND EXPRESSIVE ARTS

Because of the increasing amount of somatic-specific literature, clinical applications, and research, it is now much more common to speak of trauma memories and reactions in terms of the body. However, some of the earliest foundations for body-based approaches to trauma are found in movement-based expressive arts in the mid- to late-20th century (Halpern,

2003), including body psychotherapy, Gestalt approaches, and bioenergetics. For example, Wilhelm Reich (1994) is credited with influencing the recognition of the body within psychology and is considered a founder of the field of somatic psychology. Reich believed that the body not only reflected personality and experiences, but also was a key to restoring health and well-being. In brief, he proposed a view of the body as a physical container for the entire history of the individual. In particular, Reich emphasized that traumatic events impact the flow of energy within the body and stimulate a type of freezing mechanism he called "character armoring."

Reich's theories and techniques influenced body-oriented approaches, including Lowen's (2012) bioenergetics, Feldenkrais's (2010) structural integration, and Rolf (1990), among others. In particular, Feldenkrais proposed that a healthy self-image is connected to the entire nervous system, muscles, and sensorimotor areas of the brain. An individual's typical emotional reactions might also be apparent in specific involuntary body postures and physical tensions that increase distress. In other words, changing the body's postures and patterns of breathing and moving facilitates positive change and emotional reparation. In brief, the body serves as a representation of the individual's entire life experiences, similar to the felt sense described by Gendlin (1982) and Levine (2015). These approaches partially formed the foundation for contemporary somatic psychology, various body therapies, and the field of dance/movement therapy, underscoring the connections between the body's (implicit) experience and its relationship to emotional and executive functioning. Dance/movement therapy in particular emphasizes that movement is the primary language of the body (Gray, 2015), is related to emotions and thoughts, and "reflects our way of being human" (Halprin, 2003, p. 17).

While dance and movement are often thought to be the main forms of expressive arts that are body-relevant, all the expressive arts are actually movement-oriented and body-based. Notably, theater, dramatic enactment, performance art, and role play include the body as a vehicle for self-expression; fingers and hands are used to play musical instruments; vocal chords, various muscles and the lungs are used in singing; visual arts depend on tactile and rhythmic experiences; and even creative writing and poetry include the embodiment of sensations through words. Although each of these forms of expressive arts may emphasize a specific sensory quality and require multiple parts of brain function, it is really the body that initiates each of these processes.

As McNiff (2009) observes, "All of the arts in therapy must repossess the body if they are to actualize their healing powers fully" (p. 110). This statement incorporates expressive arts as action-oriented forms of healing engagement as well as experiences that potentially reintroduce the body to a sense of pleasure, positivity, and aliveness. To "repossess the body," any application of the expressive arts ideally begins with a bottom-up approach at the somatic–sensory level and, in particular, includes movement of some kind.

WINDOW OF TOLERANCE
AND BODY-BASED APPROACHES

After experiencing an event or series of events that are painful or horrific, just "being in one's body" can be challenging. As van der Kolk (2014) summarizes, individuals may feel too much (hyperarousal), or they may be left feeling too little (dissociation). In cases where the impact results in chronic or severe episodes of hyperactivation, individuals may need to relearn how to feel safe in their bodies. For others, it may feel impossible to stay present because of hyperawareness of one's body to the point of paralysis or reducing activity in order to avoid uncomfortable activation. Dissociation becomes one of the few ways to escape what may be perceived as terrifying sensations. Margo, a 31-year-old woman who experienced 10 years of sexual abuse as a child and subsequent sexual assaults as a young adult, explained in an initial session that "just about everything is overwhelming. I always have a hunch in my gut that something is about to happen. When I feel this [overwhelmed or unsafe], the problem is my spacing out [dissociation]. It is automatic. It makes it hard to feel anything. I wish I could feel rather than starting to space out. My body has a mind of its own." While Margo felt embarrassed that she had these episodes, her "disembodiment" was a necessary separation from her own physicality in order to survive in the moment.

While expressive arts that include movement can be helpful in releasing energy or helping to reestablish a pleasurable connection with one's body, there are several important considerations when providing a body-oriented approach. Any interventions that focus on the body can test the window of tolerance (Ogden et al., 2006) of many trauma survivors. For example, individuals who experience physical assault, sexual abuse, rape, or any type of interpersonal violence have been subjected to body trauma inflicted by another person, and that person is often a parent, caregiver, relative, or close acquaintance. Medical procedures such as surgery or invasive treatments may also leave children and adults with a lingering sense of loss of internal and external body safety. These sensations can quickly reemerge when the individual is exposed to any cues, including expressive arts, that focus on the body or stimulate one or more of the senses. Having one's body traced with a felt marker while lying on a sheet of paper, or even being in close proximity to other individuals in a movement activity, may evoke unexpected memories of abuse or cascade of distressful feelings. The somatosensory nature of expressive arts that is helpful in self-regulation can also be perceived as a form of exposure to parts of past trauma, depending on the individual's history and personal tolerance for exploration through body-related activities.

Trauma-informed practice emphasizes identifying the individual's window of tolerance and reducing the chance that traumatic memories are reinforced or needlessly retraumatize the individual. This is why it is particularly important that a foundation of safety (Chapter 5) is initially established and that strategies for grounding, anchoring, and self-regulation (Chapter 6) are available before working with traumatic memories, including procedural memories, that may be related to the body. It is also essential to provide new and more productive experiences that empower the body to overcome the traumatic event through the "embodiment" of success and competence (Chapter 9). Some of these experiences are found in sensitive application of expressive arts interventions to reinforce safety and self-regulation. Others are enhanced by experiential body-based strategies that not only calm the body, but also help individuals to re-experience their bodies as sources of self-efficacy, resilience, and new, more productive procedural memories. Thus, the first goal when working from a body-oriented approach is to provide reliable ways for individuals to move away from anxiety or withdrawal and toward the implicit sense of well-being within the window of tolerance.

The body is also a source for many different types of beliefs and values, including family, community, gender and sexuality, age, ethnicity, and religion and spirituality. Personal beliefs and sociocultural values are particularly important when inviting individuals to participate in body-based expressive arts therapies because these approaches often include touch, personal space, and eye contact. There may be proscribed rules about art expression regarding the body. For example, even a request to draw images of the human figure may not be in alignment with religious or personal values, learned ways of depicting the human body, or communication of information related to the body. Recognizing individuals' culturally relevant healing traditions supports personal beliefs and values and emphasizes the importance of self-management and ownership of one's own healing outside sessions, particularly when it comes to the body.

BEGINNING A SESSION WITH MOVEMENT: FINDING A GOOD RHYTHM

While mindfulness meditation, breath work, or other approaches are effective for many individuals, others require more active strategies to release energy trapped in muscles and the nervous system. To accomplish this release, movement is a natural starting point in any expressive arts therapy session. Trauma therapist Babette Rothschild (2011) recommends that "carefully chosen physical activity will make meaningful contributions to your recovery from trauma" (p. 115). Similarly, Perry (2009) underscores the importance of repetitive, skills-building movement rituals with children for the purpose of self-regulation and building resilience. In general, there is increasing consensus that it is important to get survivors moving and engage the body in processes not only to decrease hyperactivation, but also to enhance a sense of self-efficacy and competency.

I generally begin at a somatosensory/kinesthetic level because most of my clients are holding energy in the form of tension in their bodies. It is important to start to release this stress before the person can deeply engage in exploring emotion and narrative, higher levels of the ETC. Also, because many trauma survivors feel unsafe in their own bodies, soothing movement experiences can help individuals restart the process of feeling in control of their body.

In presenting the idea of movement-based experiences, I often say something like "We are trying to restore the good rhythms in your body that trauma stole from you." While there are many dance/movement therapy and movement-based activities, I generally let individuals show me where they are willing to begin with movement to find their natural rhythms, no matter how limited they may be in the early stages. I first became comfortable with using the simplest gestures in my work in schools with adolescents who had physical disabilities and cognitive disorders. Most of these teenagers had a good deal of emotional trauma in their histories, too. Some were only able to move a finger or hand, and others could tap or slide their feet across the floor. These gestures led to more progressive movements and expression through other art forms within the range of each individual's abilities. These initial experiences taught me to be present to even the smallest movement an individual can make because it will eventually result in other gestures and forms of self-expression. What is important to remember about the body and movement is to just simply start with basic gestures and physical sensations.

While I regularly refer individuals to trained dance/movement therapists for specific intervention, I have found that being a psychotherapist who has found healing in movement and dance for many years can be somewhat of an advantage. What is essential for the success of all psychotherapists is that they understand their own body as a source of well-being, are comfortable moving with their clients, and are enthusiastic about "getting moving" as a reparative strategy. If the practitioner is new to introducing movement to trauma-informed intervention, there are some very simple ways to start sessions with a gentle focus on the body. These simple practices help people to redirect attention, quiet the mind, reduce tension, and relax. They can also become a source for additional body-related activities and can be performed outside the session when needed. The following case example introduces a few basic practices to consider.

Case Example. Maya: Introducing Movement into an Expressive Arts Session

Maya, a woman in her early 30s who experienced childhood abuse for more than a decade, suffered from constant anxiety and hyperactivation due to intrusive memories of the physical assaults she endured. She also had just survived a fire in the apartment complex where she lived. Fortunately, she did not sustain any serious injuries, but she lost all her possessions and her residence. After the fire, Maya reported a higher level of arousal (eating quickly, insomnia, and startle responses), interfering with day-to-day functioning and increasing her overall stress.

In our first meeting, Maya told me that her mind was so agitated that she could not focus clearly enough to complete the clinic's paperwork, nor could she comprehend the informed consent document she was asked to sign. When I asked her how her body felt right then, Maya was able to say "Pretty tense," but she was not able to identify where she felt tense. Through observation, it was easy to see that her shoulders, neck, arms, and legs were tight and that her breathing was shallow. Maya also shared that she often felt so overwhelmed since the fire that she lost an awareness of her body as her mind raced and her pulse rate rose. Clearly, she needed to reduce her hyperactivation to a manageable level and be able to shift her attention to engaging with me in order to benefit from any intervention.

At this juncture, I explained to Maya that I often liked to start sessions with some easy stretches and movements. I suggested to her that we try some very simple yoga-like practices that might help her become more comfortable with her body's stress-related responses. I began this process with each of us seated in our chairs facing one another so that Maya could mirror my movements and I could mirror her movements, too. For some individuals, this close proximity may not be immediately possible until a sense of safety in the environment is established. However, Maya was comfortable with the arrangement, and so I was able to introduce the following activities that became a regular warm-up at the beginning of each session.

Tense and Release

Rather than following traditional progressive muscle relaxation where each major muscle is tightened and relaxed, I use a simpler, quicker set of directives. I first ask individuals to sit with feet flat and relaxed on the floor and to breathe in only to the extent that it is comfortable. Next, the directive is to tighten as many large muscle groups as possible by making fists, tightening face muscles, and pulling up shoulders toward the ears, holding for 10 seconds at a time, and then to exhale and release all muscles. This is repeated two to three times. Instead of making fists, flexible squeeze balls (small, squishy rubber balls) can be compressed in both hands. As with any tense-and-release exercise, the goal is to bring focus to the body through tightening muscles, followed by letting go of that tension as much as possible.

Breath, Arm, and Shoulder Movements

With Maya, it was also helpful to introduce some breathing techniques and arm and shoulder movements loosely based on yoga practices. Like that of many individuals who are anxious, Maya's breathing was obviously shallow and mostly in her upper chest. In these cases, I do not ask individuals to attempt deep breathing, but rather to just work with the breaths gradually. In other words, I invite them to inhale only as much as feels comfortable and then to gradually deepen the breathing over several rounds. I also introduced a simple arm movement—raising the arms slowly overhead on the inhale and dropping them back down slowly to the sides of the body on the exhale. A variation of this movement is to open the arms wide to the sides of the body and then raise them overhead, interlacing the fingers with index fingers pointing toward the ceiling. Yoga practitioners recognize this particular position as a specific *mudra* (gesture) that is believed to activate various parts of the mind and body. Another variation of this approach involves simple bilateral movements, such as moving each arm across the body's midline several times or moving both arms across the body midline simultaneously, targeting the large muscles in the upper body.

Self-Holding Practices

Levine (2015) describes several simple practices that are beneficial for just about any traumatized individual. I refer to them as "self-holding practices" because Levine does not have a specific name for them. They are particularly helpful to individuals like Maya who need a body-based way to ground themselves at the start of a session or require an anchor to revisit when activated or dissociative. They are a series of simple postures designed to help one's body literally "slow down" when anxious or fearful. These postures involve various placements of hands on the head, heart, and stomach along with rhythmic breathing. One is simply a self-hug (arms are crossed over the body with hands touching opposite shoulders) that settles most individuals and serves as a container for emotions and sensations. The second involves two different placements of the hands: (1) one hand placed on the forehead, the other placed over the heart and (2) one hand placed over the heart, the other placed on the abdomen. These placements can be accomplished with eyes open or closed, depending on the individual's comfort level. The point is to hold either of the placements until a shift in energy or body sensation is felt (decreased respiration, heart rate, sense of agitation). All of these self-holding practices are based on the idea that the nervous system responds to touch and that there is therapeutic benefit to altering attention and awareness. The four B's (brake, breathe, brain, and body) described in Chapter 6 as self-regulation activities are also effective holding practices that can have similar impacts on the body.

REPAIRING THE BODY
THROUGH TRAUMA-SENSITIVE OR "GENTLE" YOGA

In Chapter 5, I described one strategy for integrating a fairly simple yoga pose, with expressive arts as a way to help individuals ground the body and create an anchor. Technically, yoga is not part of the continuum of expressive arts, but it is increasingly being integrated within arts-based approaches to dealing with traumatic stress. I believe it is an important practice that needs a more central place in trauma-informed work because it is not only relevant to embodiment, but also a value-added component in multiple ways. For example, most applications of trauma-sensitive yoga support individuals' capacity to regulate physiological responses to trauma in a sensitive, gentle manner. Regular gentle yoga practice is also thought to be effective in reducing trauma symptoms through the use of breathwork, asana (physical postures), and meditation (mindfulness practice). One randomized controlled trial of trauma-sensitive yoga decreased post-traumatic stress and depressive symptoms in women after a 10-week course (van der Kolk et al., 2014). Subsequent studies on continuing yoga practices over one or more years have indicated long-term reductions in PTSD (Rhodes, Spinazzola, & van der Kolk, 2016). In brief, the addition of trauma-sensitive yoga and various iterations may be effective for individuals who have been unresponsive to other approaches to trauma symptom relief.

Many trauma specialists now believe that specific yoga practices can help replace somatic sensations of trauma, such as feeling that one's body is unsafe. *Trauma-sensitive yoga* is a mind–body approach that has shown positive effects on the physical, emotional, and mental well-being of trauma survivors (Emerson, 2015). Like mindfulness, it involves focused breath, movement, and purposeful attention (Emerson, Sharma, Chaudhry, & Turner, 2009). It includes the physical postures found in yoga, particularly hatha yoga, a gentler, less strenuous form of yoga with a slower pace. Yoga is a well-known form of stress relief with the ability to evoke the relaxation response (Benson & Kipper, 2000). As an adjunct to psychotherapy, yoga is intended to support present-centered awareness to enhance greater tolerance of emotional states. Like similar practices, trauma-sensitive yoga helps individuals to recognize the body's sensations and the mind's reactions rather than eliminating them. The goal is to become more accepting of oneself and what one is experiencing. While meditation practices are generally more cognitive, trauma-sensitive yoga encourages focus on *interoceptive* experiences—an awareness of what is going on throughout the body, not just the mind.

Trauma-sensitive yoga is a good starting point for children, adolescents, or adults and can be combined with expressive arts approaches in order to tap a variety of senses, including kinesthetic, sensory, affective, perceptual, and cognitive senses. It is an important body-oriented, movement-based approach that is an option for individuals who prefer more physically active ways to address trauma reactions. There are two important points to consider from a trauma-informed practice perspective. First, as with all trauma-informed work, it is essential to consider and respect individual perceptions of yoga and cultural beliefs about this approach. For example, some individuals believe that yoga is part of a specific set of spiritual beliefs, and so they may not want to pursue it, even though it could be helpful in ameliorating trauma reactions. In these cases, it is often best to introduce yoga practices as forms of movement to reduce stress and tap the relaxation response with individuals who may be otherwise hesitant to participate. In other words, helping professionals do not have to identify these approaches as "yoga," but can integrate basic breathing and physical postures into sessions by reframing their use as ways to address anxiety and distress. It is also essential to identify a person's window of tolerance before the person participates in any process that involves a focus on interoception and to proceed with sensitivity as to how much "body awareness" is helpful. For those individuals who have survived abuse or violence, it is particularly important that they identify their own limits regarding participation in body-based activities.

Case Example. Ron: Trauma-Sensitive Yoga with Active Military

Ron was a 29-year-old male who had returned from active combat and was on an extended military leave of absence for trauma symptoms and anger management. He was recommended for therapy when his explosive behavior resulted in a violent fight with a male officer. Ron had a past history of trauma with repeated adverse and often violent events, including his father's suicide during his adolescence. Social services documented many episodes of domestic violence between Ron's father and mother. Ron explained that he witnessed many of these episodes and that on several occasions his father severely beat him until his mother called protective services and the police to intervene. On at least one occasion, he retaliated against his father. He also admitted that his own anger was out of control, but that it served him well as a soldier in combat, allowing him to react quickly to situations that were dangerous to him and others.

Ron had an exaggerated startle response and hyperarousal as well as a tendency to react with anger and sometimes violence to what were often neutral situations. In an effort to relieve tension, he did have a fairly effective strategy—he worked out at a health club lifting weights. But despite working out to the point of exhaustion, he still did not really feel "relaxed." Ron's responses reflect what Gabor Maté (2011) notes about many hyperactivated individuals:

> For those habituated to high levels of internal stress since early childhood, it is the absence of stress that creates unease, evoking boredom and a sense of meaninglessness. People may become addicted to their own stress hormones, adrenaline and cortisol . . . to such individuals stress feels desirable, while the absence of it feels like something to be avoided. (p. 28)

Ron indicated on several occasions that feeling tense was "hard to give up" because this hyperactivation was reinforced during his military service as a natural part of response to combat. He was highly skilled at surviving extremely dangerous circumstances by being hyperalert, sleeping lightly, eating quickly, and responding with violence to defend and kill if needed.

Initially, I introduced Ron to focused breathing, body scanning, and simple postures to alleviate some of his hyperactivation. As a result, I suggested that he participate in trauma-informed yoga practice sessions along with another combat veteran at a military base program. I also participated so that I could be of assistance if needed and monitor his progress. This "quad configuration" (two individuals plus the therapist and the yoga instructor) is recommended to maximize modeling and attunement (Emerson, 2015). Ron's yoga instructor, who was well versed in trauma-informed practice, sensorimotor approaches, and some expressive arts, introduced the concepts slowly, giving Ron the opportunity to ask questions and establish a sense of control before beginning any poses or activities. Maintaining a sense of control was essential to encouraging Ron's participation in this approach; as previously mentioned, he was accustomed to maintaining a level of hyperarousal. I proposed that perhaps at least experimenting with trauma-sensitive yoga might allow Ron to find a state of "relaxed attention" and that the goal of this process was essentially to help him become more aware of himself in the present.

Like many individuals who have returned from active combat with startle responses, hyperarousal, and anger management issues, Ron was initially tense and anxious. Early sessions began with the yoga instructor simply inviting him to stand and observe his breathing, paying attention to how he experienced the breath in his body. This exercise was followed by neck and shoulder rolls and other basic yoga moves and concluded with rhythmic deep breathing. At the end of the session, I asked Ron to give me some feedback on his experiences through an exercise we used in psychotherapy sessions—using colors, lines and shapes, or mark-making on a body outline to let me know what he now noticed in his body. These images simply became visual records of his interoceptive experience of trauma-sensitive yoga and its effect on his body and mind. After the first session, Ron did note that his breathing was slower and deeper and that his body was more "at ease" than when he arrived at the session, emphasizing that feeling of ease particularly in his chest area (colored green) and also, as he said, "in my brain" (colored dark blue). He also reported that other parts of his body felt "energized" (colored yellow) (Figure 7.2).

Over time, Ron and his peer, another soldier, were invited to try more complex postures, followed by expressive arts responses in the form of drawing. While these postures challenged my physical skill set, it was important that I was present to monitor Ron's responses as part of the trauma-sensitive yoga approach. Eventually, we were able to examine many of the more difficult events of his life, including those during childhood and his recent experiences in combat through the physicality of the various poses. For example, Ron consistently cited the "warrior positions"

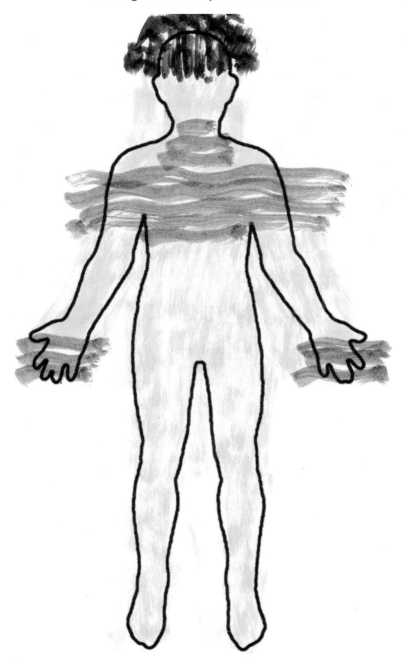

FIGURE 7.2. Ron's body image representing "at ease" in "my chest and my brain." From the collection of Cathy A. Malchiodi (not to be reproduced without permission from the author).

(standing poses where one lunges forward on one leg and arms are out-stretched) as reinforcing feelings of personal strength and courage to face whatever confronted him in life. These became a positive body resource for him when he felt hyperactivated or alarmed. Ron also was pleased that he developed new ways in "staying present," a concept central to trauma-informed yoga and similar practices. While trauma-sensitive yoga provided self-regulatory experiences, it also increased Ron's awareness of his body's responses to perceived threats, as well as his ability to simply accept these responses as they emerged. It helped him to begin the process of identifying appropriate coping responses and became a personal strategy for maintain-ing "relaxed alertness" in response to stress. In Ron's case, he was able to not only become aware of his sensations, but also find potential sources of mastery through the practice of yoga.

BILATERAL MOVEMENT AND DRAWING

The movement-based activities described in the previous section are fairly simple, which most therapists can easily implement with clients as warm-ups or grounding experiences in response to hyperactivation or dissocia-tion. However, I eventually try to encourage more active use of the body through broader movements and body-based variations of expressive arts. Bilateral movement and drawing (see Chapter 6) is another somatosensory/kinesthetic strategy that can be introduced as a warm-up to other expres-sive arts or become the main focus of a session. I first became intrigued with bilateral painting as an art student several decades ago while studying with abstract expressionist painter Robert Motherwell. Motherwell, exper-imenting with using both hands to paint large-scale calligraphic paintings, encouraged me to stay with the process of using my body's sense of rhythm to create art. Because this process instinctively felt emotionally and physi-cally reparative to me, I have continued to use it in my own art making ever since. Years later, when studying art therapy, I came across Florence Cane's bilateral drawing methods that she used as a central part of her work with children. While she believed these "liberating exercises" were essential to art making, her concepts also reinforced my belief in movement as essential to addressing trauma held in the body.

As described in Chapter 6 in reference to self-regulation, Elbrecht (2015, 2018) has written extensively about using bilateral movements through drawing, painting, and clay. In her decades of experience with an approach known as "guided drawing," she emphasizes the importance of supporting individuals' explorations of rhythm and tracking sensorimotor responses in their bodies. This extensive process of bilateral drawing and painting is outlined by Elbrecht in *Healing Trauma with Guided Drawing* (2018) and is a bottom-up approach that often generates a variety of universal shapes (Figure 7.3). The goal is not to initially identify these images; that would invite a top-down process reflecting narrative and symbols. Instead, it is important to gently encourage the individual to become aware of the somatosensory experiences associated with the drawing process. This may simply be an invitation to stay with the current movement using drawing materials or paint on paper, if the movement feels like it represents the individual's current somatic state. The therapist may also ask questions like "'How is it to direct your energy in this way?" And "How does this movement resonate in your body?" or "How do you know it needed to find this particular direction?'" (Elbrecht, 2018, p. 50). The point is to stay with the movement rather than interpret images because that will distract from the individual's body-based experience.

Because therapists may be working with individuals whose bilateral movements, drawings, or paintings often reflect tensions or pain held in the body, it is important to invite movements that shift the focus to those of self-soothing and reparative. In longer sessions that last several hours, some individuals will naturally find these rhythms on their own. Since I am

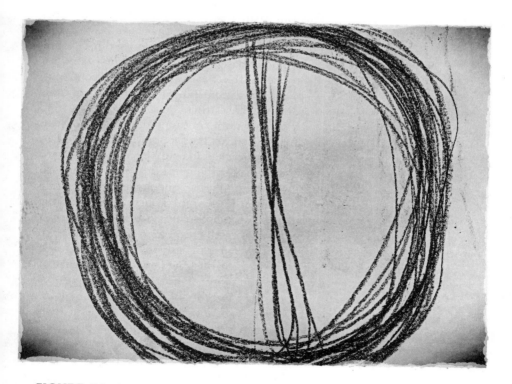

FIGURE 7.3. Participant's guided drawing of a circle and a vertical line, two universal shapes and gestures.

generally restricted by the "50-minute therapy hour," I ask the individual an important question early in the session: "What type of movement or rhythm does the body need right now in order to heal (feel calm, feel safe, or feel energized)?" In many cases, the person does not immediately know the answer to that question through movement or art expression. After all, for most of their lives, traumatized individuals have maintained protective body postures and stressful body sensations that have become part of their daily experiences. Maya, for example, could not come up with a spontaneous solution to this question. In these cases, some prompting is helpful. I may suggest taking a few minutes to relax and see if the individual can recall body movements related to soothing and pleasurable activities such as dancing, sports, or other similar experiences. The goal is to help the individual get in touch with those movements and rhythms that may have been reparative in the past—rocking or swaying, petting the fur of a favorite animal, experiences of competency that involve physical skills or moments of flow when moving felt effortless and easy.

In most situations, I find I have to invite and support people in trying a specific movement on paper with chalks to see if it resonates in the body as soothing or releasing. This is particularly true of those who have experienced interpersonal violence and repetitive events that have been so disruptive that the individual no longer has a sense of "good rhythm." While there are no universal rules about what bilateral movements work for everyone, several strategies can be effective, based on Cane, Elbrecht, and, to some extent, Shapiro's (2018) EMDR. If the individual is feeling anxious or tense, movements on paper with chalks that approximate rocking in the form of a bow (Figure 7.4) often have a soothing and calming effect. Elbrecht (2018) suggests that this is a comforting motion that may relate to the developmental need to be held and rocked like a baby. Another way to discharge energy related to tension through bilateral drawing is simply to move chalk in a vertical line upwards and branch out at the top like a tree (Figure 7.5); this technique is based on Cane's liberating exercises. While this type of bilateral drawing can be accomplished on 18″ × 24″ paper, it is especially effective when using a 36″ × 72″ sheet of kraft paper taped to a wall or a similar-size chalk board. When using any of these strategies, it is essential to check in with the individual by asking how the experience of movement is resonating in the body and if any modifications are needed. A third bilateral movement described by Elbrecht and derived from Shapiro (2018) is a horizontal figure 8 form (Figure 7.6), also known as a *lemniscate,* a configuration found in meditation and other spiritual practices. This particular movement generally helps most individuals to slow down and find a "good rhythm." In the case of dissociation, I have found it is also an effective movement for grounding and focus.

Bilateral drawing may be the focus of the entire session, or the gestural and rhythmic lines in these drawings can be a starting point for expressive

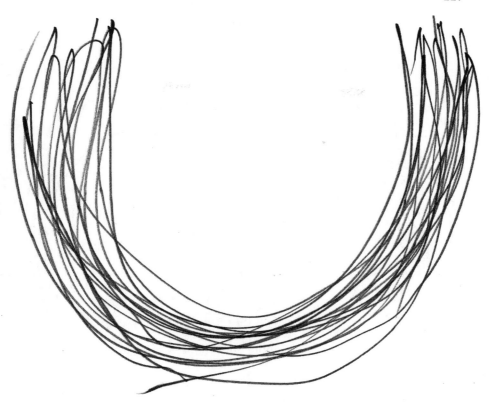

FIGURE 7.4. Example of bow shape used in guided drawing, gesture, and movement.

movement, music making, dramatic enactment, creative writing and story-telling to further explore the body's sense. In Maya's case, we eventually used some of the basic movement activities described above as prompts for gestures that eventually became bilateral mark-making on paper during some therapy sessions. Depending on the individual, relaxing or energizing instrumental music can be introduced to anchor bilateral work and encourage the person "to get moving" on paper by responding to various rhythms. As explained in Chapter 6 on self-regulation, bilateral drawing and other forms of expressive arts that involve both sides of the body also may be introduced throughout a session to facilitate relaxation in conjunction with expression of distressing memories or narratives. While not within the scope of this book, if you are a certified EMDR practitioner or use tapping as an intervention, bilateral work blends well with various forms of reprocessing therapy to support shifts in awareness.

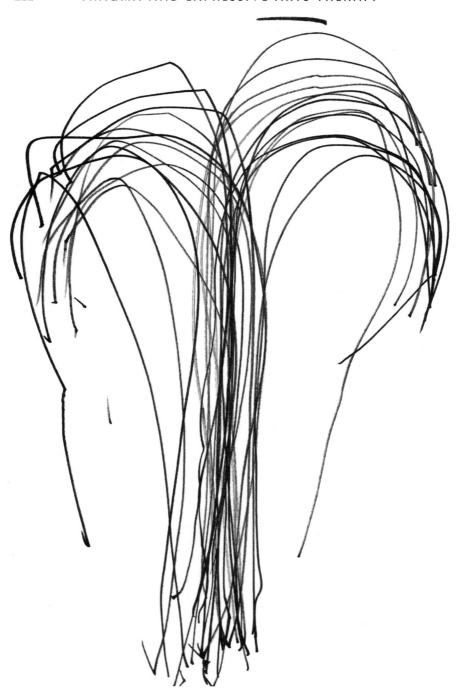

FIGURE 7.5. Example of Cane's "growing tree" movement on paper.

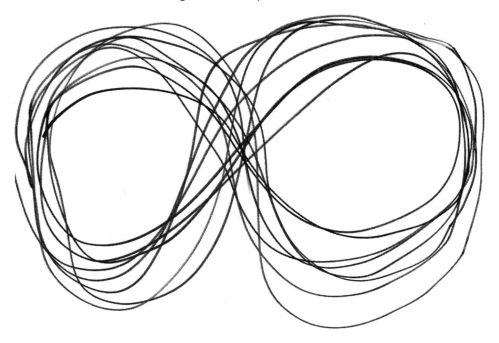

FIGURE 7.6. Example of figure eight movement on paper.

THE FELT SENSE AND BODY-BASED AWARENESS

Although the concept of the felt sense has been described in previous chapters, it is important to revisit its role and applications within expressive arts therapy as a body-based approach. Levine (1997) placed the concept of the felt sense within the framework of somatic experiencing and body-based experiences related to traumatic events. He underscored the importance of helping individuals practice the felt sense as a foundation for gradually bringing the more disturbing experiences of distress into awareness in order to begin to repair the body's sense of trauma.

Before Levine, Gendlin (1981) conceptualized what is known as the "focusing attitude," a stance of being friendly and curious toward the felt sense. During a focusing experience, individuals are invited to bring their awareness to the inside of their bodies and become "friendly" toward whatever is within their awareness. In talk therapy, the individual describes the experience (also known as a handle) by using words. For example, the felt sense could be a "clenched fist in my chest" or an image of a "person hitting my head with a mallet." The individual chooses a word to match the felt sense such as "clenched" (the fist in the chest) or "hurting" (the head being hit with the mallet).

Rappaport (2009, 2014) realized that "talk-only" might limit the expression of the felt sense of the body's awareness for some individuals, and so she integrated the concept within the framework of expressive arts and focusing-oriented therapy. In other words, the felt sense is manifested through any of the expressive arts—art, movement or dance, music or sound, writing and enactment. Gendlin (1982) describes the value of expression beyond words, noting, "More powerful than letting words come from a felt sense may be letting body movement come" (p. 35). For many traumatized individuals, moving or another form of arts-based expression is an easier way to communicate the felt sense.

In addition to tracking the felt sense of distress, after a movement activity it is also good to practice awareness of "what's working." At the end of a warm-up exercise, Maya was noticeably less anxious and more focused after participating in several rounds of tense and release activity, rhythmic breathing, and simple movement. I asked her to take a few minutes to observe her body's sense of her experience, particularly her arms, hands, and shoulders as well as her breathing. Maya noted that she was more conscious of her upper body, that her chest area felt "more expanded and energized," and that "energy was released" from her arms. I also asked her to recall how her body felt in comparison to the beginning of the session to help her learn to identify and express the difference between sensations of distress and upset and sensations of well-being, as well as to develop a conscious awareness of the body's "sense of meaning" (Gendlin, 1996).

BODY OUTLINES AND SCANS

In addition to inviting Maya to identify her felt sense before and after simple movements and exercises at the beginning of the session, expressing this awareness in a tangible form is also helpful for many individuals. Body outlines (also called body scans) are one way to go about this and are used in various ways in both trauma intervention and other settings. For example, body outlines are used for recording pain in medical patients; sometimes the patients themselves indicate their own experiences of physical pain or distress on the outlines. In trauma intervention, therapists commonly ask children and adults to depict their body's sensations of various emotions and experiences within body outline templates (see Appendices 1A and 1B for templates for adults and children, respectively). Play therapists have adapted this strategy by providing various structured ways to "color the body." Color coding is one popular approach (Figure 7.7) that includes instructions to use a specific color to represent each emotion in the body outline.

For the past decade, I have collected over 1,000 "feeling states" drawings created by clients on body outlines. This simple process is one possible way to make tangible what the body is expressing. Recently, science has

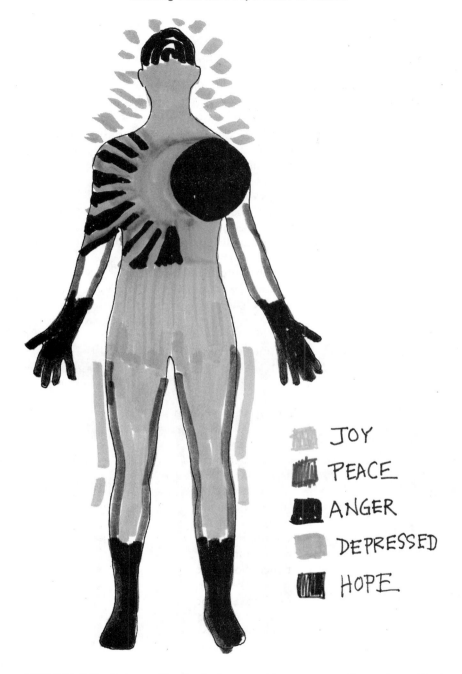

JOY

PEACE

ANGER

DEPRESSED

HOPE

FIGURE 7.7. Color-coding body image with a teenager. From the collection of Cathy A. Malchiodi (not to be reproduced without permission from the author).

caught onto what we know well in the expressive arts—that the body can literally be a "map of subjective feelings" (Nummenmaa, Hari, Hietanen, & Glerean, 2018). Researchers are using a process of "neuromapping" to identify the "human feeling space" to visually map 100 core feelings, including cognitive, emotional, and somatic sensations (Figure 7.8). This mapping is quite similar to the feeling-state drawings many expressive arts therapists have been using all along. What is potentially exciting is that the subjective feelings being systematically mapped are essentially individuals' "embodied" experiences, with very distinct commonalities in location, distribution, and energy in the participants' bodies.

Body outlines are also useful in facilitating recognition of sensations related to the body's experiences of distress. The more an individual can clearly communicate the implicit understanding of the body's felt sense to the therapist, the more the individual will feel understood. Providing opportunities for clients to authentically express how they feel inside their bodies and beneath the cognitive chatter of the mind is the critical factor in reparation and eventual recovery (Gendlin, 1996). Because body outlines can be used to help encourage body awareness via the felt sense, therapists can ask certain specific questions. These questions, as follows, should be

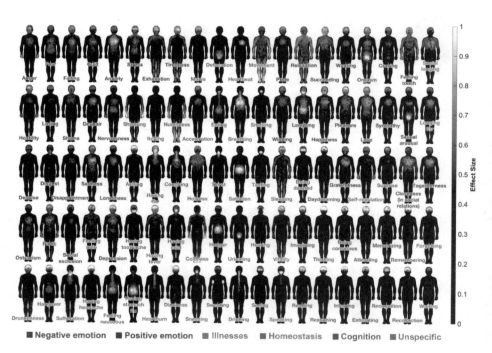

FIGURE 7.8. Maps of subjective feelings. From Nummenmaa, Hari, Hietanen, and Glerean (2018). Copyright © 2018 by the authors. Reprinted with their permission.

adapted, applied, and paced to the individual's preferences and the window of tolerance:

1. "When you experience that feeling [anger, happiness, frustration, upset, sadness], where in your body do you experience that sensation? What is happening in your body?"

2. "When you say 'I am angry [sad, happy, upset, frustrated], where do you feel those words in your body?'"

3. "How large or small is that sensation [e.g., on a scale of 1 to 10]?"

4. "When you are telling me about this feeling, what is happening inside you?"

5. "When you tell me about or imagine [a specific event, situation, person, time, or triggering circumstance], what do you sense inside your body?"

6. "After locating that sensation or feeling in your body, how are you feeling toward that sensation? What does that sensation or feeling want you to know about it? If it could talk, what would that sensation or feeling say to you or show you [image, sound, movement, enactment]?"

7. If an individual experiences different sensations simultaneously and cannot identify where that sensation is located in the body, the therapist can ask, "Which sensation are you aware of the most in this moment?"

Any or all of these questions can be used along with simple drawing on a body outline as an approach for further exploration using lines, shapes, and colors to represent the felt sense of an emotion or sensation within the body. In Chapter 3, I described a three-part approach that includes the body outline and provides an experiential example that includes working with the body's felt sense. The following example illustrates the process of sensory expression of a "worry," emphasizing how the individual perceives the interoceptive experience of where the worry is felt in the body. As in Chapter 3, the individual creates a brief written story, allowing the worry to "speak" through a non-first-person narrative:

"I am hiding deep in your body before I get activated. I lie dormant within until I am triggered. I can come to life from something someone just said, a buzzing sound, or just a feeling that something is going wrong. Until then I hide, ready to ambush. I want to express myself and look for the opportunity to be felt and recognized. Until then, I am just under the surface and ready at a moment's notice to emerge. I am seeking to be known. I am ready to cause havoc when called upon at any time of the day or night. But I also bring to you information to take action whether you like it or not.

"Once it is called forth, I burn like a fire in your stomach. I love to blow up in your gut and I make sure your fears and worries squirm with nausea like a turbulent sea. I tumble and roll. I make sure you know something is amiss. But unless you find a way to soothe this turbulent sea in your gut, I will announce that I am here in as many uncomfortable ways as I can."

With regard to individuals struggling with hyperactivation or dissociation, working with body outlines, including scanning the body for sensations, can be challenging. Figure 3.4 (Example 3 in Chapter 3) was created by a young woman who had experienced a violent physical assault and several significant losses within a year. As a result, she experienced not only frequent hyperarousal, but also terrifying bouts of nausea. She also became easily alarmed when asked to identify feelings or sensations within her body. I adjusted the experience accordingly with window of tolerance in mind. While I often ask individuals to literally scan their bodies from head to toe for the body's sense of stress or tension, I suggested a slower pace in her case. For example, I asked her to direct her attention to only a finger, one foot, or a part of her head and to be totally present to that one part of the body, while gently encouraging her to let me know about any particular sensations she perceived. On many occasions, uncomfortable memories arose, but because the focus was limited, she found she could gradually tolerate more exploration of sensations over several sessions. I also adjusted the format for the "worries" by encouraging her to draw using smaller-format paper (4″ × 4″ squares); adjusting media is one way to control and contain just how much is expressed. In this case, a small, square piece of paper is generally a safer container for depiction of powerful sensations than a larger one. To further support containment, a predrawn circle can be included on the paper, defining a structured space in which to use mark-making to represent the body's implicit sense of a worry or other emotion.

TITRATION AND PENDULATION

Body outlines can be adapted in various ways to help individuals communicate the felt sense and convey the inner experiences of distress and difficult experiences. There are many ways to keep an individual within an optimal window of tolerance when using body outlines or similar activities. One strategy I used with Maya helped her to move closer and farther away from sensations in art expressions and the body. For example, a therapist might have an individual draw a distressing sensation as seen from far above it or from a distant mountain top where one is far away and safe. Similarly, when guiding an individual to encounter "where a worry is felt in your body," it is essential to give the individual the skills needed to move away from discomfort and then closer as the person begins to tolerate more of a particular sensation.

When dealing with children, I have often used the metaphor of an owl because of its many capabilities. I describe how an owl can move its head almost completely around in a circle and can redirect its large eyes to look at something, or it can slowly turn its eyes away when needed. I might say:

> "Pretending to be the owl gives us the power to watch our own feelings, especially how our body feels inside. We can watch with full attention and if we need a time-out from watching, we can turn slowly and completely away, just like an owl does. When we are ready to look again, we can slowly turn back, but only as far as we want to and feels okay."

When working with very young children, I introduce an owl puppet with a moveable head (play therapy prop) that is particularly helpful in demonstrating this strategy.

The story of the owl and its ability to focus attention as well as turn its attention away from experiences and sensations is a good example of two important principles useful in work with body outlines—titration and pendulation (Levine, 2015). *Titration* is a term borrowed from laboratory science; it means the addition of an element or chemical carefully and often one drop at a time. In the context of trauma-informed expressive arts intervention, it is defined as the process of slowly introducing sensations via creative experiences slowly and in small amounts. *Pendulation* helps individuals to move back and forth between distressful sensations to *resourcing*—the body's internal sense of self-efficacy, resilience, and well-being. Like the owl, children and adults can learn to take in small amounts of the body's sense of trauma. They can also learn to look toward internal sensations of self-efficacy and well-being when experiencing distress, fear, or alarm.

One common expressive arts therapy approach to pendulation involves using two body outlines (a self-created or premade body outline or gingerbread figure). The child or adult is asked to think about a worry and depict thoughts and feelings on one body outline. The person is next instructed to think of a pleasant event and to use the other body outline to depict thoughts and feelings representing that positive memory. I often reverse the order of this sequence, spending more time on helping the individual find the "good sensations" before proceeding with the more distressful sensations. The therapist then facilitates exploration of the images from one to the other so that the individual experiences both uncomfortable and pleasant feelings and sensations. The overall goal is to learn that uncomfortable sensations can be tolerated and that when distress is encountered, it is possible to shift one's felt sense to memories of more pleasant experiences. If you are an EMDR or tapping practitioner, you can integrate those methods within this type of approach.

In any expressive arts approach, media or materials can be altered (titrated) to support the slow release of sensations. For example, in arts-based approaches, the size of the paper (small vs. large) is important. An index card, for example, is a small, more contained space in which one can express emotions and may be a better strategy than large paper, which is not only expansive, but also can be perceived as overwhelming for some individuals. When working with children in movement groups, I often use masking tape on the floor to create a personal space for each child. The tape marks a boundary and container within which the child can move and dance; it is also a safe space that others cannot enter without permission and provides a more limited (titrated) area for expression. Additionally, a practitioner may strategically decide to limit amounts of media, toys, and props in certain situations not only to help an individual focus, but also to reduce overstimulation caused by too many choices. These are just a few ways to apply titration to expressive arts with the distress level of the client in mind. When combined with approaches to safety and regulation described in previous chapters, these adjustments support the individual's pace and gradual tolerance for awareness of the body's sensations.

BODY MAPS AND BODY MAPPING

Body maps and body mapping are two related arts-based approaches that capitalize on the body as a theme for narratives and self-exploration. Creating life-size human figures or body tracings has a long history in the field of art therapy, underscoring not only applications with children and adults, but also the necessary precautions in applying this approach. Variations of these techniques have been modified and re-examined as creative interventions with individuals who have experienced psychological trauma and life-threatening medical illnesses, including HIV/AIDS and organ transplantation (Devine, 2008; Figure 7.9). These strategies focus on body image as not only a historical record of significant events, but also as a source for exploration of self-efficacy, competence, and personal resilience.

Body maps are generally defined as life-size human body images, whereas *body mapping* (Crawford, 2010) is the actual process of creating body maps using arts-based media such as drawing, painting, collage, or other materials. The mapping represents narratives about oneself as well as specific body experiences or memories. Solomon (2002, 2007) is credited with formalizing a process called "body mapping," applying it to work with women living with HIV/AIDS and immigrants (Devine, 2008; Mac-Gregor, 2009). Other practitioners and even artists have used it with individuals who have undergone medical procedures for life-threatening illness (Meyburgh, 2006) and HIV/AIDS (Brett-MacLean, 2009; Devine, 2008). With these individuals, the process serves as a way to explore illness, as a form of legacy and for some, preparation for death. Others note that art

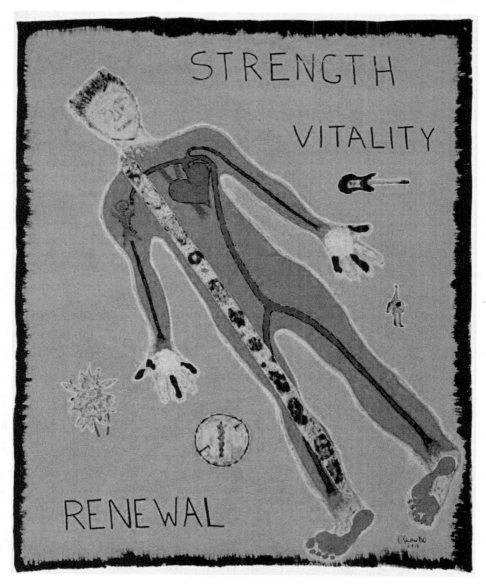

FIGURE 7.9. Example of life-size body map by an individual with an organ transplant. Courtesy of University of Kentucky Arts and Healthcare Program, Lexington, Kentucky.

therapy, narrative therapy, and body work are integral parts of body mapping and that body mapping is essentially an embodied experience (Meyburgh, 2006).

Solomon (2007) explains body mapping as a way of telling stories and creating visual images about oneself and one's life, including one's body and environment. Its intent is to help individuals gain a better understanding of themselves, their bodies and their environments, communities, and cultures. Solomon advocates use of body mapping within a group structure to capitalize on mutual support, inspiration, and ritual as part of the reparative process. While body-mapping approaches vary among practitioners, in general the individual's body is traced on a large sheet of paper in order to create a life-size self-portrait. Another participant or helping professional may trace the person's body, and in some cases, the individuals trace themselves. Participants generally stand with their backs against the paper on the wall in order to be traced; standing is a less invasive experience for most people than lying flat on the floor to be traced. Solomon's body-mapping procedure includes actual hand- and footprints; additionally, colors and symbols are painted on or around the body outline in response to specific questions about one's life, including events, challenges, and strengths.

In working with medical populations and returning military personnel, I have modified the body-mapping approach to include a variety of questions tailored to the specific needs and goals of individuals, groups, settings, and issues. The modifications are based on Solomon's work and resiliency-based variations proposed by Gastaldo, Magalhaes, Carrasco, and Davy (2012), who applied body mapping as a form of research. Depending on the size and complexity, body mapping can take several sessions to complete; with groups, the process can take 1–2 days to complete. Solomon's (2002) original body-mapping guide recommends allowing at least 5 days or approximately 30 hours to complete a body map. Because this is often unrealistic within current mental health sessions of 50–90 minutes, I have altered the process to fit the needs and capabilities of participants and specific settings. In some cases, participants can complete a life-size body map (as shown in Figure 7.9) over two to three sessions. As a variation, I also provide a large cardstock-weight paper, approximately 18″ × 24″, as an option with a series of predrawn body poses (see Appendices 5* and 6). This allows individuals to choose one or create their own on a blank sheet. It is a variation of what Gastaldo and her colleagues refer to as a "mock body map" in order to encourage and support creative expression within time-limited sessions.

Paint is traditionally provided as part of the body-mapping approach, but for a variety of reasons, I often provide collage and drawing materials. In part, this is due to limitations of the setting (office or shared space)

---

* Appendix 5 is my adaptation, incorporating the work of Solomon (2002, 2007) and Gastaldo and colleagues (2012).

where large-scale painting is often impossible. Collage and drawing materials (oil pastels, felt markers, and chalk pastels) are more easily controlled media than paint, which is so fluid; more easily controlled media again help to "titrate" the experience of working with body-related concepts through creative expression. Gastaldo and colleagues (2012) find that providing common magazine and other photo images reduces participants' frustration in locating symbols for their maps. These images include the human body (heads, various internal organs, body parts); social support (people working, helping, and interacting; people holding hands, comforting each other); various emotions (mad, sad, angry, happy, calm); and other assorted images such as food, transportation, nature, and housing. I also offer a collage box of various words, phrases, and quotes for participants who find that language best expresses their experiences. Because of the nature of creating a large body map, some important window of tolerance issues need to be considered. First, it is essential to remind individuals that it is up to them to reveal or express as much as they want. Because the process of creating a life-size body map is complex, it is imperative that the therapist plays a supporting role in helping the individual to choose and create elements and symbols. For this reason, one way to approach this process is through a good deal of structure that supports exploration as well as personal and historical resilience (life events, achievements, and relationships throughout the lifespan). This includes focusing art expression on the following components:

- Choice of a body posture to represent oneself.
- Personal history, including "where I come from" and "where I am going" (such as goals or aspirations).
- Images or symbols on the body to represent challenges, events, or obstacles that have been overcome or are in the process of being overcome (often called "marks of resilience").
- Personal mottos, quotes, or slogans and/or symbols that are sources of strength (resources).
- People and entities (pets, communities, or God or a higher power) who have been supportive (represented by photos, symbols, or handprints).
- Message or wisdom to share with others.

The following example describes the body-mapping process with a breast cancer survivor. While the experience of cancer is not commonly thought to result in trauma reactions, recent research indicates that post-traumatic stress occurs in many women during the course of treatment (Voigt et al., 2017). The majority of patients experience persistent symptoms for at least a year and develop trauma reactions in the months following diagnosis. While the degree of post-traumatic stress is generally less than that in other survivors of traumatic events, there are identifiable symptoms of distress that are disruptive and diminish quality of life. In particular, the following case illustrates how this approach supports resourcing and resilience through visual art and narrative in conjunction with body mapping.

Case Example. Petrea: Body Mapping and Medical Illness

At age 45, Petrea was diagnosed with a particularly virulent form of breast cancer. Because she had once been a genetics researcher, she knew a great deal about what a diagnosis of cancer meant and realized that the treatment would be physically exhausting and often toxic. She also knew that she might not survive due to the type of her tumor. While Petrea was stoic and realistic about the nature of her disease, she was also experiencing insomnia and severe anxiety to the point of panic attacks and occasional dissociation.

Petrea referred herself for expressive arts therapy at her hospital upon the recommendation of her internist who was concerned about her panic attacks and personality changes. In initial sessions, we worked on developing some self-regulation strategies similar to those described earlier in this chapter, with an emphasis on body movement and stress reduction. Petrea also explained to me that she had spent most of her life "holding in my feelings" and rarely sharing her emotional life with anyone, including family and close friends. The nature of her work as a physician's assistant was gratifying but consistently stressful due to the critical conditions of many of the patients she encountered. Petrea found herself experiencing various forms of workplace-related burnout similar to secondary post-traumatic stress reactions. In particular, she observed that she often felt that she might be clinically depressed, but that just underneath that depression "lurks some anger that I could never tell anyone about." To some extent, Petrea felt that her current trauma reactions were related in part to past experiences of depression and unresolved anger.

When I first met Petrea, she already had used some self-regulation strategies to reduce anxiety through breath work and progressive muscle relaxation (similar to the tense-and-release exercise described earlier in this chapter). Because she had some self-soothing capacities in place, in initial sessions I invited Petrea to use body outlines to show her depression, anger, and current feelings of panic to the extent that she was comfortable. In particular, we explored how current distress impacted her and how she experienced her trauma reactions in her body through the body outlines. This experience was alternated with her body's sense of pleasant sensations recalled from past memories and positive relationships. Fortunately, Petrea had many implicit memories of activities like skiing and friendships with colleagues. This made tangible some additional resources that she could bring into awareness when she started to feel anxious or panicked.

Because Petrea was eager to do whatever she could to reduce her panic attacks, I suggested that she keep a simple journal in between sessions to visually record specific feelings, write or draw her thoughts, or simply doodle (like the group doodle process described in Chapter 6). Because she indicated that she liked the body outline templates, she decided to use them, too, as a part of her expressive arts homework. Petrea's interest in this image-making led me to introduce her to the idea of body mapping as a possible strategy for resourcing and perhaps to "make better friends with your body" during this difficult time of the cancer diagnosis and subsequent treatments. Because of time constraints on our sessions, we decided to create a mock body map (approximately 4' × 2' in size) rather than a life-size figure and used collage and other materials. After discussing some of the elements she could include, Petrea decided to make hers into a "body map of resilience" (Figure 7.10) that focused on "marks of resilience," sources of strength, what she had learned, and family and friends who provided social support in her life. Petrea shared the following thoughts about her body map:

> "I still have trouble sorting out my feelings about being diagnosed with breast cancer. But the scariest part for me is not when I was diagnosed. It was when the treatments were completed. It was then that my panic set in. What can I do now to survive, now that the chemotherapy is over? Will the cancer come back? I also was told I might be having post-traumatic stress reactions due to this whole ordeal.
>
> Art has given me a way to express my feelings. But the body map has helped me to find my own strengths within a body that has felt violated and stressed. I did not want to relay the sadness. I wanted to express the moments of joy I have had instead."

While Petrea chose to focus on body-mapping concepts of strength and social support, other cancer survivors I have worked with often choose to directly confront how their illness has impacted their bodies through imagery. Because breast cancer can negatively impact the individual's physical sense of the body, imagery that focuses on the body may not be appropriate for those whose body image has become a source of traumatic stress. For others, however, self-expression of physical changes can be empowering, especially if coupled with resilience-based elements that "resource" strengths, social support, and post-traumatic growth experiences.

MODIFYING BODY-BASED APPROACHES

Working with the body's sense of trauma is essential, but it also can be particularly challenging when individuals have experienced interpersonal violence or assault. This final section presents some of the various

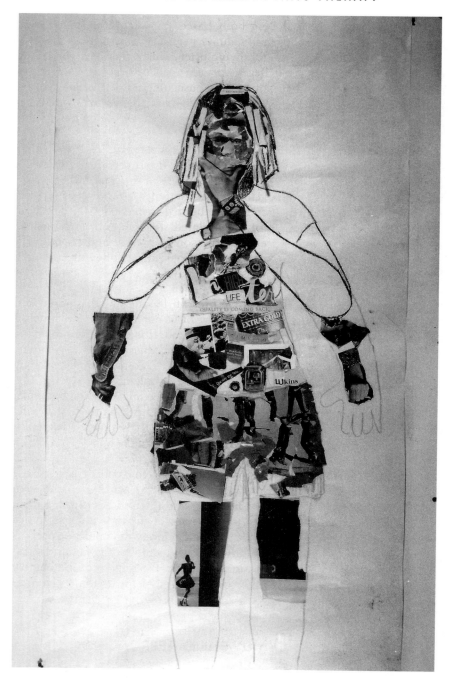

FIGURE 7.10. Petrea's "body map of resilience." From the collection of Cathy A. Malchiodi (not to be reproduced without permission from the author).

modifications used in addressing body-based sensations of interpersonal violence, while supporting the individual's personal safety, self-regulation, and window of tolerance. The following brief case examples describe how expressive arts and play are integrated into treatment with children who experienced multiple incidents of sexual abuse and maltreatment.

Addressing the Body's Sense of Trauma with Child Sexual Abuse

Child sexual abuse is possibly one of the most difficult challenges in any trauma-informed intervention. In many cases, young survivors of sexual abuse also have experienced developmental trauma (multiple adverse events during childhood), adding to concerns about how to effectively proceed. In particular, the introduction of body-related activities can be tricky and even risky because of the nature of interpersonal violence, especially sexual assault. Reinforcing the implicit experience of trauma to the body (a.k.a. "what happened") through expressive arts may generate unnecessary physical sensations and emotional reactions. The use of various body-related directives, even body outlines or gingerbread figures, should be introduced with particular sensitivity to the window of tolerance as well as to what children communicate through nondirective expressive arts and play.

Case Example. Josh

Josh experienced numerous adverse childhood events, including physical and emotional neglect and sexual abuse. He was referred to art and play therapy after being admitted to an inpatient psychiatric hospital for evaluation and treatment at the age of 10. While not much was known about Josh's early childhood, helping professionals noted that he did not have a secure attachment with his mother due to her drug abuse and relational problems with his biological father and other partners. He was in the care of his biological mother until age 7 but was removed from her custody because of neglect and several reports of sexual abuse by his mother's male partners and an uncle. Josh then lived with his aunt until he was reported to have attempted to assault a dog in the playground at his elementary school and acted out sexual behaviors toward other children. His aunt felt that she could no longer address these behaviors on her own, and so Josh was placed in inpatient care.

With children like Josh who have experienced adverse childhood experiences and been diagnosed with post-traumatic stress, human figure drawings often reflect the impact of trauma on development (Malchiodi, 2012b). Josh's quickly executed drawing of a person saying "Hi" is much more like a figure drawn by a much younger child (Figure 7.11); Josh himself appeared physically young for his age. His drawings of people generally did not include hands or feet, and the arms he drew were consistently

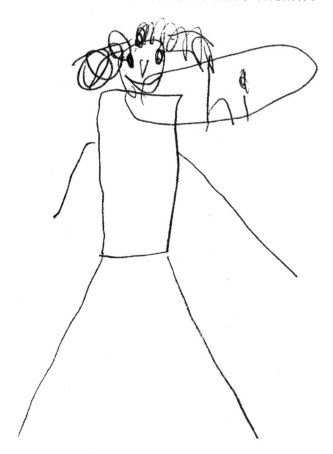

FIGURE 7.11. Josh's drawing of a person saying "Hi." From the collection of Cathy A. Malchiodi (not to be reproduced without permission from the author).

asymmetrical. While a specific meaning cannot be assigned to any of these features, drawings of human bodies by children like Josh seem to mirror the developmental disruptions that children who have experienced repeated instances of abuse, attachment problems, or neglect have survived.

Although he initially complied with my request to "draw a person," Josh told me that he did not like to draw people and could not draw an image of his family. In fact, he steered away from any sort of human figure and was uncomfortable talking about his own body at this stage in therapy. When he came to sessions, Josh preferred to work in the sandtray using mostly dinosaurs and objects, often building landscapes and terrains with sand and water. In these cases, sometimes nonbody metaphors for interoceptive experiences are a more comfortable way for children to express internal sensations related to abuse. Instead of introducing a body outline or image, a metaphor for interoceptive experiences is another way to help children express feelings and sensations through image or play activity. Crenshaw (2006) refers to this strategy as "evocative"; in other words, this strategy encourages self-expression because of the nature of the metaphor presented. Children can often come up with their own symbols that represent feelings or sensations, but Josh found this difficult. I decided to try a story commonly used in play therapy about a volcano that could speak to see if I could engage Josh in drawing it, followed by dramatic enactment or storytelling. For Josh, the volcano was easy to draw and a way to naturally convey his felt sense of various emotions related to his abuse, particularly anger. Movement and drama came about fairly naturally after the drawing through exploring how "volcanos behave sometimes." Josh practiced being "dormant," a word that he learned from me to describe "calm" or "sleeping." Of course, this volcano also had many "eruptions," and Josh and I practiced various ways to show that kind of behavior just as volcanos do in nature—shoot flames straight up the air, push lava out of the top, and then slow down as the eruption ends. I will admit that these enactments of eruptions pretty much wore me out, but they also served as a way for Josh to discharge his energy. In time, even he began to look forward to more moments when the volcano became dormant. This play-acting and movement became the basis for understanding when the volcano was likely to erupt (anger) and how to transform it into a more dormant state (self-regulation). While Josh's developmental trauma would need additional ongoing attention, he at least had begun to understand that sometimes a volcano has good reason to explode (when hurt, abused, or threatened). This realization began to help him feel less ashamed when he lost control of his impulses (sexualized behavior) and also helped him to rehearse a "calm volcano."

Case Example. Janeen

Janeen, Josh's older sister, was 8 years old when she first disclosed that she had been sexually abused by her mother's boyfriend and possibly other adult males throughout her childhood. Unfortunately, child protective services were ineffective in intervening in Janeen's situation after several reports and her own disclosure. She did not speak about her abuse again until she was finally removed from her mother's custody at the age of 9. When questioned by her case worker at that time, Janeen said, "I just want to forget what happened." She reported that she was "okay" and that she did not want to talk about the multiple incidents of abuse. In contrast, Janeen's behaviors indicated that she was having problems at school where she was often dissociative for long periods of time.

Now 12 years old, Janeen also got into fights with other children at a foster family's home and occasionally exhibited inappropriate sexualized behaviors. She also wet her bed at least once a week and had frequent insomnia due to nightmares and hypervigilance. The case worker who initially interviewed her observed that Janeen felt guilty about not being able to stop the abuse and equally ashamed of what had happened to her. She clearly needed assistance in understanding and mediating her body's responses to what she had experienced in terms of sexual abuse and her biological mother's inability to provide protection and safety.

Like many children who have had similar experiences, Janeen began coming to art and play therapy sessions and was sometimes dissociative (not in her body) and sometimes hypervigilant and anxious (too much in her body). In early sessions, I was particularly sensitive to her personal space in order to understand how she perceived adults, personal safety, and her body. With children like Janeen who have been repeatedly sexually assaulted, I always emphasize that they can talk or participate as much as they want to or not at all, make choices about where to sit or when to move around the room, and what kinds of art and play items to use. Once she chose a seat in the playroom, Janeen was practically immobilized, hunched over the art table, and mostly silent during our first session except to nod when I asked if she knew why she was going to be working with me. Because she knew why she was in art and play therapy, I simply shared that I had worked with many other children who had been hurt in some way and added, "In fact, many children who come to this playroom use drawings, toys, or figures in the sandbox to tell me stories."

While I would have liked to begin with movement with Janeen, a somatosensory approach would have been too overwhelming for her at this stage. Since she did like to draw and was comfortable using miniature toys in the sandbox, I began with more of a top-down approach. Because Janeen was so immobile, I just let her draw while I sat nearby over the first several sessions. Her first drawings were images of herself from the waist up, often in a window or behind an object (Figure 7.12), and landscape themes that included broken trees and chaotic environments. Janeen preferred not to talk about her drawings and was guarded about their content. Fortunately, she was always eager to create them at each session and seemed pleased that I was interested in them.

These drawings did provide two possible clues about trauma's impact on Janeen. The most obvious clue was in her self-portraits; Janeen never depicted anything below her waist, including legs. One could guess that this had something to do with the sexual assaults, but these images also could be saying something about her tendency to feel frozen and immobilized. Any art expression presents many possibilities for meaning and often multiple layers of communication. The other clue came from her drawings of environments in which Janeen invariably included shattered, cracked, fragmented, and tumultuous scenes. While it is impossible to put a specific meaning to these "broken" images, in my experience in working with children from violent homes, this is a common theme in drawings by those

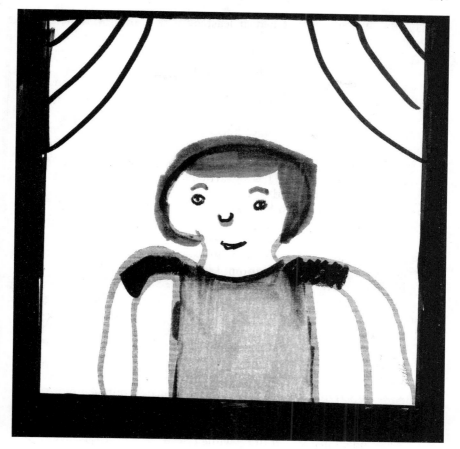

FIGURE 7.12. Janeen's self-portrait. From the collection of Cathy A. Malchiodi (not to be reproduced without permission from the author).

with a history of developmental trauma. Whereas some practitioners may place interpretations on images, I try to keep a "beginner's mind" when witnessing them, and I view them as another communication of the individual's internal sense of traumatic stress.

Because Janeen was still hesitant to step outside her safety zone of drawing, I decided to invite her to use both hands to create bilateral drawings with chalks on a large chalkboard I could place on top of the art table. Normally, I would encourage children to draw standing up, but for Janeen that was still too overwhelming. I demonstrated several different patterns she could make—arcs, circles, and straight vertical lines. If she felt that she made any "mistakes," I assured her that we could erase them very easily and she could start another drawing. Although she tried several of the movements, Janeen quickly became intrigued with making various arcs in multiple colors across the chalkboard. Pretty soon she was finally standing up and reaching with the chalks to draw on all parts of the surface—she was more active than she had been in previous sessions. When I asked her how it felt to draw with both hands, she whispered, "good" and then added, "I like making these rainbows [arcs]."

Unfortunately, I only had a few more sessions with Janeen until she was transferred to another agency for further intervention. But in those last meetings, we continued to do more bilateral movement and drawing, with Janeen eventually becoming more energetic and comfortable moving around the room. Although she still did not speak much, Janeen's eye contact with me increased dramatically and she sat erect in her chair with self-assurance on most days. Surprisingly, at the beginning of these final sessions, she regularly asked me if she could "draw the big tree on the big paper," the bilateral, liberating exercise. As her therapist, it was gratifying to see Janeen enjoy making increasingly confident and expressive movements and to reflect out loud on how much I enjoyed seeing her create these "big bold trees," several of which she took home with her to hang in her bedroom at her foster family's house. Because of our limited sessions, we never had the opportunity to discuss the multiple incidents of assault she experienced. However, Janeen's social worker later told me that Janeen was much more open to speaking about her fears and guilt about her abuse and that she provided some important details that would help protective services in their follow-up on her case. Her foster family did report that Janeen's insomnia, nightmares, and hypervigilance were much more manageable and that "big trees" became an important source of positive memories for Janeen.

CONCLUSION

Addressing the body's experience of trauma supports the necessary foundations of safety and self-regulation. This can be accomplished in many ways through expressive arts, including movement and bilateral drawing to reinforce "good rhythms," trauma-sensitive yoga, and various forms of body scans and mapping to explore sensory experiences related to distress as well as resilience. Because working with body-related sensations can be difficult for many traumatized individuals, sensitivity to individuals' window of tolerance is critical. Ultimately, the body tells an implicit story about distressful events that inform a larger and more comprehensive narrative about trauma, the subject of the next chapter.

in the environment. These sensations and reactions are a form of truth, but they also feel unreal, presenting intrusive images, smells, sounds, or other distress-inducing sensory manifestations.

I have learned a great deal from simply asking trauma survivors to explain why speaking about traumatic events may feel counterproductive, uncomfortable, or distressful. Rachel, a 50-year-old survivor of childhood sexual abuse and assault, was very clear about why talking was counterproductive. She specifically wanted to try a nonverbal approach to therapy as a result of attempting to explain to several therapists her fragmented and sensory-based memories of numerous acts of violation. After years of trying to verbalize what she recalled about multiple traumatic events, she began to feel even more guilty about what happened to her as a child and began to dissociate for extended periods of time. In retrospect, Rachel suspected that her therapists did not really believe her stories because the experiences she communicated were jumbled and disjointed and involved multiple incidents of abuse by a well-known member of her community. While she felt her therapists at the time tried to help her, she also felt ridiculed and inadequate when she was not able to explain herself. After many attempts to engage in various forms of treatment, including cognitive-behavioral and exposure therapy, Rachel decided to stop therapy altogether because talking came to be another source of trauma. As she explained to me, "I decided not to talk. Talking made me feel picked apart and vulnerable. Then I began to escape by having blackouts (dissociation) whenever I felt overwhelmed." Not surprisingly, many people report that talking about traumatic events induces the very reactions and symptoms they seek to eliminate, including hyperactivation and psychic numbing.

Some psychotherapists believe that it is not necessary to "tell the story of what happened" in order for trauma reparation to take place. For example, Rothschild (2010) clearly states that observing, exploring, or constructing the chronology of traumatic events is counterproductive and perhaps even dangerous for some individuals. In one sense, any form of memory processing that touches on trauma narratives can have adverse consequences because it can result in various degrees of retraumatization. There are also subjects who simply do not want to revisit any memories in any form, no matter how convincing a treatment approach sounds. This is particularly true in cases of interpersonal violence such as domestic violence or sexual abuse, circumstances that make it feel unsafe to share narratives even within the confidentiality of a therapeutic relationship. If a trauma is limited and acute, most people are able to provide a story if the psychotherapist is skilled in helping the person desensitize and resolve feelings. But in cases where trauma is complex, developmental, or an occurrence long in the past, there is either no recollection or no comprehensible story to tell with words for a variety of reasons.

Speechless State and Speechless Terror

One particular concept discussed in earlier chapters is especially relevant in applying expressive arts to working with trauma narratives—the lack of ability to use language to articulate stories. The "speechless state," a phrase I first learned from Lenore Terr, helped me to understand why children from violent homes were often unable to convey their experiences via language. Terr believed this condition was induced by terror during the telling or expression of traumatic events. One memorable story she told me involved a boy who was sexually abused by a babysitter when he was 4 years old and subsequently became sexually aroused during sessions with Terr. Like other children Terr saw in treatment, the boy used various toys and props to act out scenarios of abuse, coming close to losing control of his emotions and actions. As his play, he suddenly ended both activity and talking, systematically putting the toys back into a box and silently snapping on the lid as if to close off any further communication. According to Terr, this abrupt conclusion of activity was one of many examples of children's reaction to the overwhelming experience of trauma narratives that literally shut down communication in any form, but particularly language.

At the time that Terr told me about this particular case and others, we did not know what is now known about how the telling of traumatic events actually impacts the brain, mind, and body. Early neuroimaging studies of PTSD explained some of what Terr proposed, showing decreased activity in Broca's area (an area relevant to communicating experiences into language) and increased activation of the right hemisphere during traumatic recall (van der Kolk et al., 1996). These studies provided much of the initial understanding of why traumatized individuals find it difficult to use language to express what is being experienced, especially when emotionally aroused. Eventually, the term *speechless terror* (van der Kolk, 2000)—an inability to communicate that often occurs along with numbness, shock, and confusion—became a way of explaining the impact of trauma on verbalization in many individuals.

Telling Has Its Own Schedule

During many years of witnessing how children and adults express their experiences through the arts and storytelling, I have found that trauma narratives are never communicated in a specific way or on a predictable schedule. In the case of Arthur, he decided to come forward to speak to me about sexual assault when perpetrator priests began to be put on trial for their crimes and members of his religious community also came forward to seek help. Remaining silent works for a while until something in the environment or relationships triggers sensations or reactions. In play therapy, therapists speak about "taking cues from the child" and "following the child's lead." These principles also apply to work with adolescents and adults, especially in cases where physical or sexual assault or experiences of war or terrorism have occurred.

Artist Kalman Aron's story illustrates how time can play a dramatic role in trauma narratives. Decades before he spoke openly about what he saw during the Holocaust, Aron painted images related to his experiences of internment at seven Nazi camps. Because giving a Jew drawing or writing materials was often forbidden, German troops who wanted a portrait hid Aron in a locked barrack while he drew them or produced a likeness from a photograph. In return for these drawings, he was given food and was pulled out of doing hard labor; thus, by producing artwork for his captors, he was able to survive the camps.

Aron immigrated to Los Angeles in 1949 and continued to draw and paint, building his career. Until 1994, when he was interviewed by the University of Southern California Shoah Foundation about his experiences in the Nazi camps, he rarely talked about what he had seen or experienced. However, during the decades of silence, he created numerous artworks depicting his memories of those times, including self-portraits of himself in forced marches and images of fellow inmates held at Buchenwald and many other camps. In a sense, each is a visual narrative that communicates different horrific experiences lived by the artist.

One of Aron's most famous pastel drawings, "Mother and Child," sat in his studio for almost 60 years because he found he could not part with it. The drawing was created in 1951 on an oversized bedsheet and depicts a scene he witnessed numerous times in the camps where mothers tightly clutched their children as if to protect them from harm or abuse. Aron recalled that when he worked on the drawing, "I wasn't feeling. I saw it happening" (in Arom, 2017); he was unable to put into words the trauma he experienced. Later, during his interview with the Shoah Foundation, he confessed to the interviewer, also a Holocaust survivor, that while he could not speak about the content of his art for many years, he finally could talk about it, albeit with intense emotion and trepidation.

Not all individuals will respond in the way Aron did, remaining silent for decades about atrocities endured. Under different circumstances, Aron may have told his story sooner. By expressing himself through drawing, however, he did succeed in communicating something of his experiences that he was not able to put into words for decades. In expressive arts, this phenomenon occurs with clients who are able to convey implicit memories through movement, sound, enactment, or images without actually verbally articulating a specific story. In some cases, this may be due to the speechless state described in the previous section. In my experience, with the help of the therapist, a language-based coherent narrative will eventually emerge. But until then, the sensory-based expression through image, movement, sound, or enactment is all that is available for many individuals. This is often the only way to convey the body's experience of trauma, which is essential to eventually constructing and verbalizing a reparative story for "what happened."

EXPRESSIVE ARTS AS NONLINGUISTIC NARRATIVE

Most forms of trauma intervention still tend to focus on verbal expression of narratives through language. Trauma-focused cognitive-behavioral therapy (TF-CBT; Cohen et al., 2017), a well-known approach, emphasizes verbal expression of narratives as a way to help individuals make sense of experiences and as a form of gradual exposure to painful memories. The premise of TF-CBT and similar techniques is that, without offering the opportunity to communicate these narratives, memories will remain unorganized and painful. Though effective, in my experience TF-CBT does not make complete sense when it comes to expressing trauma narratives, particularly in cases of developmental or complex trauma. Changing thoughts and behavior do not consistently address the deeper somatosensory and affective layers of implicit memory that most people who have had developmental or complex trauma bring to treatment.

Earlier in this book, I outlined the four broad areas of reparation that expressive arts specifically address, one of them being the function of storytelling. Technically, storytelling is simply the social and cultural activity of sharing narratives. It usually refers to the oral communication of stories and sometimes to various ways of conveying them through theater or improvisation. Sharing stories is not an inconsequential act, whether as part of psychotherapy or within families and communities. It can correlate to decreased anxiety, connection with others, and an increased sense of self-efficacy (Fivush, Sales, & Bohanek, 2008). In expressive arts therapy, the visual arts, creative writing, and dramatic enactment are naturally conducive to storytelling, particularly declarative recollections of events as coherent narratives. But play, music, and dance also reveal stories through movement, sound, and rhythm. They convey the somatosensory nature of stories because of the nonlinguistic nature of these forms of arts expression. This implicit, embodied narrative that is at the core of arts-based work goes beyond the limits of language when we consider communication of traumatic events and the body's memories.

Levine (2015) notes that "the most salient of our memories are imbued with sensations and feelings, whether good or bad, joyful or sad, angry or content" (p. 6). Tapping into those sensory layers of communication permits natural relaxation of the mind's control and a deeper level of implicit experience to emerge that actually enhances verbal communication (Malchiodi, 2003, 2019). Jung (1989) may have intuited how this process works when he recounted his story of embodied creativity, imagination, and play in *Memories, Dreams, Reflections*. During a time of personal distress during his adulthood, Jung purposively decided to play and create as if he were an 11-year-old boy again. He used stones, mud, and other materials to build an entire village on the shore of a lake near his home. It was a conscious attempt to recover the creativity he believed he had as a child.

> I went on with my building game after the noon meal every day, whenever the weather permitted. As soon as I was through eating, I began playing, and continued to do so until the patients arrived; and if I finished with my work early enough in the evening, I went back to building. In the course of this activity, my thoughts clarified, and I was able to grasp the fantasies whose presence in myself I dimly felt. Naturally, I thought about the significance of what I was doing and asked myself: "Now, really, what are you about? You are building a small town, and doing it as if it were a rite?" I had no answer to my question, only the inner certainty that I was on the way to discovering my own myth. For the building game was only the beginning. It released a stream of fantasies which I later carefully wrote down. (pp. 174–175)

Jung understood how critical it was to engage in this type of action-oriented expression, and this experience became a turning point in how he viewed his life and work. His observations reflect much of the bottom-up expressive arts process that begins with sensory-based experiences and can be used to generate stories in nonlinguistic ways. Damasio (1999), however, explains the phenomenon through the lens of neuroscience. He articulates how any type of storytelling is a nonlinguistic process that is the result of the brain's innate tendency to categorize, choose, and integrate what we encounter when we engage with our environment. According to Damasio, storytelling begins nonverbally when we try to create a coherent image of "lived moments" within either the environment or our internalized memories. This is where we encounter the "feeling of what happens" and map these experiences in our right hemisphere, resulting in embodied implicit memories. "Telling stories precedes language, since it is, in fact a condition of language, and it is based not just in the cerebral cortex but elsewhere in the brain and in the right hemisphere as well as the left. . . . The brain naturally weaves wordless stories about what happens to an organism immersed in an environment" (Damasio, 1999, p. 189).

Similarly, McGilchrist (2009) proposes that the two brain hemispheres "collaborate and inhibit each other." In the simplest sense, one side (left) provides details and makes orderly sense of experiences, while the other side (right) provides the overall context. In storytelling, the hemispheres rely on each other to perform tasks that neither could do alone. To bring the implicit, embodied experiences into language, the left hemisphere sorts it out through words to represent these experiences. Words and embodiment come together through integration of the left- and right-hemisphere processes, incorporating tone, ambiguity, facial expressions, and metaphor with language-based narratives.

Considering these explanations for how the brain forms and tells stories, implicit narratives may be just as important as language-based narratives because they contribute the necessary elements that will eventually create coherent linguistic stories. In the case of play, for example, when verbal narratives fail to bring about reparation and resolution, it is important to help individuals get in touch with the body's perception of experiences that may be missing. Kestly (2014) proposes that in order to accomplish this, a more circular process of moving individuals from right- to left- to right-brain experiences is necessary. I see this progression as not just "back and forth" from right brain to left brain, but also as complementing the bottom-up or top-down process found in the ETC (see Chapter 3). In most cases, expressive arts begin with somatosensory and affective communication, with a goal of moving the individual toward cognitive processes that involve verbal storytelling while moving back and forth from right brain to left brain as Kestly notes. For those individuals who are caught in verbal narratives, this process may also be top-down in some cases. Because of the landslide of sensations, it can actually feel safer for some people to begin with language and work toward incorporating and integrating sensory-based experiences within narratives. This may underscore why two expressive arts processes—drawing and creative writing—are helpful when it comes to communicating narratives.

BEGINNING WITH SOMATOSENSORY NARRATIVES

For many years, I explored a structured sequence of drawing interventions with children and adults who experienced acute or multiple traumas. Over time I did not feel this was the best approach, particularly for those survivors whose stories were quite toxic, left them frozen and numb, or reinforced uncomfortable reactions. Some of them have developed drawing protocols based on principles of *memory reconsolidation* by calling forth old events through art expressions. The intention is to modify and eventually extinguish memories of trauma through additional drawings that tap resources and encourage individuals to depict images of more positive experiences (Hass-Cohen, Bokoch, Findlay, & Witting, 2018). In my experience, this approach tends to focus on thoughts rather than feelings and sensations and does not address the needs of traumatized individuals for safety, self-regulation, and body-based experiences because of the cognitive nature of drawing.

There is a place for image-based expression of traumatic events, but a structured series of drawings is not always the best fit for each individual who comes to treatment. While art expression has the advantage of capitalizing on visual images as a form of storytelling, it has limited use in expressing all the experiences that most traumatized individuals carry in their bodies that communicate the implicit stories of "what happened."

With increased understanding of the embodied nature of trauma, working with trauma narratives often calls for a multimodal approach, including the pacing and communication of trauma memories.

Levine's (1997) now famous story about his encounter with Nancy (see Chapter 5, pp. 133–134), a woman with numerous physical complaints who was referred to him, explains how memories often emerge from sensory-based, embodied recollections. At one point in the session with Levine, Nancy imagined herself running from a tiger, actually feeling herself climbing to a rock to escape the animal chasing her. From that vantage point, she could see the tiger, but she felt safe from harm. What suddenly followed was a memory of herself when she was 4 years old, and she was being sedated for a tonsillectomy. She saw herself being held down by medical personnel, who forced her to wear a mask. Nancy realized that she had indeed been trying to escape something, but she was immobilized by the doctor and nurses for surgery and hadn't been able to run away. Her overwhelming sense of helplessness and fear related to this early event were at the core of her trauma, and once these body-based sensations were experienced and released, her physical symptoms began to dissipate over time. In brief, working with the body's sense of trauma led to the recollection of a narrative that was a source of Nancy's distress.

Two personal experiences informed my understanding of how significant implicit and embodied memories of trauma can be in terms of communicating and even stimulating narratives. My first awakening about the somatosensory nature of trauma memory occurred during a dance therapy course while I was warming up for a group activity. At one point in the movement sequence, I experienced an intense pain in my right hand and arm that felt like nothing I had ever experienced in the past. I suddenly was flooded with a memory from adolescence about the loss of an older friend who was killed in combat in Vietnam. To my surprise, I started to cry spontaneously while the pain slowly dissipated from my arm. My friend's death was particularly difficult for me because I never saw him after he was drafted and sent overseas. I never had the opportunity to find closure following the loss, and I became angry about what I believed was a senseless loss of life in a war in which he never believed. I later shared this memory with the instructor, and as I did so, I also remembered the moment when I learned about my friend's death as a teenager. Distraught and crying, I went into the bathroom of my childhood home and sat on the floor, pounding my right hand against the tub. To this day, I don't know why those particular movements were associated with this memory, but I do know that they stimulated the recollection. It took more than 10 years for this memory to resurface, and at the time, it surprised me that it emerged through such a simple body-based experience.

A few years later when I was a guest lecturer at a symposium that brought together Holocaust survivors from Nazi death camps, I witnessed another remarkable example of how the body remembers, even decades after an event. The symposium included a presentation of the Nazi propaganda film *Brundibar* and several other films that children were forced to participate in while living at the Theresienstadt concentration camp. *Brundibar* is a well-known children's opera, eventually made famous by the children's performance for the Red Cross that came to visit and inspect camp living conditions. A female survivor of that camp and later Auschwitz recognized herself as one of the performers in another film showing a group of children dancing. When she spotted herself, she spontaneously got up from her seat and stood in front of herself on the film, replicating the dance she had performed as a young child while she faced the audience. The moment was so profound that I started to sob as I watched her performance in front of the film, witnessing what it must have been like to be a child forced to comply under threat of assault and murder. But I was equally stunned to see that her body remembered exactly how to perform the dance that she had performed almost 60 years ago. While her actions could be defined as a form of procedural memory, they also demonstrated a powerful implicit experience of performing for one's subjugators during extreme adverse and horrifying conditions. After she finished her performance and the film ended, she was flooded with memories of the camps and the brutality of the Nazi soldiers, and for the first time she spoke to the audience about the many children and adults who died or were murdered.

Expressive arts therapists whose core training focuses on dance and movement have provided numerous accounts of how the body expresses a narrative long before a story can be articulated with words. Amber Elizabeth Gray (2015) offers a clinical example that addresses the somatic experience of trauma and how to work with embodied experiences to support the eventual exploration of trauma narratives. Gray describes a woman, a survivor of war in Sierra Leone who had been tortured during three different detainments during the conflict and experienced the disappearance of her parents. When asked to tell the details of her story, the woman was unable to speak, crying uncontrollably. Eventually, by encouraging a positive memory involving the act of fetching water, they co-created other movements, including bathing an imagined baby and pounding millet. Gray also taught the woman how to wave, honk a horn, and rock a baby; as a result, they a co-constructed a dance with these movements. One day after they rehearsed their shared dance, the woman broke down and cried "for all I have lost." At that point, she began to spontaneously tell Gray about what happened to her family and her village and how she had been held in a rape camp for several weeks. While she still experienced freeze responses because of her trauma memories, she was able to communicate enough information to testify for an asylum claim. When Gray asked why she was finally able to speak about what happened, the woman responded, "You let me tell my story in a way I love, in dance. I felt safe to say some of the bad parts of my story after that" (p. 4).

Gray's example makes several important points about somatosensory memory. First, when terror leaves one speechless, one or more forms of expressive arts may be key to communication of narratives in the earliest stages of psychotherapy. Second, Gray demonstrates that it is essential to support and rehearse positive and strength-based experiences that reinforce a sense of well-being in the body. Movement and dramatic enactment can also help to interrupt the freeze response common to survivors who find it extremely painful and often impossible to revisit trauma memories. Using a mode for communication that was culture-relevant and resonant—in this case, dance and enactment— is also fundamental to trauma-informed practice. Third, when looking at this example through the lens of the ETC, it makes sense for many individuals to begin with work on the sensory/kinesthetic level rather than talking or even "drawing what happened," another form of cognitive activity.

Use of expressive arts as a form of communication of trauma narratives has one final advantage as well as one caution. Using art, sound, music making, movement, or enactment to recapitulate a felt sense or memories of events can be a form of re-exposure. While arts-based expression can help a person gain some distance from memories, it also can be negatively impactful if it brings up uncomfortable sensations and disturbing images too quickly and if safety and regulatory practices are not firmly in place. Expressive arts experiences will swiftly re-create implicit components of trauma narratives; it is therefore essential to have necessary regulatory, safety, and grounding procedures always in place as an initial foundation.

The following case illustrates how body-based narratives express unresolved trauma in powerful ways. It also illustrates how various expressive arts often contribute different facets of the overall narrative and how arts-based approaches can unpack both implicit and explicit stories related to trauma over time.

Case Example. Katja: The Body Tells the Story

Katja, a 28-year-old soldier recently returned from combat in the Middle East, was referred to me for help with her severe hyperactivation due to post-traumatic stress. She had witnessed the death of another soldier killed by an improvised explosive device (IED) while on a routine surveillance mission. She had been walking about 30 yards behind him when the explosion occurred. Katja was thrown to the ground, unconscious for a time, but wakened to see medical personnel dragging away the remains of her friend.

Katja was initially referred to me because she felt she was not making progress in cognitive-behavioral therapy or with medications that left her depressed and numb. She had also heard from another soldier that I didn't necessarily make people "talk about what happened," and so she told her physician that she would "give it a try." While she only had minor injuries and no head trauma, she told me in our initial session, "I think that explosion really fucked up my head in other ways." Several months later when Katja was back in the United States and stationed at a local army base, she began to have headaches unrelated to any injury. She also became anxious when anyone, including friends, came closer than a few feet from her. This sensation was compounded by overpowering feelings of anger and uncontrollable panic that she self-medicated with binge drinking and occasionally marijuana. Katja reported that she now often had long periods of emotional numbness, staring at the television in her apartment with no sense of how much time was passing.

As I note in Chapter 4, I generally begin the first session with specific questions to provide an initial sense of safety and control of the environment: "Where in the room would you like to sit, and where would you like me to sit?" "How close or far away would you like to sit in relation to me?" "Do you mind if we face each other, or would you like some other seating arrangement?" These questions are vital to understanding how individuals perceive their surroundings and how comfortable they are in proximity to me. Katja decided on a chair across the room where she could keep an eye on the doorway. This is a position many soldiers in my practice chose, not necessarily for their own safety, but to defend others from danger as part of their training. Like many of her military peers, it was apparent that Katja was in excellent physical shape. But like many individuals who are extremely fit for survival in combat, Katja was not at all relaxed in her body. While she sat far across the room from me, she was tense and hyperalert; she seemed frozen in an uncomfortable position, with her shoulders raised, neck strained, and breathing shallow and rapid.

In the first session, I introduced Katja to ways to express nonverbal embodied experiences and sensations. These types of experiences can be particularly helpful to people who are out of touch with the distress their bodies are holding. Since Katja indicated that she liked to draw, I asked her if she could show me through mark-making and colors, shapes, and lines what her sense of her body was in the here-and-now. She quickly chose a set of colored pencils from the art supplies and drew a detailed three-dimensional, opaque, brown box that she promptly titled "One Uptight UPS Package" (Figure 8.2). While I do not make any immediate interpretations of art expression, Katja's drawing seemed to reflect her body's tenseness and rigid posture. My impression was that she was indeed a tightly sealed box that had contents that would not be easily revealed.

While Katja preferred drawing to initially communicate with me, with most individuals I generally start with some sort of movement that includes mirroring to establish attunement through co-regulation. I also gently try to demonstrate and encourage playfulness to build the relationship in early sessions. Depending on the individual, this includes bilateral drawing to music, experimenting with sound and rhythm, pretending through drama or role play, and moving in space. Through building a sense of play between us, an implicit trust begins to develop and a reparative relationship

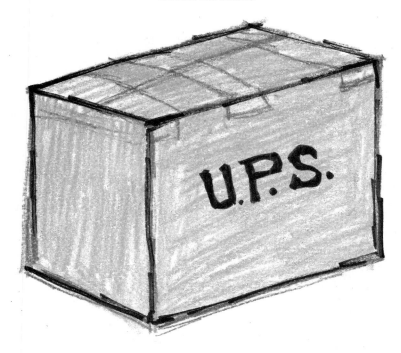

FIGURE 8.2. "One Uptight UPS Package" by Katja. From the collection of Cathy A. Malchiodi (not to be reproduced without permission from the author).

starts to form, allowing any narrative to eventually safely emerge through expressive approaches. Establishing a relationship with Katja depended on building her trust in opening up her UPS box in order to understand and work with what might be inside it.

Like other traumatized adults, playfulness was initially a challenge for Katja. She also gave me a clear message that maintaining distance was a key issue during our first session. Like Tory in Chapter 4, I introduced a prop—in this case, a giant stretchy band—to create a sense of connection while allowing for distance and control. To start, both Katja and I looped the giant stretchy band around our torsos, and I simply mirrored her movements while she kept a safe distance from me. She could easily control our proximity to each other as she experienced pulling against me while having a sense of joining with me. This became a way to safely begin to play during sessions, offering action-oriented possibilities for resistance, mirroring, and relating in a way that Katja completely determined.

As Katja started to experiment more with moving toward and away from me, I helped her to identify these changes by calling attention to them in the moment. For people who either avoid or are unconscious of what the body is telling them, talking begins the process of moving from the body's sensations to higher levels of the brain. For example, if I noticed her moving away, I simply wondered out loud, "How far do you need to move away to feel more at ease with me?" Or, "I felt you pull me by surprise. How did it feel to do that?" Katja did not always have an answer for these questions, but her eye contact and gestures clearly communicated that she was engaging with me. In this way, we began a series of nonverbal conversations through movements and eventually through talking about the space between us and how space affected her body's reactions in relation to other people in her life.

In order to support prop-enhanced movement, I also introduced music as an anchor and to help Katja self-regulate. As previously discussed, auditory cues can help anchor people in the moment and support the developing connection between therapist and client through rhythm and energy. While movement can be introduced without it, music establishes a mood—it can be used to calm and regulate, or it can bring a sense of vitality and energy into people's bodies. In the first few sessions, I started with relaxing instrumental pieces played on an iPad while we used the stretchy band. As Katja's relationship with me became more playful over time, as I did with all my clients, I asked for her input on the musical selections for movement. Some of her favorites were "Ain't No Mountain High Enough" and Motown hits that brought back positive sensory memories during less distressing times.

These initial sessions slowly helped establish a foundation for Katja to not only begin to identify pleasant sensations, but also to start to reinhabit her body in less stressful ways. But this process was not instantaneous; it took several months to work through Katja's dissociative reactions and anxiety about proximity to others. We continued to explore more of her symptoms through drawing, including movement as a regular part of the psychotherapeutic relationship. Katja took these moments into situations between sessions, gradually replacing anxiety with what I call "good rhythms" to help her "not lose it" when panicked.

Unpacking a Somatosensory Narrative

Katja's symptoms noticeably abated a bit over time, including the frequency of her drinking. She also reported that she no longer used marijuana. But she still struggled with occasional severe anxiety and outbursts of anger. Katja did notice that she was beginning to feel more comfortable when she came in close proximity to others and to me during our sessions. At one session, she decided it was finally possible for me to sit directly across from her to try some mirrored movements together. Because sharing such a close space was an indication of real progress, I mentioned it out loud. But just as we started to mirror each other's simple movements and gestures, Katja suddenly stopped and told me that she felt a distressing tension throughout her upper body. "I'm glad you noticed that," I said. "Let's start with some shoulder stretches and neck rolls instead."

Katja agreed, but as soon as we started, she reached for her neck with both hands and began to massage it vigorously. While this initially seemed like a form of self-soothing, I was alarmed to see her shoulders tense upward and her breathing become shallow and accelerated. Through several grounding techniques we had previously practiced, I quickly helped Katja self-regulate. But her dramatic reaction indicated that something important was going on that we needed to explore.

I asked Katja if she felt comfortable showing me on a body outline what she was experiencing when her hands had rubbed her neck so vigorously. She was familiar with the body outline process because she had used it several times before as a warm-up activity for other expressive arts experiences. Katja used a colored pencil to re-create the "One Uptight UPS Package" (Figure 8.2) from the initial session, placing it on the neck and shoulders on the outline.

Fortunately, we had a series of self-regulatory practices in place, including anchoring movements and music because it was time to "unpack" the contents of Katja's box. Many practitioners might ask, "Why didn't you unpack the box with Katja earlier in treatment?" This was certainly a possibility, but I prefer to let individuals pace their disclosures when possible and always after we have sufficient time to practice grounding, anchoring, and safety procedures. Most of all, having a relatively secure relationship in place is essential. In Katja's case, we were also able to practice and integrate EMDR over several sessions, and it became part of safety and grounding experiences earlier in treatment.

As we sat across from each other and looked at the drawing, I asked Katja to slowly imagine opening that box. She closed her eyes for a moment, and when she opened them, she began to slowly tell me about the contents. I interspersed EMDR at critical intervals, stopping at intervals to do focused line drawings of her breathing as a grounding technique along the way. While some soldiers choose not to talk while processing traumatic memories in this way, Katja was ready to verbally share specific details. The focus of the session was on Katja's experiences, but it is important to note that a psychotherapist also experiences somatosensory narratives during client disclosures. In this case, what Katja began to describe caused my stomach to clench and my shoulders and torso to become tense. She quietly stated that on several occasions she had been choked by fellow soldiers in her unit when they sexually assaulted her. Like many female military personnel, she had never reported them or told anyone about the assaults, hoping the memories and sensations would "just go away." Katja sobbed as she shared these traumatic moments; I was close to tears myself in listening to these stories of rape and assault of this young woman. However, this juncture in treatment would not have been possible without first building a foundation for regulation through movement and other expressive arts that helped Katja to gradually communicate her body's implicit experiences of traumatic stress.

I continued to intersperse EMDR and drawing during the session and to check in with Katja about what she was feeling in her body. At one point, she said that she felt compelled to massage her neck area again. "What do you sense now?" I asked. Rather than answering, Katja again picked up a colored pencil and drew a simple sketch of a woman wearing a T-shirt and khaki pants, facing outward with intense eyes and a powerful stance. "I was suddenly thinking I'm in boot camp again," she said after a time. "I was as strong as any of them. I could make anyone back off. But this time it wasn't fair. I was outnumbered. It wasn't my fucking fault." Katja's body was shaking, but she became almost entirely relaxed in her chair very quickly after this disclosure.

When I first met Katja, I initially suspected that she had experienced interpersonal violence at some point in her life, even though she did not disclose these assaults during intake to either her doctor or to me when I conducted a brief trauma history during the first session. Sexual assault of female soldiers is unfortunately common in the military, and I had worked with several individuals who had endured similar experiences. In subsequent sessions, we would revisit the memories of the assaults and Katja's somatosensory experiences of distress. These sessions became the turning point that allowed us to now focus on recovering her confidence in herself and her physical capabilities to meet challenges. Through expressing herself in movement, music, and art, Katja began to feel a change in her body and mind that helped her begin to release the shame she felt in being unable to defend herself in an indefensible situation.

Expressing the events associated with multiple sexual assaults was necessary to Katja's eventual recovery. But this particular disclosure did not contain all the elements of what she endured and overcame throughout our work together. Katja's trauma narratives included more than witnessing a fellow soldier's death and sexual assaults by fellow soldiers. She also eventually expressed other contextual elements that framed her perceptions of trauma. One involved Katja's sense that she was experiencing moral injury. *Moral injury* refers to personal harm to an individual's moral conscience that often results in psychological, social, cultural, and/or spiritual shame. While by definition moral injury is not pathology, it is relevant to the trauma-informed principle that a normal human response to a traumatic event may include shame, guilt, humiliation, indignity, and dishonor. In Katja's view, she experienced an egregious transgression by peers who betrayed her by forcibly raping her. She also indicated that she would have disclosed the sexual assaults when they occurred, but like many female soldiers she felt she could not "trust the system." Katja explained to me, "I felt like the system was raping me all over again." This is a common observation I have heard from many female soldiers who have endured similar interpersonal violence from their peers. In sum, while expressive arts provide opportunities to communicate multiple implicit and explicit narratives, reducing reparation to a few target memories is not only inadequate, but may also overlook the individual's humanity as a trauma survivor.

DRAWINGS AS NARRATIVES

Johnson (Johnson, Lahad, & Gray, 2009) proposed that of all the individual creative arts therapies, art therapy might have a unique role in gaining access to imagery related to trauma narratives. This observation was based on the early work of van der Kolk and the use of patient art expressions by Greenberg and van der Kolk (1987). The art therapy community also picked up on the idea that encoding of traumatic memories may be a visual process for many individuals, and thus art expression could offer a means to bring these memories and associated stories to consciousness.

Out of all the arts-based possibilities for telling stories, client-generated drawings are probably the most easily integrated into psychotherapy by most practitioners. Art expression is not only useful with children; most adults I have worked with have used drawing to communicate parts of traumatic experiences that are not easily expressed with words. Because drawing is often directly related to storytelling through images, it may more effectively tap declarative memories, particularly timelines of events. However, the sensory nature of drawing materials (color, size, smell, or texture) can bring out episodic and implicit memories as well. Recall the story of the group of adults who experienced sexual abuse as children described in Chapter 5. In that case, simply introducing new boxes of crayons stimulated disclosure of numerous memories related to traumatic events related to abuse and neglect due to the tactile, visual, and olfactory characteristics of the media. While each individual in that group had experienced sexual abuse as a child, many "feeder memories" (Shapiro, 2018) emerged that were related to the traumatic events and early childhood.

To my knowledge, Pynoos and Eth (1986) first introduced the idea that a structured interview that includes drawing and talking about what happened might play a role in trauma recovery in their work with child witnesses to homicide. Their protocol was used with over 200 children in a variety of clinical settings and included homicide, suicide, rape, accidental death, kidnapping, and school violence. It involved three general stages: a drawing, storytelling, and discussion of the actual traumatic situation. The interview was designed to enable the practitioner to "gain insight into the child's understanding of the event and to characterize the behavioral and emotional responses in order to provide specific professional support to the child soon after the trauma" (Pynoos & Eth, 1986, p. 306) and required only one session to complete. The researchers conceptualized a method for acute consultation to assist the child in functioning immediately following a psychologically traumatic event. The method was based on the premise that the mode of witnessing violence is largely visual; thus, drawing might be the most appropriate vehicle for expression. This hypothesis was based on Piaget and Inhelder (1969), who observed that drawing should be considered as being "halfway between symbolic play and the mental image" (p. 54). Although the interview had a specific structure, it also allowed therapists to follow the child's lead and cues and to address feelings and disclosures as necessary. Many years later, Steele and Raider (2001) expanded this interview to include a series of drawings focusing on not only the incident, but also "before" and "after" the event witnessed to assure child participants that the incident was no longer happening.

The single-session interview developed by Pynoos and Eth was an important contribution to understanding the role of trauma narratives in psychotherapy for several reasons. In particular, their choice of a free drawing to begin a structured interview showed how image-making might serve as a stimulus for verbalization when words might be difficult or unavailable. In subsequent years, several studies demonstrated that there is indeed a connection between drawing and an increase in verbal communication (Gross & Haynes, 1998; Lev-Weisel & Liraz, 2007). The introduction of drawings also introduced the idea that visual expression might be a useful reference point for discussion throughout a session, depending on the child's interest or ability to use it to describe a story about the traumatic event.

In adapting this one-session drawing protocol in my early work with child witnesses of domestic violence, two other possible advantages emerged. One was the importance of initiating sensory activity (drawing) to counteract the passivity often experienced as the result of a traumatic event. The introduction of drawing could possibly help to reverse the sense of helplessness, support relationship, and even enhance mastery to some extent (Malchiodi, 1998). Another advantage was, with the help of the therapist, children can begin the process of reframing their perspective from passive witness to a more empowered stance. Many of these same observations have been made in studies with adults. For example, Harel-Shalev, Huss, Daphna-Tekoah, and Cwikel (2017) studied drawings created by Israeli women who served in the military to see if their images helped them to communicate elements that were not verbalized, including undisclosed stress responses. They specifically chose drawings not only to help participants communicate distressing narratives they might not otherwise share, but also to convey implicit and embodied stories, "vividly expressed, without mediation" (p. 509) and to provide a sense of empowerment through an action-oriented tasks.

RE-ENACTMENT OF TRAUMA NARRATIVES THROUGH ART AND PLAY

Children commonly express stories they cannot communicate with words not only through drawings but also through play. *Post-traumatic play* is a term now used to describe both the recurrent memories and the re-enactment common to children who are distressed by single incidents or multiple traumatic events. In "Forbidden Games: Post-Traumatic Child's

Play," Terr (1981) first used the term to describe the play activity of children who have experienced traumatic events, but not the resolution of emotions associated with those events. In studying a small group of children who had experienced different traumatic events, she concluded that repetition of play-based narratives with toys, through enactments or in drawings, was a distinctly prominent feature. Terr explained:

> The play of traumatized youngsters is far less elaborate than the imaginative play of nontraumatized children. In post-traumatic play there is simple repetition of the experience or simple defensive elaboration, such as identification with the aggressor, undoing, and passive into active defenses. . . . There is little opportunity for variety; the traumatic situation was real and ended badly (overwhelming the child's ability to cope). The play creates anxiety, because it almost literally recreates the traumatic event. The more the play fails, the more anxiety is generated because the child perceives that he/she cannot find effective mechanisms to deal with the trauma even in retrospect. (pp. 746, 757)

In contrast to normal play, which leads to pleasure, satisfying expression, problem solving, and learning, post-traumatic play is often anxiety-ridden and constricted, repetitive, rigid, and without resolution. Post-traumatic play fails to allay distress in that it attempts to deal with an actual external event rather than an internal experience.

I first learned the basics of trauma memory and post-traumatic art and play through Terr's (1981, 1990) research on the stories that child survivors of the Chowchilla kidnapping told and later from Gil (2006). Both Terr and Gil found that each child's story was idiosyncratic—what might be horrifying for one child was not disruptive for another. Within Terr's theory of post-traumatic play, repetitions of similar content occurred, but each repetition of events and memories was special to the individual. As mentioned previously, Gil (2016, 2017) expanded Terr's original concept, making an important delineation between what she defined as "stagnant post-traumatic play" and "dynamic post-traumatic play" (Table 8.1). Stagnant post-traumatic play may leave a child retraumatized, dissociative, hyperaroused, or feeling hopeless and helpless. In contrast, children who engage in dynamic post-traumatic play are less rigid, interact more freely with the therapist, take a more active role on their own behalf, and are generally more emotionally relieved after expressing narratives through play activities. Their play leads to more empowering narratives and repair of trauma reactions. Gil (2017) takes these definitions a bit further by stating, "I view posttraumatic play as a type of play . . . that can be categorized more accurately as a form of child resilience" (p. 4). Thus, these narratives are efforts to manage traumatic memories and as such, fit into the conceptual framework of trauma-informed practice.

The differences in the two types of play Gil describes can be subtle but are discernible in children's play and art expression, with careful

TABLE 8.1. Differences between Dynamic and Stagnant Post-Traumatic Play

Dynamic post-traumatic play	Stagnant post-traumatic play
• Affect becomes available.	• Affect remains constricted.
• Physical fluidity becomes evident.	• Physical constriction remains.
• Interactions with play becomes varied.	• Interactions with play remain limited.
• Interactions with clinician become varied.	• Interactions with clinician remain limited.
• Play changes or new elements are added.	• Play stays precisely the same.
• Play occurs in different locations.	• Play is conducted in the same spot.
• Play includes new objects.	• Play is limited to specific objects.
• Themes differ or expand.	• Themes remain constant.
• Outcomes differ, and healthier, more adaptive responses emerge.	• Outcomes remain fixed and nonadaptive.
• Rigidity of play loosens over time.	• Play remains rigid.
• After-play behavior indicates release or fatigue.	• After-play behavior indicates constriction/tension.
• Out-of-session symptoms may remain unchanged or peak at first, but then decrease.	• Out-of-session symptoms are unchanged or increase.

Note. From Gil (2006, p. 160). Copyright © 2006 The Guilford Press. Reprinted by permission.

observation and experience. The point is that children whose narratives do not result in positive resolution signals that they may need more purposeful, direct intervention from the therapist. The following vignette provides an example of a child's stagnant post-traumatic art and strategies to redirect toxic narratives.

Case Example. Rosa

Rosa was 7 years old when she, her mother, and her younger brother arrived at a domestic violence shelter. Rosa's mother, Tasha, was only 15 years old when she gave birth to Rosa, at which time Rosa's biological father abandoned them. For the next 7 years Rosa lived in public housing in a large midwestern city in an environment dominated by drug abuse, neighborhood violence, and poverty. Tasha was also physically assaulted by several boyfriends whom she brought into the home. Reports from child protective services indicated that Rosa was sexually abused on several occasions, but the details of the incidents remained unclear. Social services and law enforcement documented numerous domestic violence events, and in one case, Rosa was a witness and a victim of physical brutality.

In the course of her talk, she shared some of the trauma-related challenges she faced as a child—grandfathers who died in refugee camps; a cousin who died because of inadequate health care; a friend who died in a plane crash because firetrucks did not have water; repressive governments that normalized a daily sense of fear; and times when food was rationed. Although these experiences were part of Adichie's narratives, she also emphasized that they were not the sum of her life story. In fact, there are resilience-relevant narratives (Chapter 9) that are not catastrophes and are just as important. In Adichie's view, even though Africa is often a land of crises ranging from violence to poverty and illness, there are always stories about joy, dignity, and hope.

Adichie delineates a core principle within the context of trauma-informed work—individuals bring multiple stories of disempowerment as well as empowerment to treatment, and these stories exist within a larger context. Most therapists understand that the people they see in treatment are composites of multiple stories. However, when it comes to trauma, many practitioners often believe that a particular target memory is essential to integration and recovery. In Rosa's case, her trauma narratives that included multiple adverse events became an overall life narrative rather than stories of discrete events. I was able to address the specific narrative Rosa presented through her drawings and introduced grounding and regulatory strategies in the short term. But to begin to identify and address her life narrative that included developmental trauma, disrupted attachment, and inconsistent parenting often requires long-term intervention that is inclusive of context. For example, caregiver functioning also impacts a child's post-traumatic adaptations and often is as significant as any traumatic event that is enacted through art or play. If I had been able to continue working with Rosa, helping her and Tasha to express and organize narratives within the context of their relationship would have been a next step in addressing Rosa's post-traumatic art, play, and stories. It is critical that Tasha or a significant caregiver eventually become involved in the treatment context in any effort to develop positive attachment and strengthen the relationship that had been compromised during many years of abuse and other adverse events.

WRITING AS A TOP-DOWN APPROACH TO NARRATIVE WORK

Although expressive arts open up multiple opportunities for bottom-up work, trauma stories can emerge from top-down, linguistic approaches found in the cognitive level of the ETC framework. For some individuals, starting with writing as a form of narrative is the most comfortable place to begin. I often become aware of when a client can benefit from this approach during initial sessions if someone brings in journals or even fragments of writing to share with me. While I read what they have entrusted with me, in most cases the writing is quite powerful and raw; reading it out loud would be emotionally overwhelming for them. However, the simple fact that they have decided to let me read it is important because it tells me that this is one way they feel comfortable with self-expression of what are often deeply painful experiences.

Pennebaker and Smyth (2016) have done the most extensive research on the value of writing in mediating emotional distress. They began by exploring whether or not a sampling of individuals had experienced a traumatic sexual experience before the age of 17. In one study, 15% of the participants indicated that they had—an unexpected but important finding. Pennebaker and Smyth also discovered that these individuals were also more likely than other participants to have physical health problems. That discovery led to subsequent studies to help understand this correlation and whether any specific type of intervention might be effective.

Pennebaker and Smyth (2016) eventually concluded that experiencing traumatic events could be related to poor health outcomes, specifically when traumatized individuals kept the trauma a secret. In order to understand how "telling about traumatic events" impacted health, they compared two volunteer groups of college-age students. One group was asked to write about something that troubled them emotionally. The second group was asked to write about a nonemotional topic, such as what they would be doing over the next few days. These groups engaged in these tasks for 15 minutes at a time for 4 consecutive days and were told that their writing was confidential and anonymous. The only other instructions they were given were as follows:

> I want you to write continuously about the most upsetting or traumatic experience of your entire life. Don't worry about grammar, spelling, or sentence structure. In your writing, I want you to discuss your deepest thoughts and feelings about the experience. You can write about anything you want. But whatever you choose, it should be something that has affected you very deeply. Ideally, it should be something you have not talked about with others in detail. It is critical, however, that you let yourself go and touch those deepest emotions and thoughts that you have. In other words, write about what happened and how you felt about it, and how you feel about it now. Finally, you can write on different traumas during each session or the same one over the entire study. Your choice of trauma for each session is entirely up to you. (Pennebaker & Smyth, 2016, pp. 16–17)

What Pennebaker and Smyth found was striking. Those students in the group who asked to write about emotions were much less likely to visit the university medical clinic over the next 6 months than the group that simply wrote about facts. Additional studies using data obtained from participants' blood samples found that those who engaged in the emotional writing task had more aggressive immune systems than the control group.

When Pennebaker and Smyth and others first began to study writing, it was thought that it might help individuals overcome emotional inhibition. People who suppressed a traumatic memory might find resolution in expressing themselves about their trauma through writing. While this may be true, there seem to be multiple mechanisms that yield benefits. For example, writing helps individuals organize thoughts and sensations into coherent narratives. In constructing stories in this way, many people break free of ruminating and mental cycling about traumatic events and thus are better able to regulate emotions. Also, when individuals open up through writing about trauma, they seem to be more able to talk with others about it. This may suggest that writing can reinforce the necessary social interaction that supports healing over time.

This research suggests that there are several things to consider when introducing writing about trauma-related experiences to individuals:

• *Timing.* Many of Pennebaker and Smyth's studies indicate that people who write about a traumatic event immediately after it occurs can feel worse, including showing elevated blood pressure and heart rate. Many possible reasons account for this outcome, including the fact that some individuals are not prepared to face deeply troubling experiences such as traumatic events. Pennebaker and Smyth (2016) recommend waiting a couple of months after a distressful experience before introducing writing.

• *Consistency.* Studies indicate that writing for a specified period of time each day, as well as writing nonstop without inhibition, is important. However, "more" may not be "better" in terms of amount of writing. Studies have concluded that people should not write about a horrible event for more than a couple of weeks.

• *Distancing.* The overall goal in writing about traumatic events is to gain psychological distance from these experiences. Pennebaker found that shortly after the terrorist attacks on September 11, 2001, public blogs communicated significantly more negative emotions and increased psychological distancing. While negative emotions in the blogs decreased to pre-attack baselines, the presence of psychological distancing remained elevated over the following several weeks. With this finding in mind, individuals who prefer language over other forms of communication may find that a writing-based approach helps them in ways that other expressive arts approaches do not. In particular, it may help some traumatized individuals see their situations more objectively, detach from memories, or construct reparative and coherent narratives.

GETTING PAST IMPASSES IN TRAUMA NARRATIVES

Katja and other individuals who have been subjected to interpersonal violence or even an extremely distressful event do not or cannot easily verbalize their implicit experiences or explicit memories of events. There are many reasons that individuals "clam up" during disclosure of distressful sensations or stories (Malchiodi & Crenshaw, 2017). The following strategies can help alleviate these impasses, including ways to use expressive arts as creative interventions during sessions.

Using Non-First-Person Language

As mentioned in previous chapters, using "non-first-person language" is one way to ease the distress of talking about sensations, feelings, or experiences for some individuals. Recent studies on "self-talk" provide some evidence for how psychotherapists should direct individuals to speak or write about what might be anxiety-producing experiences that emerge during expressive arts therapy. These studies indicate that non-first-person self-talk improves emotional regulation through self-distancing and reduces self-focus in the moment. Just to be clear, first-person talk involves using pronouns such as "I," "me," or "my." In contrast, non-first-person pronouns are "you," "it," or a name (including your own name). A good example of non-first-person positive self-talk would be "Keep going, Cathy, you are doing great. You have this" (something I repeatedly say to myself before facing an audience of 1,000 people to prevent stage fright). While athletes and others have applied non-first-person self-talk to enhance performance and confidence, variations of this type of talk may be effective in other situations as well, including those that involve painful memories or distressing events.

Two recent studies demonstrate how this simple strategy may help individuals to self-regulate and reduce stress when verbalizing difficult narratives. One study (Moser et al., 2017) indicates that referring to oneself in the third person may lead people to perceive themselves in ways that are more similar to how they think about or perceive others. In other words, this simple shift can help individuals get some psychological distance from stressful experiences and thus can be helpful in emotional regulation. A second study evaluated how brain activity (functional magnetic resonance imaging [FMRI]) differed in participants who reflected on distressing experiences using first- and third-person language (Kross et al., 2014). When using non-first-person language, participants showed less activity in the brain region related to distressing emotional memories when using third-person self-talk, indicating better emotional regulation. In both studies, researchers concluded that non-first-person talk generally improves heart rate variability and healthy vagal tone. This physical response is relevant to trauma intervention, positive attachment, and emotional regulation.

As previously noted, expressive arts easily support opportunities to shift perspectives through projection (shift from first-person to non-first-person communication) or what is often referred to as *refraction* (parallel communication). In other words, helping individuals safely distance themselves from the experience being conveyed is most important.

Starting a Conversation about the "Unusual"

Often therapists do not know where to start when they are talking to individuals about their drawings or expressions. When I am at a loss for where to start, I ask myself, "What seems unusual, emphasized, or important in this image [object, movement, sound, enactment]?" This observation can be used as a point of conversation and dialogue. While it can be particularly effective with preschool and school-age children who sometimes emphasize elements of their drawings through size or characteristics, it can be a way to begin a conversation with adults, too. The following example illustrates how a child's drawing with an unusual feature became an effective starting point for dialogue with the girl and led to details of an abusive situation in her home.

Case Example. Leah: Details of Sexual Abuse

Leah was an 8-year-old girl who was referred by child protective services for art and play therapy because of possible sexual abuse after her classroom teacher reported what she considered inappropriate sexual behavior at school. Her social worker suspected that Leah had been abused by a family member, but she was selectively mute, especially when asked "who hurt you" or "who touched you." Her parents were cooperative with protective services, but English was their second language and the social worker who handled the case did not feel that they really understood why child protective services was concerned about their daughter.

I was asked to work with Leah to see if she might provide additional information about what happened through art and play. Like many children within her age range, Leah depicted an X-ray view of her home with her in it that showed many details within her parents' two-story house. When I asked about the drawing, Leah eagerly explained that the house had two floors and pointed out that on the second floor there were several bedrooms and two bathrooms. On the first floor was a family room with a large television and a kitchen with what Leah said was a refrigerator. The refrigerator struck me as unusual and too large in comparison to the rest of the drawing's contents. The television also seemed quite prominent, but of course many families have large flat-screen TVs in their homes. At the start of the session, I asked Leah a couple of general questions about her picture. She politely responded to each of my queries but did not volunteer any stories beyond what I specifically asked her. I then pointed out the refrigerator that was so prominent in her drawing. Leah's whole composure began to change in that instant, as if I had finally recognized what was important to her in the picture. She told me at that point that everyone in the family went to that refrigerator before they left the house in the morning. Following Leah's lead and mention of the routine activity in the kitchen, I asked her if she could name the people who went to the refrigerator before they left the house each day and what they took out of it. Leah said her mother and father, who left the house first, took out milk and eggs for breakfast; her two older sisters, who went to high school, came to the kitchen next to make their lunches. When I asked who was left after that, she answered that there was an older brother who often overslept and was late for work. He rushed to the refrigerator to get a "red drink" (energy drink in a can) and left to catch a bus. Finally, when I asked, "So is anyone still at home besides you?" she quietly said that only she and her uncle, who was unemployed and stayed home to watch her.

Although it became obvious that Leah's uncle might indeed be the perpetrator, this first session led to additional art and play sessions that eventually confirmed that he was sexually assaulting her during the day after everyone else had left for work or school. As it turned out, the television in the drawing did play an important role in the eventual details of Leah's experiences. The uncle turned it on for her to watch cartoons while he assaulted her. I learned from Leah and her drawings and play activity that she "disappeared" (dissociated as an adaptive coping response) when her uncle was "hurting me." While her disclosure led to additional, long-term intervention, fortunately elements in Leah's initial drawing helped her to tell "what happened" with important details to help me and her protective service worker to intervene.

Redirecting the Trauma Narrative

In the television series *Mad Men,* lead character Don Draper says, "If you don't like what's being said, change the conversation." This quote reminds me of another common impasse in therapy—young clients who are stuck in a nonproductive narrative similar to stagnant post-traumatic play and cannot, for whatever reason, move on to a more hopeful, reparative story that leads to recovery. Although helping professionals unconditionally accept what individuals communicate during sessions, as Terr (1990) originally explained, there are situations when children in particular "get stuck" and cannot get past a particular story or memory while in treatment. In a positive sense, many of these children are not hesitant to talk and are actively engaged in communicating with their therapists but are really not getting any closer to resolving what is troubling them. In acute traumatic events, some may eventually resolve their feelings and distress, especially with the help of parents and caregivers. But in many cases, like the one below, a parent becomes concerned that a child is not making progress. The child is, in fact, experiencing emotional pain and may even become retraumatized by retelling a story over a series of sessions.

Case Example. Josh: Stuck in a Narrative

Josh, age 10, was referred to me by his dad, Neil, because of a car accident in which Josh's friend Tom, also 10 years old, was admitted to the hospital because of his injuries. Josh and his father sustained minor bruises but no serious injuries. The accident was the unfortunate result of a young woman who was distracted and ran a red light, hitting Neil's car. At Neil's request, I made several home visits, instead of office visits, to work with Josh and his father about the trauma. Before my first home visit, Neil reported to me that Josh was obsessed with repeating the story of the accident and had even re-created the car crash in drawings he made at school. His teacher confirmed that Josh had become very distracted since the accident and was unable to concentrate on class activities. Josh also worried incessantly about Tom, even though he visited his friend in the hospital and at home and understood that he was recovering and would return to school soon.

When I initially met with Josh, I told him that it was okay to talk about what happened and that I would like to learn more about his experiences. Josh recounted the accident in great detail and also described what happened when he and his father followed the ambulance with Tom in it to the hospital and other important events associated with the car crash. He even asked me if I wanted him to repeat the story or had any questions. As Neil reported to me by phone, Josh's retelling of the accident never left him relieved, but in fact made him more anxious and sometimes even breathless. Most importantly, the repetitive narration and drawings about the incident were increasing Josh's level of distress. In this case, it was important to consider ways to "change the conversation" without denying Josh the chance to tell his story and be heard.

In a subsequent meeting, I worked with Josh on his body's sensations related to his anxiety and fears by using "colors, shapes, and lines" to show me on body outlines where he had these experiences. We also practiced several routines to help him calm down while at school and before going to sleep at night. However, Josh continued to want to talk about the accident again and showed me "what happened" through several drawings about the major events during that day. I suggested to Josh that we ask his father to join us in the session if that was okay with him, explaining that I thought his father also might need to share in the storytelling because he, too, might be upset about what happened on that day. When Neil joined us, I explained that Josh and he shared an important story and that maybe it would help to make a special time to tell it and then, like placing a book on a bookshelf, to put it away until another time when it could be told again. Because Josh had created detailed drawings about the accident, those drawings would become part of the storytelling each time the story was told.

At this juncture, Josh, Neil, and I also co-created a ritual for the telling of the "accident story" between this session and the session next week. First, after the story was told, the drawings would be placed in a large envelope and put on a shelf (I pointed out one shelf that had books and magazines on it in the living room). The envelope would stay there until it was time to talk about what happened again, and Josh would have to ask his father to retrieve the envelope from the bookshelf and have his father participate in the storytelling with him each time. I suggested that at this point it did not matter how many times the story was told, but that the ritual of the storytelling (father and son together, retrieving the envelope, sitting down to look at the drawings and tell the story, placing the drawings back in the envelope and putting it back on the shelf) was important.

During the next few days, Neil and Josh followed the plan each night after dinner. When I arrived the next week for Josh's session, I again listened to the story and reviewed the drawings with him. But this time after the recounting of the accident, I asked him to tell me more about his friend, Tom, who was about to return to school, something that pleased Josh. In particular, I asked Josh if he could show me any photographs of himself and Tom together. As it turned out, there were quite a few photos to share because, as Josh said, "Tom and me hung out together a lot." I suggested that if it was okay with him and his father, we could add these photographs to the envelope for now and that perhaps he could make some new drawings at this session about some of things that he and Tom did together before the accident. In other words, I was actually asking him to create images of things when the accident "was not happening" and also to include photographs of the memories about the many positive times Josh and Tom experienced together. While a few more sessions were necessary to redirect Josh away from the dominant trauma narrative, he gradually became less focused on the story of the car accident. In part, his father's perseverance with reinforcing the limits of retelling the story and the storytelling ritual was extremely helpful. However, the integration of other experiences and events through images in the form of drawings and photos, along with storytelling, broadened the narrative to include the many positive things that Josh had in his life, especially with his friend Tom. The "conversation" then moved away from the accident to positive talk that included good memories and thoughts about the future.

In Josh's case, introducing another art medium would have been another way to change or redirect nonproductive narratives. Because Josh really enjoyed drawing and sharing what he created with me, I continued with it as the main form of expression. As previously mentioned, introducing a three-dimensional material like modeling clay or Play-Doh opens up possibilities for making adaptations to a story through malleable media and rearranging elements. New objects or entities such as helpers or first responders, for example, can be introduced to create different endings to stories or to play out themes of rescue, recovery, and self-efficacy. The sandtray provides another way to make images through arrangement of miniature figures that the child can easily move around and manipulate. Dramatic enactment (discussed in more detail in Chapters 9 and 10) with puppets or role play is another option. In brief, the therapist can suggest elements to add to a child's story, or the therapist can ask, "If you moved that figure over here, what would be different about the story you have told me?" The point is not only to allow children to retell their stories, but also to strategically invite them to redirect the story by the position or arrangement of objects in the sandtray or other media.

FAMILY NARRATIVES

Families pose an interesting challenge when it comes to trauma narratives. Over the years I have worked with numerous families who experienced a natural disaster; families who have a seriously or terminally ill child; and families with one or more adults or children who have experienced interpersonal violence. I often think about how I can help families to communicate family stories and particularly how they approach challenges or crises as part of the work on trauma. As in work with individuals, I also think about how to help them develop regulatory skills within the family and how to establish a sense of safety in their bodies before we begin to address any collective trauma through expressive arts. The same principles of getting people moving rather than allowing narratives to become frozen and stuck apply. I therefore try to introduce playfulness within the mix of coaxing narratives as soon as possible within the family's window of tolerance.

Rather than asking for a narrative about a specific trauma, I take a slightly different approach when working with families. Family groups generally include children of various ages, and any expressive arts process has to meet their developmental needs. But I also try to provide ways to safely express stories without directly focusing on what may be a story that the family feels they need to protect or are not ready to disclose.

In working with families, I try to use metaphors that help stimulate the imagination. While it is optimal to help them find their own metaphors, a traumatized family may not have the capacity to come up with one on their own. In most cases, however, if presented with one and given some support to explore it, most families construct meanings through a metaphoric theme. This is especially true if an action-oriented approach like expressive arts is part of the process. The goal is to provide an engaging and playful experience that allows for a sense of "controlling the narrative," even though, in most cases, some or all of the trauma story may emerge through arts-based expression.

Living Together on an Island

"Living Together on an Island" is a strategy I learned and adapted from Landgarten (1981) and is often an evocative metaphor for how individuals "survive together" when they are under stress. Family members are invited to draw the outline of an island on a large piece of paper and then co-create a drawing of how they would manage living together on that island, including what they would need to survive and thrive as a family unit. The theme of this activity generally becomes a metaphor for how the family sees their various roles in coping with challenging or adverse events. It also generates a story about how the family reacts to challenges to solve (or not solve) problems. To relieve the obstacle of drawing self-images of each family member on the island, I provide each person with toy figures such as a plastic animal or a familiar cartoon character to represent themselves. This "non-first-person" option makes the experience less threatening because participants can "talk" and interact through the animal or character. The advantage of the toy figures is that they also engage children and can easily be moved around the island for storytelling and role-playing purposes.

To guide the process, I often introduce playful questions to help generate responses, including movement, sound, dramatic enactment, and song:

- "What are the laws or rules on your island?"
- "What is your island's motto or favorite saying?"
- "What is your island's favorite song? Do you ever dance to that song?"
- "If I made a movie of your island, what would be the title of the film?"
- "How do you send and receive messages from other islands?"
- "Who visits your island?"
- "When a storm comes, what do all the animals [inhabitants, cartoon characters] do to stay safe?"

This strategy is particularly effective with families who have undergone the stress of a child or adult family member with a life-threatening illness such as cancer. I have often witnessed these families literally camping in the patient's hospital room for days and weeks during multiple crises and medical interventions. During this time, they have little contact with extended family, friends or colleagues and dispense with all familiar routines. Siblings of pediatric patients may feel isolated from parents or caregivers, sensing that the critically ill patient requires the parents' full attention. They may also harbor their own fears and worries about illness and death, silently suffering with insomnia, nightmares, cognitive difficulties, and anxiety. In a way, the family often forms its own "island," separate from previous normal day-to-day interactions with friends, work colleagues, and, in the case of siblings, classmates because of the needs of the identified patient and the unpredictability of the patient's illness.

Scribble Chase

"Scribble chase," a concept based on Lusebrink (1990), is another example of a multilayered strategy that helps families and groups generate stories about themselves or life events, including traumatic ones, through art expression, improvisation, movement, sound and musicality, and storytelling. It was first described as a way to explain the various levels of the ETC because it starts with a very sensory/kinesthetic activity, moves to a perceptual experience, and ends with communicating a narrative. I use it because it involves playful, spontaneous responses and challenges participants to improvise with the therapist's prompting and support.

To begin, two people in the family share one piece of paper, and one "chases" the other's scribble with a marker or pastel around the paper for a couple of minutes, resulting in a playful and spontaneous maze of lines. The dyad reverses the process on a second piece of paper, and the other person "chases" while the other participant "leads." Each person then looks at scribble on which he/she was the leader of the chase and adds color, shapes, or lines to create several images. The dyads share these images with each other and eventually with the other family or group members. From these images, they choose several (five is a good number) to use in creating a group mural or image (Figure 8.5). The participants are encouraged to add anything they want to in order to create a story with the chosen images. The final process can include telling a story about the mural or using one or more of the expressive arts (movement, sound, song, dramatic enactment) to communicate a narrative. To encourage sound and musicality, I have a set of various percussion instruments. Children's toy instruments, including bells, tambourines, xylophones, drums, clappers, and kazoos, usually engage most families in playfully sharing "sensory-based" stories.

In using this process, it is important that the therapist exhibit a playful attitude. Like all traumatized individuals, each family member needs support and prompts from an enthusiastic facilitator to take risks and express. While the intended outcome of this activity is to develop and perform a story through sound, gesture, or enactment, an important social engagement experience for the family is at the core of the process through play and implicit interactions. Arriving at a narrative is only part of what is a multilayered experience that provides opportunities to reinforce attachment and attunement between family members through expressive communications.

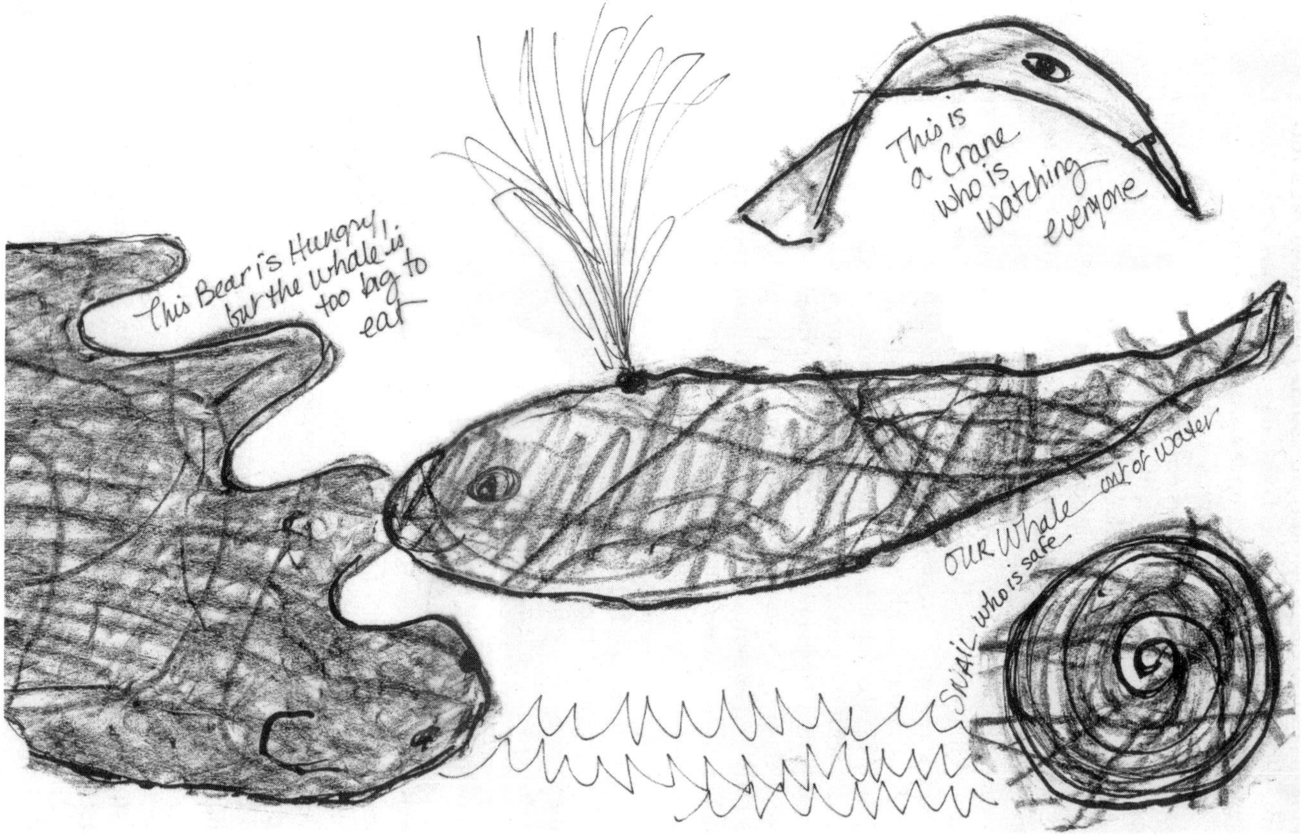
This Bear is Hungry, but the whale is too big to eat
This is a Crane who is watching everyone
OUR Whale out of water
SNAIL who is safe

FIGURE 8.5. Scribble chase group mural. From Malchiodi (2012b). Copyright © 2012 The Guilford Press. Reprinted by permission.

ATROCITIES MUST BE TOLD AND WITNESSED

Whether families or individuals are involved, art expressions are almost always important forms of storytelling. Drawings in particular are powerful vehicles for narratives because of the multiple layers of declarative and implicit stories embedded in them. In each case, these images never fail to impress me in terms of what they communicate and what individuals say about them. While I have been a witness to countless trauma stories via drawings, one particular experience relates to the importance of art-based expression for all individuals subjected to unspeakable atrocities. This experience taught me not only how traumatic events can dramatically impact visual communication of narratives, but also their essential role in empowering survivors when traumatic events are extreme.

In February 2005, pediatrician Annie Sparrow and Olivier Bercault traveled to refugee camps on the Chad–Sudan border where more than 200,000 individuals were trying to escape genocide in the Darfur region of Sudan. They gave paper and crayons to children so that they could draw while Sparrow and Bercault talked to their caregivers. To their surprise, without any prompts, the children drew shootings of civilians, tanks firing on villagers, and military helicopter and Antonov and MIG planes dropping bombs on adults and children. In the weeks that followed, these scenes were repeated in hundreds of drawings by children from approximately age 8 to 17 (Figure 8.6). Many children depicted specific attacks they had witnessed, showing huts and villages burning, the rape of women and girls, and the shooting of adults and children.

In 2007, I was asked to review and provide an opinion on the content of some of the children's drawings for the International Criminal Court. For the first time in history, the court had accepted 500 art expressions depicting the conflict in Darfur as contextual evidence for war crimes trials being held against Sudanese officials. While it is difficult to evaluate drawings without hearing from the art makers themselves (Malchiodi, 1998), what I saw illustrated very clear narratives with astonishing details about what these children had witnessed and elements that could not be simply imagined. Originally, Sparrow and Bercault believed that the drawings formed a compelling case against Sudanese governmental officials as complicit in the Darfur crisis and violations of the laws of war. In reviewing these drawings and creating my report, my mind and body still shudder from memories of what I witnessed through the eyes of children. The horror, mayhem, and brutality depicted by these children was impossible to ignore. The detailed visual narratives in many of the art expressions recorded what was seen, felt, and heard during violent and barbaric ethnic cleansing. Ultimately, these drawings formed not only a body of evidence, but also a collective trauma narrative comprising detailed memories of multiple atrocities. It was an unsolicited account of what these children believed was taking place in Darfur (Hill & Aradua, 2013). As an art therapist and psychologist, I

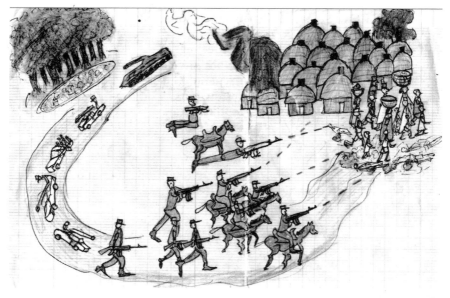

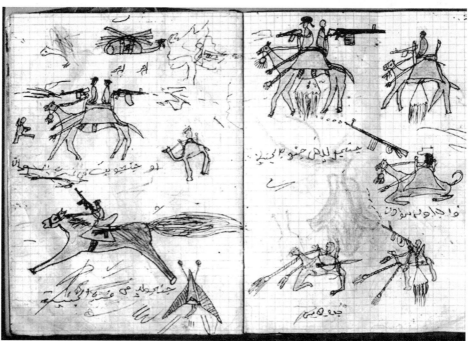

FIGURE 8.6. Child's drawings of genocide in Darfur. Courtesy of Human Rights Watch.

categorize this type of art expression as "spontaneous" because the children were not asked to specifically recall their experiences with the genocide, nor were they asked to draw their feelings about what happened.

These children's drawings exemplify two principles that Herman (1992) identified regarding trauma reparation and recovery. The first is that adverse events must be communicated and witnessed. While the witnessing usually comes from the psychotherapist, the public now constitutes the witnesses to these children's visual narratives via the Holocaust Memorial Museum in Washington, DC, and through a documentary film on their drawings. As I witnessed how trauma survivors used the arts to communicate trauma narratives, I began to have a deeper understanding of Herman's emphasis on restoration of social order in addition to the individual's own reparation and healing. She also observed that the inability to disclose trauma stories due to denial or need for secrecy is often at the root of psychological trauma. This tells me that we must give traumatized individuals every possible channel to express what many individuals cannot or will not communicate with words.

CONCLUSION

Expression of trauma narratives through declarative means such as drawing or writing or implicit experiences such as movement or gesture, dramatic enactment, and sound or music are central to the process of reparation via expressive arts. No matter how these narratives are conveyed, in each case they provide individuals with ways to communicate multilayered perceptions and impressions of traumatic memories. More importantly perhaps, expressive arts help traumatized children, adults, and families generate stories that can be witnessed and thus be both heard and seen.

But trauma narratives related to brain and body–based memories of distress are not the only stories that need to be communicated in order to support repair and transformation. It is also necessary to address declarative and implicit narratives related to resilience—the source of strength, mastery, and self-efficacy. Resilience as both an explicit and embodied experience is essential to trauma recovery and is the subject of the next chapter.

CHAPTER 9

Resilience

ENHANCING AND EMBODYING
MASTERY AND COMPETENCE

Toby, who turned out to be one of the most difficult cases I have ever encountered, arrived at my office unannounced one late afternoon. A 27-year-old young woman, she knocked lightly on the slightly opened door and poked her head around the corner asking, "Are you the art therapist?" I responded with a "yes" and asked her if I had missed a scheduled appointment with her. Toby shook her head and said, "I have all these drawings and collages with me and I just need to talk to somebody about them. I am a biology student, I'm not an artist, but I just keep making a lot of them." She did have "a lot of them"—she emptied two knapsacks each containing a dozen sketchbooks onto my desk. Each was completely filled with mostly crayon drawings and magazine collages. When I asked her how she got started with all this creative expression, Toby replied, "I walked into a store one night and bought my first sketchbook and crayons. Still not sure why I did this. But that is why I am here to see you."

Toby helped me to learn much of what I know about resilience and how expressive arts support it. The images I witnessed in those sketchbooks on that day were viscerally disturbing, and I immediately recognized that she needed support to address whatever was distressing her. But despite the unsettling content of those images, Toby had found a way to survive for the moment through action (making art images) and efficacy (coming to my office). Creating those simple images and taking the risk to share them with me were acts of resilience that eventually turned out to be life-changing for her.

In talking about trauma, it is difficult to discuss the term *resilience* without sounding trite. Resilience has become a ubiquitous concept in psychotherapy and trauma treatment associated with the idea that if one has enough of it, one can survive any adversities in the long run. Without a doubt, all the children and adults I have seen in my practice are resilient in some way. Many people I see in treatment actually seem to be functioning well on the surface—they hold jobs, they go to school, they maintain friendships. They have survived adversity, and they also have a lot of practice in falling down and getting up on their feet again. The innumerable ways that traumatized individuals meet challenges demonstrates their resiliency in devising strategies to cope with circumstances and events that are often horrifying, inescapable, or unconscionable. The fact that each of them, like Toby, even makes the journey to see a helping professional, commit to therapy, and take the risk of self-expression is an indication of a degree of resilience. But the strategies that make them seem resilient in some areas are not working in others, particularly in how well each is coping with trauma.

Trauma-informed practice emphasizes that practitioners are inclusive of resilience as a factor in reparation and recovery. Bringing the concept of resilience into sessions does provide opportunities to introduce less pathology-driven frameworks for reparative work. Despite what is known about it through research and clinical observations, it is not easy to restore, support, or enhance resilience, especially in those who are most traumatized. However, there are some practical as well as innovative ways of introducing and supporting it through expressive arts. These possibilities come not only from what are typically known as resilience factors, but also from the unique qualities of expressive arts themselves—the bottom-up continuum of practices that focus on sensory-based, embodied methods to support mastery and competence.

THE FOUR WAVES OF RESILIENCE

There are many accepted definitions of resilience, including the popular adage stating that it is the ability to "bounce back" from adversity. Siegel (2014) echoes this commonly used phrase, noting that it "can be defined as having flexibility and strength in the face of stress and possessing what is needed to rise above adversity, learn from experience and move on with vitality and passion" (p. 18). Many individuals have protective factors such as a supportive family and caregivers, the ability to self-regulate, and the personal initiative and temperament to indeed "bounce back" from most distressful events.

Wright, Masten, and Narayan (2013) explained what they consider four distinct phases or waves in resilience research. In the earliest of these conceptualizations, those individuals who seemed to fare well were labeled "invulnerable" (Anthony & Cohler, 1987) and were said to have inborn superpowers. Fortunately, we realized that this conclusion ruled out the possibility of resilience for the vast majority of individuals, implying that they might be incapable of overcoming childhood trauma and adversity. This initial wave was followed by a second wave of research that focused on developmental contextual influences in addition to personal factors. The third wave translated the basic science of resilience into actual interventions to promote resilience and establish guidelines for prevention approaches to reduce the impact of adversity. Finally, the fourth wave focused on "multilevel dynamics and the many processes linking genes, neurobiological adaptation, brain development, behavior, and context at multiple levels" (Wright et al., 2013, p. 30). As a result, resilience is now studied from many perspectives ranging from genetics to social interactions.

Masten (2001) may provide the most widely accepted summary of resilience, saying:

> Resilience does not come from rare and special abilities, but from the everyday magic of ordinary, normative human resources in the minds, brains, and bodies of children, in their families, and in their communities. . . . The conclusion that resilience emerges from ordinary processes offers a far more optimistic outlook for action than the idea that rare and extraordinary processes are involved. The task before us now is to delineate how adaptive systems develop, how they operate under diverse conditions, how they work for or against success . . . and how they can be protected, restored, facilitated, and nurtured. (p. 235)

This is obviously a more hopeful view of resilience than was first envisioned and transforms the belief in resilience as a "superpower" to one of "ordinary magic." While Masten refers to children in her work, Bonanno echoes similar conclusions about adults who have experienced trauma: "What is perhaps most intriguing about resilience is not how prevalent it is; rather that it is that we are consistently surprised by it. I have to admit that sometimes even I am amazed by how resilient humans are, having worked with loss and trauma survivors for many years" (2009, p. 47; see also Bonanno, 2004).

Brooks and Goldstein (2015) added the importance of mindsets in supporting resilience. In their work with children, they classify this as a set of assumptions that individuals make about themselves and others and that these assumptions in turn influence behavior and actions. According to these researchers, a resilient mindset includes these critical factors: feeling loved and accepted; efficacy in resolving problems and making informed decisions; recognition and enjoyment of one's strengths; feeling comfortable with peers and adults; and a belief that one can make a difference.

RESILIENCE IN THE CONTEXT OF SOCIAL AND ENVIRONMENTAL CHALLENGES

In introducing resilience through expressive arts therapy, I often ask myself, "How can I possibly encourage individuals to be resilient when overwhelming challenges of environment, socioeconomics and disempowering political structures exist in their lives? And how can I encourage anyone to engage in the arts as a form of empowerment?" In part, my beliefs about how expressive arts support resilience come from personal experiences of growing up in a single-income household and a family that faced multiple socioeconomic and other stressors. I know how the arts helped me literally untangle emotions as a child and adolescent despite limitations and that music, dance, theater, and visual art became my source of strength during trauma and loss (Malchiodi, 2019). But while my belief in expressive arts as a form of resilience may be personal, it is equally derived from evidence of their long tradition as agents of health and well-being, self-selected universally by humans throughout history in how they have been used to address adversity. This evidence for expressive arts as resilience-driven endeavors is not at all new; it comes from both ancient and contemporary applications of the arts for healing purposes (Arrien, 2013; Dissanayake, 1995) and it is instinctive (Kandel, 2012). Humans have continually turned to the arts as an act of resilience when confronted with physical, emotional, social, and spiritual challenges in life (Malchiodi, 2015a, 2019).

In Chapter 2, I introduced the concept of healing-centered engagement (Ginwright, 2018) as an important piece of the trauma-informed focus on empowerment and strength-based approaches. While many practitioners are enthusiastic about this principle, putting it into practice continues to be far from easy because of contextual barriers within the frameworks of trauma-informed practice that include sociocultural, environmental, and political concerns. For the most part, psychotherapeutic services take place in clinics, agencies, or offices far removed from the individual's actual day-to-day challenges. The gap between the current mental health system and the ideals of trauma-informed care is one issue that many researchers fail to note in their discussions of resilience. Strength-based concepts of empowerment, open dialogue, and self-efficacy are at best difficult to implement, and ultimately, enhancing resilience is only possible when the larger context of the individual is considered.

Carla Page (in Treleavan, 2018), the past director of the Audre Lorde Project, a center focused on lesbian, gay, bisexual, two spirit, trans, and gender nonconforming people of color, defines resilience as

> Being able to transform inside of perhaps the worst conditions, but still on a cellular level being able to respond, intervene or transform what has been done to me or us . . . to remember that we deserve dignity, honor and a way to look at how we can sustain our well-being, in a society that has almost normalized our physical, emotional and spiritual degradation. That, in and of itself, is collective resilience. (p. 125)

This is a more nuanced perspective that reinforces the notion that attention to resilience within the context of psychotherapy will not eliminate oppression or inequality. Page's statement indicates that ultimately all therapists must recognize what supports the individual's safety, self-regulation, and well-being within the individual's larger context. While we may not be able to change this context, we must at least begin to grasp the wider challenges that involve more than simply identifying strengths and assessing trauma symptoms.

EXPRESS YOURSELF: AN EXAMPLE OF RESILIENCE-BUILDING IN CONTEXT

There are many effective expressive arts programs that support resilience and provide trauma-informed, healing-centered engagement for individuals who live in oppressive, violent, or otherwise challenging neighborhoods and environments. They deliver arts-based services that these individuals might not receive through traditional clinic or agency, and they do so in ways that are community based. Express Yourself (EXYO) is an example of this type of programming and consists of two nonprofit youth arts organizations, one based in Beverly, Massachusetts, and the other formerly in Milwaukee, Wisconsin. As forms of healing-centered engagement, these programs extend multidisciplinary arts studios into their respective communities and into residential treatment programs, locked hospital units, correction facilities, alternative educational programs, and out-of-school programming for traumatized youth. Participants come to EXYO from a variety of backgrounds, mental health, and experiences of traumatic stress, including experiences of isolation and lack of meaningful connection to others. Individuals become immersed in all the arts—music, dance, theater, and the visual arts—with the goal of a culminating performance for family, clinicians, peers, and the community at large.

EXYO immersive arts-based experiences (Figure 9.1) are designed to sequentially build upon each other during the course of many weeks of programming and to emphasize consistency, commitment to participation, respect for peers and artistic process, and creativity open to all levels of collaboration (youth, artists, guest artists, and support staff) leading to artistic excellence. In particular, the collaborative approach between artists, youth, and guest artists helps youth to learn from each other, resolve differences effectively and peacefully, and work together toward common goals. Warm-up activities begin in a circle (including theater games, drumming, singing, and movement exercises) in order to establish a familiar routine into the deepening of artistic work. Each group has a structured plan with room for adaptation and adjustments based on participant dynamics and relevant to the eventual production of a culminating performance for the public. Each group provides the opportunity of both process engagement and the gift of being seen and heard by a circle of peers. The staff members become co-creators with the youth, providing structure, boundaries, and opportunity to engage. There is an underlying principle of unconditional

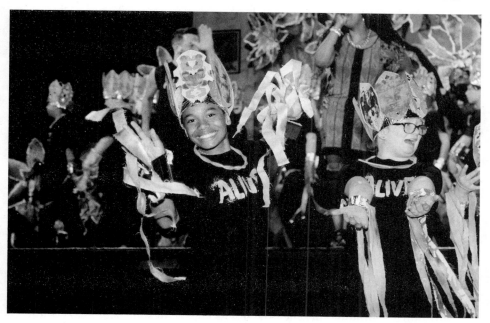

FIGURE 9.1. Express Yourself Program participants performing on stage. Photo by Mike Dean. Courtesy of Express Yourself Milwaukee.

care and safe boundaries, and all artistic staff have training in youth development and specific principles of the EXYO model that ensures consistency and builds trust.

The EXYO's overarching objective is resilience—it seeks to help youth perceive themselves as active contributors in their community and establish meaningful friendships and relationships among participants through the arts immersion. The collaborative team approach encourages engagement matching their individual needs while building connection to the group process. EXYO addresses the complexity of participants' unique challenges, while offering direct experiences of inner strength and resilience and creating positive connections between self, peers, facilitators, and caregivers. An annual culminating "grand performance" reflects participants' year of artistic exploration and self-discovery. Every aspect of the show—the set, the music, the dancing, the videos, the spoken words—is the result of hundreds of individual contributions from youth working in the studio, in the community, and in treatment and corrections facilities. Being celebrated for their successes is often something new for these youth; for the adults in their lives, the performance offers a way to see their children as an important part of an exceptional event. The audience's overwhelming support and encouragement supports the participants' experiences. It is a memorable and joyous time for these youth who often are not accustomed to being seen in a positive light. The program therefore creates a space for them to be celebrated for all that is right about them rather than criticized in terms of pathology, challenges, and problems. They experience what it is like to be part of a standard of artistic excellence, performing side by side with artistic staff and guest artists who inspire expanded trust in themselves and others.

Jimmy is a good example of a participant in EXYO programming. He was brought to the EXYO studio with a group of young people from various agencies in the community. His history included mental illness in his family and bullying by his classmates. In addition, his home life was fraught with inconsistency, violence, and broken attachments. Jimmy himself had a history of multiple hospitalizations and home placements.

Initially, Jimmy was very anxious and unsure about whether he wanted to be at EXYO, constantly looking at his peers in the room alert to whether they accepted him. An EXYO artist brought him to the main table while the group was forming. She invited him to work on a small art project and to help her complete the preparation for a subsequent group activity. During the group session, the artist and Jimmy sat together in the circle for the warm-up activities; he watched the others engage in some ice-breakers and soon found himself cautiously joining in the activities. After the circle broke up, the group dispersed to the visual arts area. Jimmy found his spot at the table and engaged in the art making, still keeping to himself and working parallel with his peers. The group ended with a circle song and a simple dance. Jimmy followed along, still staying close to the artistic staff with whom he was now familiar. Over the weeks of groups as different modalities were introduced, Jimmy became less dependent on the artist staff support and began making peer connections and friends. In the annual performance, Jimmy's art from the initial session was part of a larger set piece, and he participated in a dance and drum performance as well as the finale, happily engaging with his peers. Over many years, EXYO (both in community studio and in mental health facilities) has been a constant place for social support and belonging for Jimmy. The consistency of the program created a bridge for him that was inclusive of his individual needs as well as his community and context.

Programs like EXYO bring the therapeutic benefits of expressive arts directly into communities through sensory-based experiences of synchrony and co-regulation, arts-based mastery, and actual theatrical performance. The potential of establishing "communal rhythms" (van der Kolk, 2014) through all the arts within a normalizing environment where participants learn to work together truly captures all the identified factors that support resilience. However, the model for healing-centered engagement described here is not always available to all individuals, and many psychotherapists may not have access to this type of programming for their clients. But there still is an important takeaway for those working in more traditional office and clinic settings. The experiences of mastery and competence provided through programs like EXYO demonstrate that the embodied nature of the arts is an important component of resilience and one that can be integrated within any psychotherapeutic setting.

RESILIENCE IS LEARNED THROUGH THE BODY

Currently, most psychotherapeutic strategies for resilience-building still tend to be more "talk-oriented" and top-down, focusing on cognitive changes rather than implicit experiences. For many years, the majority of my work has been directed toward developing resiliency programming for active military personnel and their families, including children and adolescents. Multiple branches of the military have integrated resilience research and many principles of positive psychology based on the work of Seligman (2007) within this type of programming. Supportive and consistent relationships that lead to development of self-efficacy, confidence, positivity, and hope are undeniably part of what forms a foundation for resilience throughout the lifespan. Optimistic self-talk and cognitive-behavioral approaches also help many individuals.

However, what I discovered in designing and developing these programs over a 10-year period is that not everyone can be "talked into" experiences of confidence, mastery, or competence; it also has to become a felt sense in the body. This is where I believe the more bottom-up, nonlinguistic expressive arts have a distinct role in supporting resilience. While the mind can be influenced to include various components of a resilience mindset, clients have taught me that there is much more to it than simply changing the brain, particularly when it comes to overcoming trauma. In other words, when the person can say, "This is not just a thought I am thinking but it is a feeling that I sense and perceive in my body," I know that individuals really feel resilient at a deeper level. Their bodies literally become convinced of competency, mastery, and self-efficacy. While I have witnessed this change in children and adults as they begin to overcome traumatic stress, I actually learned this from a unique personal experience in mastery and empowerment.

Many years ago, I went through a series of traumatic events that shook me in ways I had never experienced in my life. Unfortunately, the impact of those events was compounded by the illness and death of my father and a suddenly tenuous financial situation in our family. Seeing my father's sudden decline sent me into a constant state of helplessness as I watched a man who had always been vital begin to deteriorate so precipitously. I decided to see a therapist for some help, and I also enrolled in a dance class to get myself moving and become part of an additional community. But in being completely overtaken by so many challenges, I knew I needed something pretty dramatic to help me regain my confidence and the trust I had possessed in the not too distant past.

I sought to do something that would challenge me in a completely different way—I decided to learn to fly a small airplane. Unlike many people who fear being thousands of feet above the ground, flying always had positive connotations for me. I have always enjoyed commercial flights, even when encountering turbulence, and I loved traveling in small propeller planes to more remote airfields. As a child, I had always been fascinated by airplanes and the idea of being high above the earth. In fact, my father used to take us to the closest commercial airport to watch takeoffs and landings. In those days before heightened security became the rule, you could go into the terminal and sit in an observation deck to watch air traffic. When we did not go into the actual airport, my father would park the car near the end of the runway where we could actually feel the vibrations of large planes landing above us and see them taxiing into their gates. My mother rounded out my aviation fantasies with the biographies of Amelia Earhart and astronauts whose flights took them into what at that time was considered outer space.

Believe me, learning to fly a small plane was a challenge at first. I was not young when I took on this challenge, and I am pretty sure that no one thought I would follow through and reach my goal. But I persisted through learning instrumentation, how to file a flight plan, listening for my callsign, and make pre- and post-checks of the aircraft, as well as many hours of practice on a flight simulator. I learned through the skills and focus it takes to become a proficient aviator through endless touch-and-go routines (takeoff and landing, followed by an immediate takeoff). I could begin to sense my flight instructor becoming more confident in my abilities, despite some occasional terse commands from him when I was coming in too "hot" (fast) on final approach to the runway. It may have taken me a little longer than most to make the necessary solo flight for my certification, but I eventually could finally call myself an aviator.

It took many hours of incredible focus, a form of mindful engagement where complete attention is required. You just simply cannot think about anything else during the time you're in the air flying an aircraft. Along with this highly developed focus comes a sense of empowerment when you begin the takeoff sequence, eventually lifting off the ground on climb out. A sense of mastery comes with learning to accomplish the most difficult part of flight, which is landing the plane and "sticking" it to the runway. One might think that all the complicated technical components and maneuvers I learned helped to increase my resilient mindset. But in retrospect, that is only one part of what I believed changed within me to support a renewed sense of resilience. It was the embodiment of competence that I internalized as a felt sense. Like all pilots, I learned the importance of knowing the "feel" of the aircraft during flight, takeoff, approach, and landing. Your instruments, the tower's instructions, and your own technical knowledge of course are essential. But there is an embodied intelligence that informs a pilot of when things are going well and also when something just doesn't "feel right." You actually feel it in your body, which gives you additional information not found through instrumentation or the control tower and gives you the confidence to do what is necessary in the moment.

Let me be clear here—I am not suggesting that everyone recovering from trauma must adopt such a dramatic measure to overcome it and restore resilience. But the principles I learned from this experience informed my views of how we become resilient through the felt sense of what it is like to become competent through mastering a skill or activity. Because the expressive arts and play involve the actual experiences of mastery, they not only support an internalized competence, but also provide the necessary sensory-based moments that contribute to the felt sense of efficacy and empowerment.

The strategies described in earlier chapters of this book for building relationships, enhancing self-regulation, and developing an internalized sense of safety are essential foundations in addressing resilience. The expressive arts can be applied in several ways to support resilience, providing strategies that capitalize on bottom-up processes over more language-driven approaches, naturally tapping a felt, body-based sense of mastery and competence.

SETTING THE STAGE FOR RESILIENCE: RECLAIMING THE ABILITY TO PLAY AND LAUGH

Although the expressive arts involve imagination and the creative process, an ability to play, whether with music and sound, movement, enactment, or art materials, is at the core of self-expression. Throughout most of my work with individuals who have experienced traumatic events, the ability to engage in spontaneous play has been compromised. This is particularly true for those who endured chronic abuse and adverse events as young children. Recall Christa whose story I shared in several parts of this book. Because of multiple experiences of interpersonal violence, she never could quite bring herself to let go and just play with me or her brother. With children and adolescents who have developmental trauma, the ability to play freely often is missing, or it becomes distorted as reflected in their chaotic and unsatisfying stagnant post-traumatic play. Adults who have endured multiple adversities throughout life begin to believe that it is no longer possible to feel joy, enjoy humor, or play without inhibition. They may also have internalized the thought that playing equates to laziness or is simply a "waste of time."

The moment that children and adults can play and laugh with me through expressive arts, even if just fleetingly, is one of the benchmarks

I look for not only in reparation, but also as a manifestation of personal resilience. While one's therapeutic persona can gently communicate a sense of playfulness, there are other ways to manifest a playful atmosphere even in clinical settings. As full disclosure, I am not a play therapist by credentials and thus do not have a lot of the typical toys and props in my office that are found in play therapy rooms. But in the various spaces where I have seen clients in over the years, I always have at least a few specifically selected playfully humorous images on the walls. One poster that has traveled with me ever since I worked with children in shelters is one of three bulldogs wearing shower caps while in a bubble bath in a tub. When I am showing young clients around my office, I often stop and point to it, and if a child seems curious, I ask, "Well, what do you think about these silly dogs wearing shower caps and sitting in a bubble bath? Have you ever seen something like this before?" Generally, I don't get much of a response during an initial session, but as our relationship forms over time, those three bulldogs in a tub eventually get a giggle or a funny comment.

Another image I have prominently displayed on my desk is that of a toddler dancing across a large sand mandala created by Tibetan monks in a train station. Sand mandalas are sacred symbols and take many days to create through painstaking, detailed work. While the photograph of the dancing toddler is whimsical, the story behind it is profound and evocative. The Tibetan monks had been working on the sand painting for several days and were only halfway finished with their work. The child simply slipped under the rope surrounding the mandala during a time when the monks were not there and began to dance in the sand, thus destroying all the work that had been accomplished. In response, the monks laughed out loud when they saw what had happened; they smiled and simply started their work all over again. As we talk about this image and story, the message that many clients come to understand is that it is okay to laugh even in the midst of tragedy. Also, many narratives, including those of resilience and even playfulness and humor, can exist along with those that may be adverse.

Humor, and particularly laughter, are not formally included in the continuum of expressive arts therapy, but they have been a large part of my practice for decades. I try to sensitively infuse humor mainly in the form of carefully focused storytelling and by being gently playful during movement and other activities. There is also a physiological impact is inherent to laughter, especially the deep-belly laughs that come with experiencing humor with others. Moreover, humor stimulates multiple physiological systems that decrease levels of stress hormones and increase the brain's reward system (Savage, Lujan, Thipparthi, & DiCarlo, 2017). Laughing is a visceral experience that literally shakes the body, reminiscent of what Levine means when he speaks of "shaking off the trauma." In expressive arts therapy, this is a particularly natural way to create that experience while working on reparative and resilient behaviors.

Throughout previous chapters, I have emphasized the importance of play in establishing psychotherapeutic relationships. For Katja who was a survivor of multiple sexual assaults and who witnessed the death of a fellow soldier, reclaiming her own competence as a highly skilled and physically and mentally strong individual was not possible until she could safely play with me during sessions. In Katja's case, being able to resource a sense of play through self-regulating music provided her first significant moment of mastering panic attacks, a turning point in her own sense of competence and self-efficacy. For traumatized children and particularly for those who have endured multiple adverse events, introduction of ways to play and discover pleasure in one's body is an essential foundation for establishing the body's implicit sense of mastery.

LEARNING TO BELIEVE IN HELPERS

Fred Rogers of *Mr. Rogers' Neighborhood* fame said, "When I was a boy and I would see scary things in the news, my mother would say to me 'Look for the helpers. You will always find people who are helping.'" Research tells us that social support is a key factor in enhancing a sense of resilience (Masten, 2011). Those individuals who experience secure and positive attachment early in life with an adult caregiver learn to believe that helpers exist when adversity strikes. As it turns out, this is an important belief throughout one's lifespan when one is encountering traumatic events.

I learned a great deal about how children's confidence in adult helpers impacts resilience in the weeks and months after the terrorist attacks on September 11, 2001. During that time, I interviewed approximately 150 classroom children near New York City and in the Midwest and West Coast of the United States about their drawings of "what happened" and what they were experiencing after the attacks. The drawings and trauma narratives were remarkably similar and almost always contained images of the Twin Towers being hit by airplanes (Figures 9.2 and 9.3). There were a few variations, often depending on what type of media images children were exposed to on the day of the events. For example, while most children simply drew the buildings being struck by airplanes, children in one classroom I visited who saw televised images of people falling from the Towers included that element in their drawings (Malchiodi, 2011, 2013).

Fortunately, other elements that form a larger context emerged in most of the children's drawings I encountered. During my interviews, I noticed that in most cases, "helping adults" such as firefighters, police, or medical personnel were included in the drawings and storytelling. In talking with these young people, I came to believe this was indicative of their confidence that adults were there to assist and protect those who were hurt or in danger. While their images illustrated the actual disaster, they also conveyed the sense that help existed. In hindsight, this could be viewed as arts-based

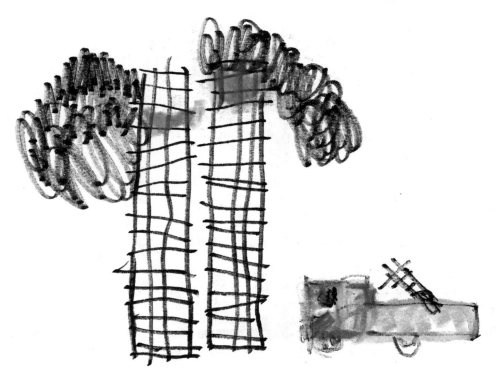

FIGURE 9.2. A child's drawing of the Twin Towers disaster on September 11, 2001. From the collection of Cathy A. Malchiodi (not to be reproduced without permission from the author).

evidence that may correlate to the low rate of post-traumatic stress reactions in children who directly witnessed the event. The majority of these children had caregivers who provided stability, supporting their sense that adults were present to assist and that life would eventually return to normal. Despite the mental health community's immediate concern that children in particular might experience long-lasting traumatic stress after the terrorist attacks, even those who were most exposed to the disaster seemed to do well in the long term.

In contrast to the terrorist attacks of 2001, children's drawings about their experiences with Hurricane Katrina, a storm that devastated New Orleans and surrounding areas of the U.S. Gulf Coast in August 2005, nonverbally conveyed quite different narratives. While the events of September 11, 2001, were dramatic and wide reaching, Katrina left a different imprint owing to the nature of the event. The children drew images in which rescue and helpers were noticeably absent; instead, they portrayed attempts at self-preservation and scenes depicting rising waters and dangerous predators

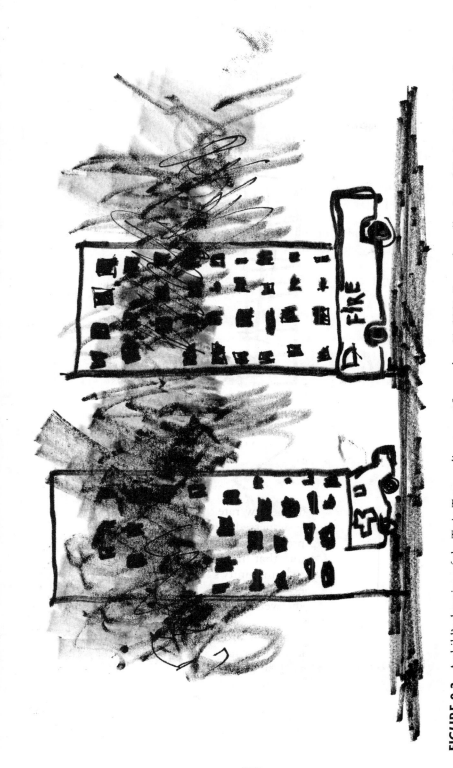

FIGURE 9.3. A child's drawing of the Twin Towers disaster on September 11, 2001. From the collection of Cathy A. Malchiodi (not to be reproduced without permission from the author).

(Figure 9.4). What was communicated initially without words accurately captured the sense of abandonment, helplessness, and hopelessness that was felt when, in the aftermath of Katrina, assistance did not arrive in a timely fashion.

For those who have experienced multiple traumatic events with adverse outcomes, it is not easy to believe that helpers will arrive to provide support. Belief in rescue is also elusive for those individuals whose experience of trauma occurs within an ecology of social injustice where help has been unavailable and barriers such as racism and inequality exist. In essence, the experience of Hurricane Katrina highlights the very real societal challenges many children, adults, families, and communities experience on a regular basis. Despite considerable obstacles in some cases, addressing social support is a necessary element in enhancing resilience.

The psychotherapeutic relationship contributes to establishing a sense of social support, albeit in a limited way. Brooks (2010) calls this the "charismatic adult" who instills the idea that hope and optimism are possible

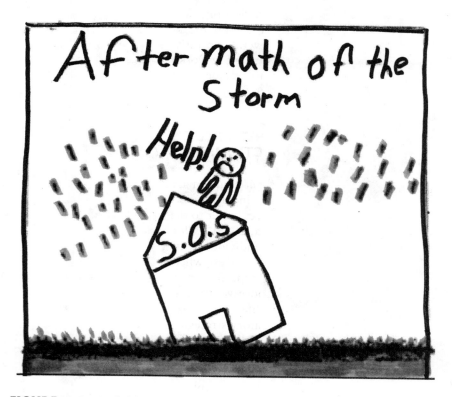

FIGURE 9.4. A child's drawing of the aftermath of Hurricane Katrina in 2005. From the collection of Cathy A. Malchiodi (not to be reproduced without permission from the author).

outcomes despite adversity. When the relationship is successful, individuals do remember that help is possible. Consider the example of Christa (Chapter 4) who recalled my relationship with her years after she had received art and play therapy with me. But in order for a positive helping relationship to endure beyond the session room, additional support systems are essential. Fortunately, expressive arts are uniquely suited to this because they often take place in groups and extend into communities, outside the clinics and mental health agencies. In my experience, re-entering a community is an essential part of resilience-building as well as trauma reparation. Programs such as EXYO described earlier in this chapter are an effective way to not only expand meaningful social support, but also provide necessary opportunities for self-efficacy through therapeutic arts. Chapter 10 describes several similar arts-based programming for adults. While these opportunities may not be available to everyone, an expressive arts group is the next best alternative, particularly groups that include participant interaction such as dramatic enactment, singing or making music with others, and group movement or art-making experiences.

As demonstrated in the next section, strengthening the child–caregiver relationship is another avenue to support both positive attachment and strength-based experiences. Several expressive arts strategies that psychotherapists can incorporate and adapt in working with traumatized children are explained, including how to include caregivers within resilience-based approaches.

THE THREE C'S: CALM, CONNECTION, AND CONFIDENCE

In working with children, I often focus on arts-based intervention through a three-pronged model that incorporates the most widely accepted approached to support resilience. I refer to these as "calm, connection, and confidence" (Malchiodi, 2015a, 2019). *Calm* refers to the basic goal of all treatment, which is to help the individual learn to self-regulate and feel safe while developing skills to reduce stress when faced with upsetting events. *Connection* is the most important element in all strength-building intervention; social support and positive attachment are central to resilience throughout childhood and the lifespan. It also could be called *co-regulation* because it capitalizes on regulatory strategies between either therapist and child or caregiver and child. Finally, *confidence* refers to a sense of mastery that supports an internal locus of control and the belief that one can successfully address challenges. These three areas and applications of trauma-informed expressive art therapy are explained in more detail throughout the following case example of a child client who experienced an acute traumatic event and whose treatment included approaches capitalizing on these resilience-enhancing strategies.

Case Example. Kaitlyn: Supporting Resilience after an Acute Trauma

Kaitlyn, a 9-year-old girl, sustained several dog bites while in her backyard. She was playing on a swing set when a large dog running loose in the neighborhood attacked her from behind without provocation. The dog first bit her on her back, dragging her from the swing for 20 feet while Kaitlyn screamed for help. By the time a neighbor and Kaitlyn's mother reached her, the dog had bitten the child several times on various parts of her body. Another neighbor quickly came to the scene with a gun and captured and killed the dog within the proximity of Kaitlyn and her mother. A few minutes later an ambulance, fire truck, and police cars arrived on the scene. Kaitlyn was placed on a stretcher and rushed by ambulance to a local hospital along with her mother. The nearest hospital was 15 miles away, making the experience even more tense and frightening for both mother and child. Approximately 30 minutes later, Kaitlyn was admitted to the emergency room for surgery to address her wounds. Despite the seriousness of multiple dog bites, she was in stable condition by the end of the day and medicated to address the pain and possibility of infection.

Kaitlyn was expected to make a full recovery, but her wounds required that she remain in the hospital for several weeks. I first saw Kaitlyn on the third day of her stay at the hospital and met with her and her mother in her hospital room. Because of the nature of her injuries and medical treatment, Kaitlyn had to remain in a stationary position, propped up by pillows and semirestrained at our first meeting. It was obviously uncomfortable and stressful for her because she was previously a physically active child. Compounding her distress, Kaitlyn was also fearful of the many medical procedures she was subjected to, even though she understood that the doctors and nurse were trying to help her recover.

Kaitlyn's mother reported that before the incident and hospitalization her daughter tended to be "shy" and did not seek out support or help from teachers or other adults. She had been told by a counselor at Kaitlyn's school that her daughter was "somewhat overly constrictive" in her behavior and tended to be more withdrawn when stressed than hyperactive. When I asked Kaitlyn's mother how Kaitlyn expressed her feelings when distressed, she said that often her daughter would say simply, "I'm fine" or, in many cases, "I don't know." Kaitlyn's mother added that it seemed that after her divorce her daughter's communication was less spontaneous and she had difficulties expressing anger, sadness, or worry. Additionally, Kaitlyn often displayed "pleasing behavior," attending to the needs and emotions of her mother or other family members before her own.

Initial Sessions

In my first meeting with Kaitlyn at the pediatric unit, it was obvious that many aspects of her hospitalization, various medical procedures, and physical restraints were uncomfortable and upsetting to her. But instead of openly communicating her pain and frustration, Kaitlyn responded to her situation by remaining quiet and withdrawn. I respected Kaitlyn's response as an adaptation to an abnormal situation rather than a defense and allowed her to displace her emotions to something external (e.g., to speak to me through a puppet or cartoon character) than to communicate directly about her feelings and experiences. At the same time, in order to enhance Kaitlyn's resilience, it would also be essential to help her identify how her body responded to stress and worry, strengthen positive attachment with her mother, and provide experiences of mastery.

In my next session, Kaitlyn was able to engage in some free play with a set of family puppets I brought to her bedside along with some art materials. As the puppet play progressed, I began asking her if she could speak for any of the puppets and, if so, what the puppets would say. Kaitlyn puzzled over the request for a few minutes, but then suddenly picked up the girl puppet and said, "She did something very bad . . . 'cuz why would all this bad stuff happen?" She also volunteered that "she always felt crummy because she thought she messed up mom and dad staying together." When I asked her to tell me a little more about that, she said, " 'Cuz this girl did things like burn the waffles in the oven and made a mess in the bathroom. Bad stuff happened to her." Kaitlyn clearly expressed self-blame not only for the dog attack, but also for her parents' divorce. In addition to the stress of hospitalization, she had numerous worries about previous experiences and ruminated about them.

Because Kaitlyn seemed interested in the brightly colored drawing materials I brought to her bedside, I asked her if she would like to draw a picture of any of the puppets. Without hesitation, Kaitlyn took a set of the marking pens and paper and drew an image of her mother, writing "Mom is the best," and made a reference to her mother's favorite sports team (Figure 9.5). As her style and enthusiasm indicated, it was obvious that she loved and even admired her mother; she depicted her with positivity and did not blame her mother for not rescuing her from the dog attack.

During the first week of Kaitlyn's hospitalization, I had the opportunity to meet with her mother separately on two occasions. Kaitlyn's mother was understandably distressed by the dog attack, the injuries to her daughter, and the subsequent hospital stay, which would probably require many outpatient follow-up visits over several months. I noticed in these meetings with the mother that she tended toward pessimism in her perceptions about herself; she commented that "things just never seemed to work out for me" and "I sometimes believe that I am not loveable," referring to her divorce from Kaitlyn's father. Like Kaitlyn, the mother lacked confidence and blamed herself for the event, offering that "when the dog attacked Kaitlyn, I thought what a terrible mother I must be, a real jerk and failure. I think she must hate me for not being a better parent when this happened." In considering Kaitlyn's puppet play responses, it was clear that both mother

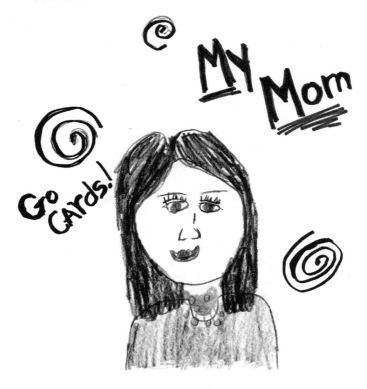

FIGURE 9.5. "Mom is the Best!" by Kaitlyn. From the collection of Cathy A. Malchiodi (not to be reproduced without permission from the author).

and daughter felt responsible for all the "bad stuff" that happened and that the mother felt like a failure as a parent.

Kaitlyn's mother was surprised when (with Kaitlyn's permission) I showed her Kaitlyn's drawing of her. She remarked that after the dog attack she could not believe that her daughter thought she was "the best mom." Despite this strong perception, Kaitlyn's mother appeared noticeably relieved after looking at the drawing. I suggested that if Kaitlyn was in agreement, they might display the picture in the hospital room and after discharge, in a prominent place in the home where both mother and daughter could see it regularly to serve as a positive reminder of their relationship. This simple illustration is a good example of one of the inherent values of art expressions. In this case, a simple drawing served as a sensory-based, visual reminder that can cue positive responses between sessions.

While there were many issues to address in terms of Kaitlyn's psychosocial needs, post-injury, and subsequent trauma reactions, the following sections describe how the expressive arts therapy approach was used to support resilience in Kaitlyn and her mother. In brief, these strategies include enhancing self-regulation and stress reduction, reinforcing positive connection between parent and child, and increasing a sense of mastery through expressive arts and play. Although three areas of specific intervention are discussed, most of the sessions addressed multiple goals (self-regulation, connection, and mastery) of treatment, with resilience as a core objective.

Calm: Supporting Self-Regulation

In Chapter 5, self-regulation is explained as a core strength (Perry, 2015) embodying a set of internal skills that include the abilities to be able to calm oneself when upset and to help oneself "feel better" despite obstacles and challenges. Self-regulation also includes the ability to manage experiences on emotional, cognitive, social, and physical levels. While some children who are unable to self-regulate present as disruptive and are labeled hyperactive, other children like Kaitlyn may appear withdrawn, quietly perseverating, and ruminating without relief.

In general, resilient individuals are effective self-regulators; that is, they are able to remain calm under pressure and quickly adapt to new challenges. Because self-regulation can be practiced, both children and adults can learn this skill to manage stress after traumatic events and to enhance the ability to master new stressful situations successfully. Expressive arts experiences can be self-regulating, in and of themselves, if the activities are perceived to be self-soothing and engaging for the art maker. The repetitive, sensory-based qualities of specific arts-based interventions can therefore help relieve stress and enhance the relaxation response.

For children and their caregivers who are struggling with trauma responses, enhancing resilience begins by introducing ways to reduce stress and effectively self-regulate in the earliest stages of trauma intervention. A major goal of expressive arts therapy with hospitalized children like Kaitlyn is to provide ways for them to decrease distress and frustration and increase their sense of calm and control (Malchiodi, 2013). In most hospitals, professionals known as *child life specialists* provide specific self-regulating art and play interventions. In Kaitlyn's case, child life staff members were available to help her understand medical procedures through medical play with syringes, bandages, toys, and props. My role became to offer additional intervention through the use of arts and play and related methods of self-regulation. My particular goal was to develop strategies that Kaitlyn and her mother could practice at home after the inpatient stay ended. Enlisting parents and caregivers in supporting self-regulation is central to reinforcing this skill because caregivers play a pivotal role in overall success.

I initially taught Kaitlyn some child-friendly ways to use breathing to calm herself when she felt upset. We practiced breathing deeply "like a sleeping bear," "buzzing like a bee," and "roaring like a lion" from our bellies. Although in the earliest part of her hospital stay, Kaitlyn was limited to her bed, I strategized ways to gently get her moving to disrupt any possible freeze response that might be developing. I helped Kaitlyn learn how to make a cardboard butterfly that she could balance on the end of her finger when she needed distraction from anything that was upsetting (see Malchiodi, 2014b) and that would at least get her hands and arms moving while in bed. Because it was important to include Kaitlyn's mother in some of the sessions, I taught both of them how to make "tangle doodles"—simple mark-making with colorful felt pens in various familiar, easy designs and patterns based on a formal method called Zentangle® (Krahula, 2012) that is perceived as an enjoyable, relaxing activity. After Kaitlyn and her mother had a chance to experiment with various designs individually, I introduced the idea of making a joint tangle doodle by tracing their hands overlapping each other on a piece of paper and filling in the spaces with whatever lines and shapes they liked (see Chapter 6 for a similar example). This activity not only created another opportunity to engage in relaxing mark-making, but also served as a symbolic gesture of connectedness that both parent and child seemed to enjoy.

The experience of tracing her hand inspired another drawing by Kaitlyn in the next individual session with me. She asked me if she could trace her hand on paper and surprised me when she asked to show me how to "draw a dog's face." She carefully and quietly colored the image, asking for a pencil at the end to draw one more part—a chain on the dog's collar (Figure 9.6). When I asked her to tell me about the picture, she quietly answered that "dogs need to be chained 'cuz they can hurt people if they are running around. This dog has a strong chain [pointing to the chain in the drawing]." I did not push her to tell me more about the dog image as relating to her experience with the dog that hurt her. Instead, I observed that "sometimes dogs are not chained and they can roam into other people's yards. But if this happened and the dog hurts someone, it was not the person's fault that she was hurt by the dog. I think it is pretty smart that you thought to put a chain on your dog in your drawing." While it would take many sessions before Kaitlyn really believed that she was not the cause of the dog's attack, she did nod with a slight smile when I mentioned her way to keep the dog restrained by her imaginary chain.

At this point in therapy, I introduced the concept of "thought catching" (see Chapter 6; Seligman, 2007) as an additional self-regulation strategy because both Kaitlyn and her mother tended to self-blame when negative events occurred, automatically perseverating on adversity. In order for both to be able to self-regulate and reduce stress responses, it was critical to help them identify thoughts (thought-catch) that led to negative feelings and how these emotions felt in the body. I adapted a process for Kaitlyn and her mother that would direct them to an awareness of the felt sense of distress as it impacted their bodies. By using simple body outlines, I asked them to "catch their worry thoughts" and to show me through mark-making and colors, shapes, and lines "where the worry is in your body and what does it look like." Because Kaitlyn's mother responded well to top-down processes

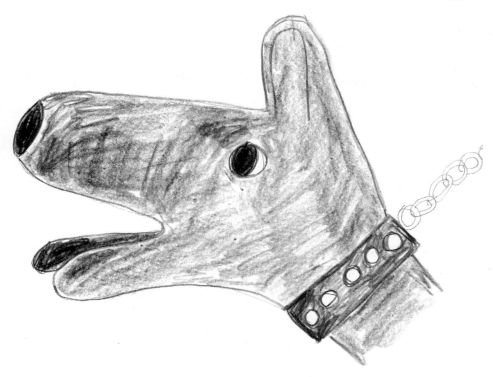

FIGURE 9.6. Drawing of a dog on a leash by Kaitlyn. From the collection of Cathy A. Malchiodi (not to be reproduced without permission from the author).

that started with thoughts and verbalization, this approach was particularly helpful for her rather than beginning with feelings or sensations. Over several sessions, this activity helped both child and parent recognize when they were engaged in negative thinking and how to identify those feelings in their bodies, providing each with the opportunity to apply self-regulation activities to "catch their thoughts" and reduce stress reactions.

Connection: Strengthening Attachment and Co-Regulation

The presence of a stable, nurturing parent or caregiver is widely accepted as a foundation for instilling and supporting resilience in children. While Kaitlyn did not feel abandoned by her mother during the dog bite incident, Kaitlyn's mother certainly expressed distress about not being available quickly enough to stop the dog from harming her daughter. For this reason, it was essential to create sessions that focused on strengthening a sense of positive, secure attachment between parent and child. Expressive arts and play also became a way for me to model effective communication and activities that Kaitlyn's mother could use with her daughter in between sessions and after therapy was terminated.

In using arts and play-based activities to support resilience through positive connection, the concept of *attunement* is a key part of intervention. Well-attuned caregivers can detect what their children are feeling and experiencing, recognize nonverbal communications, and respond appropriately through verbal, tactile, and other means to reduce children's distress. Good attunement is also related to an experience of *reflexive convergence* in which two people "feel felt" by each other (Siegel, 2012). It promotes flexibility in response to stress and positive attachment, key experiences related to the development of resilience.

Arts-based intervention can be applied in many ways to reinforce attunement and reflexive convergence between parents and children. Some of these strategies involve simple movement activities that incorporate mirroring, rhythm, and synchrony between parent and child, reinforcing not only connection but also co-regulation. Once Kaitlyn was mobile again and had her doctors' permission to move about freely, I taught her and her mother a 7-minute workout for co-regulation that we practiced at the beginning of each joint session. It included sensory integration techniques that I had learned and modified, such as elephant stomps (marching by lifting your knees as high as possible); cheetah runs (running in place as fast as you can, like the fastest animal in Africa); bear walk (hands and feet on the floor, shifting weight right and left); and starfish jumps (jumping jacks as fast as possible with arms and legs spread wide).

Dyadic art and play therapy are also good ways to encourage interaction because parents and children can experience each other through many different sensory-based channels, including visual, tactile, movement, rhythm, and auditory channels. For example, the "two-way scribble drawing" is one simple way to structure a dyad art experience; parent and child simply create a scribble together on one large piece of paper with crayons and felt-tip marking pens or oil pastels. I often make the activity into a game by instructing the parent and child to take turns being the leader in a scribble chase across the paper. If the child is the leader, then the parent follows the child's scribble on the paper with a marker or chalk. I also introduced bilateral drawing (Chapter 7) to them. It turned out to be one of the experiences they enjoyed more than any other arts-based ones during our sessions together. To add rhythm to the activity, I helped Kaitlyn and her mother develop a playlist of different songs to play while they created two-handed drawings on paper and chalkboards. Bilateral drawing quickly became a regular activity that they repeated at home on a white board with felt markers in between sessions.

When I noticed that Kaitlyn perceived the "scribble game" as too childish, I invited her and her mother to co-participate in arts and play activities that focused on topics relevant to trauma reparation. In one session, I asked them to co-create an environment or world in a sandtray for a small toy animal (in this case, two rubber ducks) where the animal could feel happy, cared for, and safe. This particular approach was used to open up a conversation about feelings of safety that had been compromised by the dog attack and about what steps could be taken to "feel safe" in the future if another distressing event occurred. It also provided an opportunity to help this dyad reflect the resilience skills they already possessed but perhaps did not recognize. This session helped Kaitlyn and her mother to finally talk about what security, comfort, and nurturance meant to them. In particular, this experience helped Kaitlyn's mother identify ways she could be a more effective parent when tending to Kaitlyn's needs for consistent reassurance and validation of feelings.

Finally, strengthening the connection between any caregiver and child is more about the process itself than about any specific arts-based directive to induce positive attachment and enhance resilience. I introduced many different, yet simple, creative activities to Kaitlyn and her mother that emphasized mutual and reciprocal engagement and provided opportunities for both collaborative and parallel art making (individual art making during the same session). Through collaboration, both parent and child strengthened their abilities to resolve problems and develop coping strategies together. In working individually while in session together, Kaitlyn and her mother were able to express their personal perspectives to each other. In brief, telling a story about one's art not only validates one's worldview, it also promotes attunement and reflexive convergence through eye contact and verbal and nonverbal communication through creative, playful experiences.

Confidence: Enhancing a Sense of Mastery

Confidence means many things in terms of enhancing and restoring resilience. It is essentially children's feelings of capability, safety, trust, and positive attachment despite acute trauma (as in Kaitlyn's case), loss, or multiple adverse experiences. While self-esteem is often seen as key to confidence, it is really a sense of mastery that is most important. Ultimately, the goal of confidence-building is to help children perceive themselves accurately, so that when adverse events that are not their fault occur, they will feel competent and worthwhile.

In working with parent–child dyads like Kaitlyn and her mother, identifying and increasing personal resources for coping with current and future stress or crisis are essential. As mentioned in Chapter 5, the Israel Center for the Treatment of Psychotrauma (2014) developed the building resilience intervention (BRI) model that encourages the development of resilience in children and parents in its ongoing trauma intervention programs with survivors of terrorism and war. This useful program can be adapted to any stressful situation. In the BRI model, children are encouraged to focus on their strengths while expressing their experiences of bombings and life-threatening circumstances. One of their arts-based resilience-building activities directs children to invent a device to deal with rocket bombings; children depict imaginative devices that vacuum up missiles and send them out into space, or they invent safe places that can escape the missiles' detection. The goal is to enhance the sensory experience of personal empowerment through active, hands-on participation.

I used a similar approach with Kaitlyn and her mother, helping them to talk about "what happened." At the same time, I asked them to explore via art materials what they had learned since the dog attack. While it is important to provide any traumatized individuals with the opportunity to communicate their memories of and feelings about what happened in terms of traumatic events, it is equally important to ask them how the experience may have helped them to learn or discover new things. Otherwise, clients are left with only the sensory aspects of the trauma and cannot identify how they have survived and thrived since the crisis or loss occurred. In joint and individual sessions, Kaitlyn and her mother creatively brainstormed various ideas. In particular, they emphasized their need to develop a plan of action if another unexpected event should ever occur. This eventually became a collage of images for their actual plan of action. The pair included a picture of a swing set that they decided could be moved closer to the house where Kaitlyn's mother could see her; they also included a whistle for Kaitlyn to wear to sound a distress signal or, as Kaitlyn decided, to "scare off animals." Her mother also added an image of a church and people. She decided that developing a larger network of social support for herself from members of her church and neighbors would improve her own resilience, thus helping her, as she said, "to be a stronger mom for Kaitlyn."

Kaitlyn and her mother particularly enjoyed using various forms of movement and gesture to communicate feelings and body-based experiences throughout most of our sessions. In order to support resilience, I asked them to "strike a pose" that conveyed strength and confidence. Sometimes we practiced the simple yoga stance called Tadasana (also called mountain pose; see Chapter 6) to evoke those feelings. On other occasions we made the experience more playful and created "superhero masks" of popular characters like Superwoman and Wonder Woman. Kaitlyn and her mother wore the masks and pretended through various poses to have specific powers that could neutralize anxiety, sadness, or guilt. I photographed them in these poses and printed them so that they could have images of themselves in these strong, confidence stances. Eventually, I included the experience of "resourcing" (Levine, 2015) to pendulate between difficult feelings related to traumatic stress and strength-based ones by using movement or gesture to move back and forth between each. This was an important turning point in Kaitlyn's and her mother's treatment. They finally began to be able to recognize how their bodies felt when stressed, anxious, or sad and realized that they could use their "strength poses" to reinforce their sense of confidence when overwhelmed.

The point of this movement-based activity and similar arts-based activities is to move beyond talk and capitalize on experiencing self-efficacy, personal resources, and coping strategies through the senses. While we could have simply talked through a plan of action for the period following their treatment, action-oriented strategies not only make the hard work of therapy more pleasurable but also provide positive tactile and kinesthetic experiences that give participants the "felt sense" of mastery. In the case of this mother–daughter dyad, the two created a tangible image that they took home and placed in a prominent spot to serve as a reminder of their plan and the resources they had developed to meet future challenges.

Termination and Graduation: Recapitulating the Three C's

In our final sessions together, Kaitlyn, her mother, and I used art and play experiences to recapitulate the resilience goals of "calm, connection, and confidence." These sessions also provided Kaitlyn with the opportunity to reauthor or reframe the dominant narrative of the trauma story and experience events in new ways (Malchiodi, 2012a; see Chapter 10 for a more detailed discussion). I find that narrative approaches are a good complement to resilience-based work when they are integrated within overall expressive arts and play therapy interventions because they infuse storytelling into the termination process. One particular story that is useful with children who have experienced a life-changing trauma involves the butterfly life cycle. The story draws on the metaphor of a caterpillar changing into a butterfly as a way to demonstrate how things eventually change after a crisis. Butterflies created from cardboard, caterpillar puppets, and a paper bag "cocoon" can be used as props to tell the following story (adapted from Goffney, 2002). I modified it for Kaitlyn, explaining to her that I wanted to tell her a special story about our work together at the hospital and in outpatient therapy:

> "Do you know where butterflies come from? They start out as eggs and become caterpillars before they become butterflies. Going through a bad experience is like the birth of a butterfly. Before the butterfly is ready to fly free in the world, it has to go through many changes. While all these changes happen, the caterpillar [a prop made from the finger of an old glove] stays safe in its cocoon [keep the caterpillar in a paper bag].
>
> "When we go through a bad time, we can feel pretty scared. Sometimes the only way we can feel better is to stay in our cocoons for a while. While you were in your cocoon, you learned a lot about many different thoughts and feelings. As time went by, you did not need that cocoon as much as you did at first. All of us eventually want to spread our wings and fly again [the caterpillar breaks out of the cocoon and

becomes the butterfly]. Your butterfly learned many new things while in its cocoon, including things it can do to feel better if something upsetting happens."

While I had a little more of the story to tell, Kaitlyn asked to stop for a moment so that she could make another butterfly to come out of the cocoon. The original butterfly used in the story was part of an activity on self-regulation (balancing a cardboard butterfly on one's finger tip). Kaitlyn wanted a second butterfly to emerge from the brown paper bag cocoon. She wrote the word "Mom" on the new butterfly to include her parent as a key part of the narrative, and so we decided to rewrite the story once again to include both butterflies emerging from their shared cocoon to fly together. In a subsequent termination session with both Kaitlyn and her mother, Kaitlyn enacted her butterfly life cycle and included two butterflies, one for herself and one she had made for her mother. While Kaitlyn and her mother still had some challenges to overcome, it was clear that their relationship was strong and that they both had mastered the initial traumatic event that brought Kaitlyn to the hospital.

Finally, during our last session, I strategically presented a children's story called *Shoot for the Moon* (Humphrey, 2011), a tale about a real dog named Rudy who helped his owner learn some important positive lessons about life and resilience. Rudy the dog offers several simple messages about bouncing back from adversity such as "don't be afraid of your shadow," "stretch yourself," and "just roll with it." One lingering area of mastery that Kaitlyn struggled with involved her understandable fear of dogs. Even though she had concluded that the dog that injured her was a "very, very bad dog," she also wanted to have a dog of her own one day. The story of Rudy whose messages encourage the reader to believe that change is possible helped Kaitlyn, her mother, and me to have a conversation about the future, with hope and strategies for continuing to build confidence and a sense of safety. The story provided a "virtual therapy dog" in this final therapy session and ended with Kaitlyn's drawing of her own dog and herself standing together (Figure 9.7).

SELF-COMPASSION: MINDFULLY ENHANCING RESILIENCE

Most of what I introduced to Kaitlyn and her mother to enhance regulation, connection, and mastery also stressed the importance of being in the moment rather than ruminating about the past or worrying about the future. The expressive arts help direct attention on the here-and-now because they are natural manifestations of mindfulness practices. That is, when one is focused on drawing, making sounds or music, or moving in synchrony, one is being mindful in the moment of that activity or process.

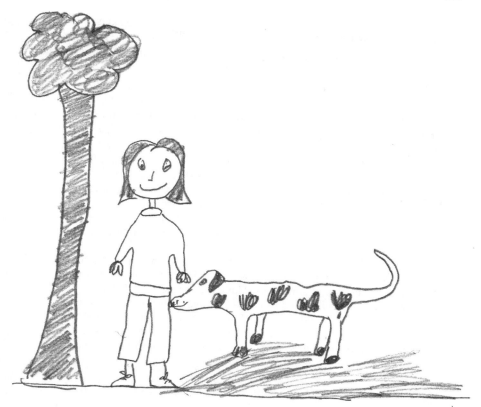

FIGURE 9.7. Drawing of Kaitlyn and her wish for a dog of her own. From the collection of Cathy A. Malchiodi (not to be reproduced without permission from the author).

As previously described, mindfulness involves conscious awareness of what is happening in the here-and-now rather than memories or ruminations on the future, both of which may lead to upset and suffering. By paying attention to the present moment, including moment-to-moment interoceptive experiences and thoughts, we shift from fear-laden responses and cognitions, which frees up possibilities for conscious choices, flexibility, and actions. "When you have enough energy for mindfulness, you can look deeply into any emotion and discover the true nature of that emotion, if you can do that, you will be able to transform that emotion" (Hanh, 2011, p. 89). To me, this is an essential experience that allows potential actions and changes to emerge that enhance resilience. In fact, traumatized individuals often find it easier to be compassionate, curious, and comforting to others and unable to provide themselves with the same kindnesses (Fisher, 2017).

Clearly, cultivating compassion, particularly self-compassion, is an important and perhaps necessary piece in trauma reparation. It emphasizes the "experiencer" of the experience, with the goal of bringing kind and loving awareness to the traumatized individual, calling on what is essentially the person's own internalized caregiver. Like mindfulness, the goal of practicing self-compassion begins the shift from negativity to a more open and accepting stance, allowing new behaviors to become achievable.

Kristen Neff (2019), a major researcher in the area of self-compassion, summarizes it as follows:

> Having compassion for oneself is really no different than having compassion for others. Think about what the experience of compassion feels like. First, to have compassion for others you must notice that they are suffering. If you ignore that homeless person on the street, you can't feel compassion for how difficult his or her experience is. Second, compassion involves feeling moved by others' suffering so that your heart responds to their pain (the word compassion literally means to "suffer with"). When this occurs, you feel warmth, caring, and the desire to help the suffering person in some way. Having compassion also means that you offer understanding and kindness to others when they fail or make mistakes, rather than judging them harshly. Finally, when you feel compassion for another (rather than mere pity), it means that you realize that suffering, failure, and imperfection is part of the shared human experience. "There but for fortune go I."

Like resilience, self-compassion requires attention not only to an individual's sociocultural context, but also to the person's trauma history, including experiences of assault. The trauma history often predisposes individuals to feelings of guilt and shame that disrupt the capacity to feel compassion for oneself. That is why, in using the expressive arts and play to develop self-compassion, I try to use what I call "one-off" strategies. A simple one that I described in Chapter 5 involves caretaking a rubber duck and creating a safe place for it. For individuals like Toby whom I discussed in the beginning of this chapter, this became a way to experience sensations of compassion that she could not allow herself to have because of her shame and guilt about multiple sexual assaults. Later in her treatment, Toby also began to internalize compassion through group expressive arts therapy where she could express compassion and empathy for others and, in turn, experience it from others through musicality, art, storytelling, and movement. Group work is a way of sharing the common humanity that Neff and other researchers note develops self-compassion through knowing that one is not alone in having similar feelings, thoughts, and perceptions. It is the experience of "interbeing" that Thich Nhat Hanh (2011) cites as the core of self-compassion.

There are also important physiological changes associated with the experience of self-compassion. Research suggests that it may be a powerful trigger for the release of oxytocin, which is strongly associated with feelings of trust, calm, safety, generosity, and connectedness. In contrast, self-criticism appears to have a very different outcome and one that generally increases the stress hormone cortisol. Generating feelings of self-compassion actually decreases our cortisol levels. Rockliff and her colleagues (2011) asked participants to imagine receiving compassion and feeling it in their bodies. Every minute they were told to allow themselves to feel that they were receiving great compassion or loving-kindness. The participants imagined these statements had lower cortisol levels than those in the control group. The study concluded that the safer people feel, the more open and flexible they can be in response to their environment. This effect is reflected in how much their heart rate varies in response to stimuli. In receiving compassion, participants' hearts became less defensive. Recent studies using the drug MDMA (methylenedioxy-N-methylamphetamine; also known as ecstasy), in combination with psychotherapy, appears to be a promising avenue that supports structured experiences of self-compassion as a treatment for severe post-traumatic stress (Mithoefer et al., 2019).

EXPRESSIVE ARTS APPROACHES TO SUPPORT SELF-COMPASSION

To date, few expressive arts approaches have specifically targeted the development of self-compassion and its role in addressing traumatic stress. One approach, focusing-oriented art therapy (Rappaport, 2009), which is described in Chapter 6, intentionally cultivates self-compassion through use of visual arts as the chief component, along with a "focusing attitude." Rome (in Rappaport, 2009) defines the focusing attitude as "akin to the Buddhist virtue called maître—lovingkindness or friendliness directed toward oneself. It is a potent and at times quite magical way of making friends with oneself" (p. 63). The qualities of an open heart are the foundation of this attitude, which teaches the practice of friendly curiosity, "being friendly, accepting and keeping company" (Rappaport, 2009, p. 199) to learn unconditional presence and equanimity of emotions. In a focusing-oriented approach, this practice is the basis for learning how to accept one's felt sense, moment to moment, and it is key to compassion for the body's experience of traumatic stress.

The focusing attitude can be practiced and communicated through any of the expressive arts but is possibly most easily introduced through art expression. Using whatever relaxation protocol the individual is comfortable with for self-regulation invites an awareness of someone or something that embodies kindness, acceptance, and compassion. Again, I like to use a one-off approach, asking the individual to imagine giving kindness, acceptance, and compassion to either a pet or animal, a child (real or imaginary), or a person in need. The goal then is to sense these qualities within one's body. At this point, I invite the person to show me, using a body outline with colors, lines, shapes, or mark-making, where that experience is felt. Rappaport (2015) suggests that if an image for this felt sense emerges, drawing or other materials can be used to express it on paper or by creating a collage or object.

Because everyone needs a slightly different way to experience self-compassion, I have modified several different approaches and have combined them with movement and/or visual arts. For many people, these approaches are more effective because they are perceived as accessible and easily mastered with the help of the psychotherapist. I also "assign" many of the experiences described in the following section as self-compassion homework between sessions. Because these are positive experiences, they can also be "tapped in" through positive installation methods by practitioners who integrate EMDR into their sessions.

Placing One's Hand over One's Heart

Levine's (2015) Somatic Experiencing provides many powerful approaches to enhancing resilience in traumatized individuals. These methods often incorporate principles of self-compassion. Levine's practice of placing one's hand over one's heart while breathing gently and with loving-kindness is a way to support self-compassion. This practice can be combined with either a memory of being cherished by another individual (friend, partner, teacher) or imagining a special moment of caring or love for someone else. The goal is to allow these feelings to be experienced within the body and to try to stay with them for a few minutes. If it seems helpful, I often ask individuals to use colors, shapes, lines, or mark-making on a body outline to capture what the sensations felt like through imagery. That image can then be used as a point of reference to recapture the sensations of loving-kindness at other times.

Receiving a Compassionate Visitor

I regularly introduce the idea of an "imaginary compassionate visitor" as one way to experience compassion. This can be someone whom the individual knows, but in many cases, it is an imagined entity with a loving presence that is wise, caring, and empathetic. For those individuals who have a difficult time conjuring up such an entity, some coaching may be required to identify characteristics that embody a compassionate presence. Similar to Rappaport's (2009) arts-based strategy to represent the focusing attitude, I have clients create actual cardboard figures of these visitors not only to make details and characteristics tangible, but also for use in storytelling and particularly role play and enactment. The latter may include sharing worries or distress with the visitor, experiencing what it is like to be unconditionally understood and accepted, and imagining what words of encouragement or support one would hear.

What I am trying to evoke through this experience is the individual's own self-care system that may be offline due to the impact of traumatic stress. Although this approach is resilience-focused, if effective it also often has a calming impact on the individual and can become a resourcing image to mediate distress.

Extending Loving-Kindness to What Is Unlovable

Loving-kindness is also known as *metta,* and in Buddhism it is defined as a way to open one's heart and mind even when one is experiencing pain and suffering. It is part of a practice of wishing all sentient beings well, no matter what we think or feel about them. This includes extending the same loving-kindness to ourselves. There is a tradition in metta of saying the following phrases or variations of them:

- "May I (you) be safe from harm."
- "May I (you) be happy."
- "May I (you) be healthy."
- "May I (you) live with ease of well-being."

These phrases can be repeated as needed to make an impact, or they can be adapted to directly express loving-kindness to the difficult or unlovable parts of the self. For example, if personal shame is a dominant feeling, one might use a phrase like "May my shame find soothing and peace." I sometimes combine repetitions of these reparative phrases with regulatory body movements such as holding one's hands together and swinging them gently back and forth or a rocking butterfly hug (arms crossed, left hand on right shoulder, and right hand on left shoulder). As individuals work with this practice, they often naturally modify their phrases to focus on any current "unlovable" parts of themselves and find their own movements to complement the phrases.

Practicing Awe

Expressive arts are one of the best ways I know to encounter the phenomenon known as "awe." The experience of awe is not particularly rare, but it is often perceived as mysterious and hard to describe. To me, it falls into one of those truly body-based sensations that lets us know we are truly alive. Awe comes from many sources, including the birth of a child, elements of nature like the Aurora Borealis, the ocean, mountain peaks, or the giant redwoods, or human-made structures like the Great Wall of China and the Taj Mahal. Whatever it is that evokes awe often leaves us grateful and humbled, momentarily shifting our attention away from ourselves and into an experience of something much larger and transcendent. It also can help us to perceive ourselves in more positive ways and expand our world-views (Bai et al., 2017), and it is linked to decreased inflammation in the body (Stellar et al., 2015). Allowing ourselves to regularly and deeply experience awe connects us to something greater than ourselves in the moment and naturally moves us away from distress.

When I speak to individuals in treatment about awe, I often share an experience I have every time I hear a particular guitar riff at the end of David Bowie's "Starman." Each time I hear it, I feel a sudden surge of transcendence and joy that are so powerful my body tingles. Music is one way that many people feel awe, and it is generally an easy way to get regular exposure to the feeling of awe, once music that brings on the feeling is identified. The arts (visual, music, dance, and theatrical performances) can bring about awe in some people. This is possibly why some doctors are now prescribing visits to museums and encounters with nature (parks and gardens, walks in a forest). While less intense, even photographs or images can approximate the experience of awe.

In "practicing awe" for longer periods of time, whether through an image or through consistent exposure to awe-inspiring sensory-based experiences, the goal is to help the body deepen its ability to tap these resilience-enhancing sensations when necessary. Whether through music, enactment, or imagery, the sensation and embodiment of awe can also be strengthened within the brain and body by using positive install methods found in EMDR (Shapiro, 2018).

SELF-COMPASSION AS A CULTURAL PRACTICE

Because the concept of self-compassion is derived from culturally based spiritual practices and beliefs, applications to psychotherapy often bypass this source within the framework of trauma-informed work, losing the true meaning of mindful self-compassion. Of course, one way to learn the practice with the necessary depth of understanding needed to apply it comes from some form of mindfulness on a regular basis. This can be in the form of meditation, various mindfulness routines, or yoga. But learning from those who live these principles has given me a much deeper understanding of what it takes to integrate the concept in a meaningful way through expressive arts.

Dharma Creative Art Therapy Program

The Dharma Creative Art Therapy Program (DCAT) is facilitated by Kotchakorn Voraakhom and Prim Pisolaybutra, trauma-informed expressive arts practitioners and artists. Their unique program is located in Thailand and is based on the Buddhist *Dharma* practice, which has been integrated with self-expression through drawing, painting, molding clay, and other methods. Dharma principles, including meditation, ritual prayer, and self-compassion form the core of the approach. This particular program was designed for individuals facing terminal illness. The goal is to help these individuals live in the present and to practice awareness that death reflects the impermanence of being, a foundational belief in Buddhist Dharma. Buddhist activities, including morning–evening chanting, listening to Dharma, and use of nature, are part of the therapeutic environment.

Part of DCAT's effectiveness derives from integrating Buddhist principles within a framework of group interaction. Voraakhom, Pisolaybutra, and their research team have captured the practice of self-compassion through culturally resonant expressive arts adapted for the purpose of supporting resilience and addressing the trauma of end of life, including the following:

Gratitude Gestures and Hand Postures

Simple body movement is emphasized as a way to communicate feelings, particularly as ways to express gratitude and to accept support from other participants. This also includes staff who take a moment to reflect on group members through simple nonverbal gestures and hand movements. By implicitly expressing gratitude and acceptance, participants also experience a felt sense of these forms of compassion in their own bodies.

Clay Talk

After meditation, participants are given three pieces of clay with different textures. They are asked to touch the clay with both hands and reflect on their feelings toward each texture (soft, medium, and hard). They are also asked to manipulate and knead the clay as if it were their new friends. They then shape the clay into three subjects in the following order: (1) a self-symbol; (2) a representation of a person they miss or are thinking of in the moment; and (3) a gift they yearn for. By sharing these experiences, the participants are encouraged to listen deeply to each other and also to express kindness to themselves through the gift they most want for themselves.

Hoo–Hung–Mum

"Hoo–Hung–Mum" are sounds created from three different parts of the body: "Hoo" is the tone created from the head; "Hung" is the tone created from the nose; and "Mum" is the tone created from the chest. As participants vocalize each sound, they create a vibration in the different parts of the body and are asked to concentrate on these vibrations as a form of body meditation. Then, participants are asked to pick a meaningful word and write it down on paper, keep it in their minds, and repeat "Hoo–Hung–Mum." In the process, participants form new meanings by connecting the meaningful word in their minds and the rhythmic vibrations from their bodies. For those who have been dealing with body trauma due to illness, this activity can be adapted to help individuals communicate self-compassion to parts of the body that have been impacted or disabled by medical treatments.

These three approaches, while culturally resonant in Thailand, can be adapted in ways that may help any individual understand and practice self-compassion. Just as with any other application of expressive methods, it is essential that when arts-based strategies are integrated with concepts such as compassion that they make sense within the individual's or group's contextual framework.

INTERGENERATIONAL RESILIENCE

In Chapter 2, the concepts of intergenerational trauma (transmission of negative consequences across generations) and historical trauma (transmission of oppression and atrocities aimed at a specific group or culture) were presented as important pieces of trauma-informed practice, particularly exploring the impact of transgenerational trauma on the individual, families, and communities. While vulnerabilities have dominated the study of trauma across generations, the idea of intergenerational transmission of resilience has inevitably emerged (Jackson, Jackson, & Jackson, 2018; Southwick, Bonanno, Masten, Panter-Brick, & Yehuda, 2014). Also, if as trauma-informed practitioners we view trauma reactions as normal, adaptive, and often creative responses to adversities and survival, then these responses are evidence of resilience.

Many individuals, particularly those who endured developmental trauma or multiple experiences of interpersonal violence, may find it difficult to identify the thread of resilience in their intergenerational history. As I looked back on the dominant narratives in my family of origin, I eventually came to realize that I had inherited two distinctly different narratives. One was clearly related to intergenerational trauma and emerged from my mother's side of the family. While I never exactly knew the details of this storyline, in retrospect I recognized that it included multiple adversities, including abusive experiences, addiction, illness, and losses. Even as a child I began to recognize the threads of these traumatic storylines, especially in my mother, but also in my maternal grandmother and aunts and uncles who embodied an unspeakable sadness and hopelessness.

My father's side of the family presented a very different narrative, but it, too, included many stories of adversity and hardships. But my felt sense of these stories is very different in comparison to the maternal side of my family. During the 1920s and at the age of 10, my father was selected to make the journey from Italy to the United States to live with members of the Malchiodi family who had moved to America at the beginning of the 20th century. My father's parents were invited by their U.S. relatives to send one of their children to reside with them in Brooklyn, New York. This was seen as an opportunity for at least one of four siblings to advance and enjoy what was considered a better life than the impoverished farm life he led in the original small village of Grondone, Italy. My grandparents had to make the difficult decision as to which child to send. Because of cultural traditions, the eldest male child, my uncle Nicola, could not make the journey because he was expected to care for his parents. My aunt Vittorina was the only daughter and very young at the time; she could not be sent because of gender, age, and expectations to stay close to her parents. This left two other siblings who were twins—my father, Giacomo (James), and my uncle Luigi (Louis). The decision was eventually made to separate the twins and send my father to live in the United States with an aunt, her husband, and their children.

While this separation was undoubtedly traumatic for my grandparents, my father thrived as a result of that decision. During my childhood, I only heard positive stories of the opportunities he experienced as a result, including work as a laborer in a steel mill and the ability to build a home for my mother and the family. The separation from his parents was difficult, but he reframed it as a life-changing narrative in which he was given chances to move ahead personally and financially—opportunity that would never have been possible in the family village. By the time I was an adolescent, I clearly knew what narrative I wanted for myself and my future. My father's story was one of resilience that gave me a way to envision a personal narrative quite different from the limitations of my neighborhood, gender, and socioeconomic influence.

Not everyone is fortunate to actually embrace their family's resilience in this way, but I believe it does exist to some extent within all families, including those who have experienced intergenerational or historical trauma. The challenge within the process of psychotherapy is finding whatever small threads of resilience that are part of this intergenerational resilience narrative and try to capitalize on those threads to mediate and revise trauma stories over time. The following section describes an expressive arts approach that can be adapted to explore intergenerational resilience with clients.

Creative Genograms and Resilient Family Histories

Most psychotherapists are familiar with how to construct a genogram of an individual's family of origin (McGoldrick, Gerson, & Petry, 2008). Expressive arts therapists often look at this process in a slightly different way by integrating various arts-based processes into the mix. Schroder (2015) has explored the various ways therapists can help clients create visual genograms by using various media and approaches. As she notes, it is a visual process that helps most individuals "show up" through metaphoric vocabulary in a comprehensive way that encompasses layers of family history and relationships. Gil (in McGoldrick et al., 2008) provides a play therapy variation, capitalizing on the three-dimensional nature of toy miniatures in a sandtray. "The symbolic nature of the miniatures make them a fascinating tool for drawing out unrecognized family characteristics and patterns in a fanciful format . . . projection occurs when clients infuse objects with emotion or personality traits; [the process] creates a safe enough distance in which to begin to acknowledge, understand, or address personal issues" (p. 261).

My mentor family art therapist Shirley Riley (2004) convinced me of the importance of infusing expressive arts into the genogram process. Riley often spoke of how art in particular expanded her understanding of families' belief systems, saying, "The free form of the genogram and the use of color to indicate emotional attachment added greatly to their personal statement and gave life to the many persons involved. I could better enter their worldview when I saw the complicated relationships and cultural implications" (p. 37). Riley also impressed upon me the need to understand how improvisational techniques could help families literally enact a creative genogram and how one could work with those body postures to "re-story" a family's dominant narratives. Similar to Gil's miniatures, Riley suggested that re-creating family members and generations in nondrying colored clay was an effective way to do this. Because of the malleable and moveable nature of clay objects, the therapist and the individual can actively rework the pieces representing family members and revise various configurations, relationships, and dynamics and add new elements to the family history to make changes to the narrative.

While I might help an individual to create a genogram to explore generational family characteristics that are related to current traumatic stress, there is another way to approach this if we accept that resilience is also a thread within traumatized family histories. Pipher (2019) elaborates on the value of these types of family stories, noting that these can be stories of adventure, actions for the greater good, strength-based memories, survival against the odds, special abilities, and even moments of humor in the face of tragedy. However, it is not always easy to get traumatized individuals to believe in a "resilience thread" within what often seem like trauma-laden memories in families of origin. Toby, whom I described at the beginning of this chapter, is one such person who struggled with the idea of a resilient thread in her family history. She experienced developmental trauma in the form of multiple physical and sexual assaults by family members and later abuse by clergy in her church. To survive, Toby ran away from home at age 15 and was raised in foster homes until she was able to support herself and complete a college degree in a medical profession. By the time she was a young adult, she began to have severe panic attacks and dissociative episodes that brought her to my office and, eventually, into long-term treatment for trauma.

Like many individuals, Toby also found it hard to come up with any particular person who might have given her the strength-based skills to commit to and stay with treatment, hold a job while experiencing distressing trauma-related reactions, and survive day to day. In these cases and if it seems appropriate, I sometimes give a personal example to help individuals imagine that their personal genogram contains a resilience narrative. I share the information that I have a paternal grandmother whom I never met because she lived in Italy and died before I was old enough to travel to see her. The fact that I never met her in person did not stop me from imagining what she might have been like and what she may have contributed to my personality and worldviews. I was told that she raised four children and endured the loss of twins during childbirth and later a 6-year-old son in an accident. It always struck me that she must have been an incredibly strong woman to have faced the death of several children and to live in a small Italian village in a remote area with very little in terms of comforts. These few details have helped form some of my own perceptions of the source of my own strength to endure life's harsher moments as well as my beliefs that resilience is part of my "family tree."

As Toby and I explored what she knew of her family history, a dramatic piece emerged—some of her ancestors were of Cherokee descent. Among the Cherokee people, there is a generational story of historical trauma that is quite dramatic—the Trail of Tears, a series of forced relocations of Native Americans from their ancestral homelands that began in 1830. Although she did not have any specific stories about how her ancestors must have struggled to survive, in one session we speculated about it, conducting some Internet searches to obtain more details about the Cherokee tribe and the atrocities they experienced.

The following week when Toby came in for her regular appointment with me, she brought one of her art journals to show me a collage she had made with images, including a map of the actual relocations and the Trail of Tears migrations. She also read a written entry from her journal to me about her collage: "Suddenly I had a sense of connection to everything and everyone that contributed to who I am and how I got here to work with you. I have now read a lot about the 'Trail of Tears' that my ancestors had to go through, how they were forced from their land. In a way, the abuse forced me on my own trail of tears to escape more harm. But those ancestors, they made it. I think that must be the strength I have and why I am still alive today."

To capture this story, we decided to use a gourd (Figure 9.8), a material culturally relevant to Native Americans, to represent the ancestors who contributed to Toby's intergenerational resilience rather than a more

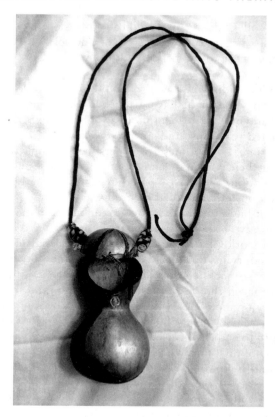

FIGURE 9.8. Toby's intergenerational resilience depicted through a decorated gourd. From the collection of Cathy A. Malchiodi (not to be reproduced without permission from the author).

typical creative genogram with drawing materials or collage. Inside that small gourd, Toby placed various painted seeds and natural objects to symbolize the entities whose courage and strength she believed she inherited. In the case of capturing resilience that comes in the form of a powerfully, worldview-altering story, making it special becomes part of the ritual of honoring the individual's discovery of a new narrative of strength.

As we continued to explore this story and the contents of the gourd over several sessions, Toby and I enacted the entities by improvising what each might communicate through words or postures (similar to the strength poses described in the previous section). My goal with these expressive explorations was to help Toby slowly redirect attention from what had predominantly been a narrative about traumatic events that dominated her family history for several generations to one that also contained resilience in the form of courage, stamina, and hope. The enactment, improvisation, and power poses, in addition to storytelling, helped Toby to begin to accept this resilient narrative as a felt sense that she could call forth in her body to counteract distressful sensations related to her abuse.

In reality, individuals never actually know what may have contributed to the parts of them that know how to survive and eventually thrive. Intergenerational resilience is just a concept, but it is one that can be useful to explore with some clients. While Toby was unable to identify any specific family members relevant to a resilience narrative, in looking back at her cultural ancestry she was able to discover some connections between that ancestry and her own abilities to survive adversity. Putting together her self-discoveries in the form of visual imagery and enacting intergenerational stories of resilience helped Toby to begin to embrace and embody a sense of strength and efficacy.

CONCLUSION

Resilience is undoubtedly an important piece in the overall process of trauma reparation. If adversities do impact individuals' capacities for mastery and competence, then it follows that we need to focus on those strategies that enhance self-efficacy and hope in the future. Many factors make resilience-building challenging, including social injustice and other barriers. However, using arts-based strategies to help children, adults, and families express and explore it in action-oriented ways holds many possibilities for psychotherapeutic changes. These possibilities not only include transforming cognitive beliefs about one's efficacy, but also provide necessary sensory-based experiences that contribute to an embodied sense of mastery and competence.

Supporting and enhancing resilience in any form is also predicated on the ability to imagine new narratives for one's life, post-trauma. This is a critical step because without the ability to transform distress-laden narratives, one has not completed the final step in trauma reparation—making meaning by imagining a new story for one's life, the topic for the last chapter of this book.

CHAPTER 10
• • • • • • • • • • •

Meaning Making

IMAGINING NEW NARRATIVES
FOR BRAIN AND BODY

Because making meaning of life experiences is integral to being human, it is key when it comes to trauma recovery. The experience of any profound psychological trauma challenges what has previously been meaningful in life for survivors. Recovery from trauma means developing a new understanding and worldview that attributes new meaning to what was experienced. This may feel unattainable for those who experienced multiple or complex events, but it is necessary to renew a healthy sense of self and reframe life stories that have been ruptured by traumatic stress.

Possibly the most referenced source regarding post-traumatic meaning making is Viktor Frankl, a psychiatrist who described his experiences in a concentration camp during World War II in the seminal *Man's Search for Meaning* (1963). As motivation for staying alive, Frankl chose to share his food, provide emotional comfort to other prisoners, and focus on the love of his wife and family who were also prisoners. Tragically, most of his family died by the end of the war. Frankl also held a vision for the book he would eventually write about why some individuals survive extremely adverse conditions while others do not:

> We must never forget that we may also find meaning in life even when confronted with a hopeless situation, when facing a fate that cannot be changed. For what matters is to bear witness to the uniquely human potential at its best, which is to transform a personal tragedy into triumph, to turn one's predicament into a human achievement. (Frankl, 1963, p. 135)

Frankl concluded that an individual's discovery of meaning for events and life gave them hope and resiliency. Within his concept of logotherapy, he observes that there are two ways to find meaning in life: (1) creating something new and (2) experiencing other human beings through their individuality and uniqueness. These principles resonate with the foundations of expressive arts therapy because creating something new is a core practice and what is created is shared with and witnessed by others, whether the psychotherapist, group, or community.

In addition to Frankl's concepts, there is a third meaning-making component that is unique to expressive arts therapy. Talk therapy is one way to communicate new meanings, but in order to be transformative, individuals must experience them at somatosensory and affective levels, too. Verbalizing these new narratives may be a necessary part of reparation, but I don't believe we cannot simply talk individuals into making meaning of traumatic events for two reasons. First, all stories that become the foundations of any meaning making begin as nonlinguistic expressions before they become language-driven (Damasio, 1999). Second, these stories are generated through the multilevel process of somatosensory, affective-perceptual, and cognitive-symbolic communications found in the expressive arts—the three levels of the ETC described in Chapter 3.

Finding and embracing a new narrative after trauma is one of the most difficult challenges for individuals in the process of recovery and integration. For psychotherapists, it is not easy to facilitate because internalized stories can be tenacious and longstanding diagnostic labels may have become part of a person's identity for years. Also, the brain, mind, and body have become accustomed to the sensations associated with traumatic stress and associated memories. For many people, these sensory reactions have become so familiar that they ironically are difficult to release and replace with healthier responses.

For this reason, the practices described in previous chapters—relationship, regulation, safety, body awareness, and resilience—are essential for most individuals in order to create new narratives for one's life. Equally important in this phase of reparation is the recovery of a sense of playfulness and pleasure in brain, body, and relationships with others. This includes the process of resensitizing the body to experiences of joy and aliveness and restoring imagination through expressive arts. Reconnection to others is also a key factor in finding wholeness because new meaning is ultimately created through relationships with others and within community. These three reparative functions—resensitization, restoration and reconnection—are the core principles emphasized in this chapter.

To more fully explain how the expressive arts support meaning making, I circle back to four authors whose work guided my thinking throughout this book: Lenore Terr, Judith Herman, Peter Levine, and Bessel van der Kolk. Each provides a key component that explains how the expressive arts repair and ultimately can help traumatized individuals form new narratives and become whole. These key components include (1) supporting moments of transformation, (2) altering trauma-laden stories, (3) rejoining community, (4) resensitizing the body, and (5) imagining new narratives.

SUPPORTING MOMENTS OF TRANSFORMATION

In my earliest work as an art and play therapist, Lenore Terr taught me what it takes not only to identify what caused trauma reactions, but also what brings about actual transformational moments. In her work with children, she believed that there is always something that impels that individual to change, either over a period of time or sometimes in an instant. This moment of change becomes a palpable and recognizable turning point in that individual's life. The therapist, according to Terr (2008), may recognize what one did to effect the transformation, but in many cases, may just grasp that there has been a "magical moment of change" due to one significant event or a series of interventions.

At some point during the course of psychotherapy, we may visually witness a positive emotional change in a child or adult or hear a shift in a narrative from an individual who is in the process of discovering new meaning, post-trauma. In expressive arts, there are unique moments of transformation related to the characteristics of expressive arts themselves. I may see someone enter my office with some "new moves," a sense of humor, and a palpable, playful energy that was not apparent in previous sessions. Other times the moment of change appears in the form of a written or visual journal entry that the individual is excited to share because it contains something hopeful or exhilarating. Sometimes I see a new set of symbols appear in an art expression, hear a more assertive beat on a drum, or witness a fresh configuration of miniatures in a sandtray. While there is no universal reason for the appearance of these expressions, the shift or magical moment of change that Terr spoke of is apparent through new self-assurance, positive affect and a change in content of what is communicated.

As most individuals move through the expressive arts therapy process, inevitably one or more of the arts—movement, musicality, image-making, play, creative writing, or enactment—becomes a regular part of communication. For example, some people take up creative writing, visual journaling, painting, yoga, or tai chi, singing, or another practice as a regular part of their lives. They also may adopt a medium as an avocation because it has become a form of self-regulation to reduce stress, or they want to continue their exploration through one or more art forms as a regular self-care practice. But sometimes a form of expressive arts brings about transformational experiences that lead to even deeper, long-term engagement in the arts that results in a new identity and thus, a source of new meaning for existence.

Case Example. Ray: Creating a New Identity Through the Arts

Ray, a 37-year-old combat veteran who served in Iraq during the siege in 2005 at Fallujah, self-referred to the clinic because of post-traumatic stress and depression. After a neurological evaluation, doctors at the clinic believed that a traumatic brain injury was partly the cause of his mood disorder, stress responses, and some memory issues. But Ray also believed that he was depressed before he enlisted in the Army and his head injury and that his struggles may have started as far back as adolescence.

Because of his depressed mood, Ray had quite a bit of difficulty becoming engaged with expressive arts, although he continued to regularly keep appointments with me. When clients get stuck in moving forward with expressive methods, I often try to help them identify what kinds of expressive activities may already be a part of their lives. Like many soldiers referred to me, Ray was pretty sure he never did anything more than draw or sing while in elementary school. By the third session, however, he remembered something that answered my question, offering, "Well, I used to whittle things. You know, get a stick and carve into it with a pocket knife." As we got further into this memory, Ray shared that most of the time this activity took place on the back porch with his father, a veteran of the Vietnam War. As it turns out, it was an extremely pleasurable memory for Ray. As he explained, it was a time when he felt close to his father, who often was distant due his own traumatic stress, depression, and alcoholism.

Since the clinic did not permit what would be defined as a weapon (a pocket knife) onto the premises, I arranged for several at-home sessions with Ray and asked if his father could be present to show me how they went about whittling. Both Ray and his father enjoyed instructing me in how to select the right wood for carving and some of the basics of the craft while we all sat together on the back porch of Ray's home. In the process of showing me how to master a piece of wood with a pocket knife, they began to share some of the deeper stories of not only their relationship but of their experiences with traumatic stress and depression. It was as if the repetitive motion of carving a stick or a block of wood began the flow of words, and significant memories and stories emerged. These moments of recall not only allowed these two individuals to strengthen their relational bond, but also to share time together that ultimately became transformational for each of them as veterans of military service with traumatic memories of active combat.

While many positive outcomes emerged from these sessions, another equally important change in Ray began to take place. He started to see himself as a competent wood carver and, as I reflected to him, a developing artist with a unique style. To my surprise, Ray took my approbation seriously and asked me to help him find ways to learn more about sculpture, with the goal of studying with someone who could help him become even more proficient in wood carving. While he continued psychotherapy with me and visits to his psychiatrist to address his depression, we also found a way for him to pursue art courses that were free to veterans at a local university.

A few months after we ended our meetings, a neighbor told me about a military veteran who had announced that he was "looking for any fallen or dying trees" for his new wood-carving business. I was not surprised that it was Ray and that he had already produced two large-scale carved pieces in a nearby community where many trees had fallen or were uprooted due to an extreme windstorm. He had carved the remaining trunks and stumps into life-like animals to the pleasure of the homeowners and the neighborhood that now had beautifully executed artworks instead of fallen trees on their streets. He also employed a couple of veterans as assistants and was conducting a weekly wood-carving class at his church. Ray had revised his life story from our initial whittling sessions on his back porch to something that obviously included artistry, creativity, and purpose. While he maintained scheduled visits for medications for his depression, his main focus was now clearly on something that he loved to do and that gave him the chance to contribute in a larger, more meaningful way.

In Ray's case, becoming an artist enabled him to take shattered and fragmented trees and sculpt them into objects of beauty and aesthetic value and, in doing so, alter his life story in a profound and impactful direction. Not everyone who comes to expressive arts therapy sessions ends up as an artist but, in my experience, a surprising number of individuals do continue to mature as artists in some way. The magical moments of change that Terr described have one important thing in common—they all involve helping individuals alter trauma-laden stories into life stories with new and reparative meaning.

ALTERING TRAUMA-LADEN STORIES

Of all those authors who describe the process of reparative meaning making, Judith Herman (1992) most clearly identifies the components of psychotherapy that make this possible for trauma survivors. Central to the final stage of her three-part model is the emergence of a new sense of self, a worldview of the future, and a redefinition of oneself within the context of relationships and the environment. It is during this stage that the experience of traumatic stress ceases to be the organizing principle or centerpiece of one's life. In sum, the trauma is no longer the only story that defines the individual. While many therapists refer to this process as recovery, it is really an experience of integration because it does not mean the complete absence of feelings and thoughts about the traumatic experiences. It means being able to live life without these feelings, thoughts, and sensations controlling one's life; it is a reconciliation with oneself. Herman notes that now the "task is to become the person she wants to be. In the process she draws upon those aspects of herself that she values most from the time before the trauma, the experience of the trauma itself, and from the period of recovery" (p. 202). Essentially, this is where the necessary integration takes place that makes new meanings possible.

Since the time I first read Herman's three-stage model in the 1990s, my worldview of each individual has included this conceptual framework for reparative meaning making as a psychotherapeutic goal. Talk therapy certainly provides an effective way to help individuals transform trauma-laden stories. For those who find words difficult, expressive arts provide a way to go beyond words or may be the necessary catalyst to stimulate verbal narratives. But in order to introduce arts-based approaches to support meaning making, it is important to set the stage for individuals to begin to revise trauma-laden stories and reclaim the life stories that trauma events have ruptured.

Narrative Therapy and Clients' Storytelling Rights

While there are many ways to help individuals tell and transform stories, I find that narrative therapy is one approach that is resonant with expressive arts. Narrative therapy focuses on the process of meaning making directly through the individual's life story (White & Epston, 1990). Like expressive arts, it involves externalizing the presenting problem. Most therapists are probably familiar with the core belief that the person is not the problem; rather, the problem is the problem (White & Epston, 1990). That is, the idea of separating distress from the individual's internalized experience is central to narrative approaches. The ultimate goal is to help individuals see the problem-laden dominant narrative as a smaller part of the whole self and to recognize that individuals are multifaceted in terms of culture, context, and the sum total of life's experiences (Denborough, 2016; White & Epston, 1990). What I value about narrative therapy is the central premise that, while individuals cannot always change the stories that others have about them, they can influence the stories they tell about themselves. With sensitivity and support, life stories can be reworked and reframed over time.

Narrative approaches become particularly important when individuals are ready to revise the trauma-laden stories that, according to Herman, need to be transformed in the final stage of reparation. These trauma-laden stories often appear to have been literally written by others and to be deeply embedded as tenacious forms of "private logic," the highly personalized worldviews due to trauma described in Chapter 8. As with any of the practices I have described, telling stories with the goal of transformation requires specific support when we consider what can be lifetimes of traumatic events. In these cases, the "Charter of Storytelling Rights" developed by narrative therapist David Denborough (2016) is one way to communicate the idea that individuals have the right to create stories of their own lives and to reclaim and revise their meaning:

> Article I. Everyone has the right to define their experiences and problems in their own words and terms.
> Article II. Everyone has the right to have their life understood in the context of what they have been through and in the context of their relationships with others.
> Article III. Everyone has the right to invite others who are important to them to be involved in the process of reclaiming their life from the effects of hardship.
> Article IV. Everyone has the right not to have problems caused by trauma and injustice located inside them as if it were some deficit in them.
> Article V. Everyone has the right to have their responses to hard times acknowledged. No one is a passive recipient of hardship. People always respond. People always protest injustice.
> Article VI. Everyone has the right to have their skills and knowledge of survival respected, honored and acknowledged.
> Article VII. Everyone has the right to know and experience that what they have learned through hard times can make a contribution to the lives of others in similar situations. (p. 9)

Denborough's list not only resonates trauma-informed practices, but also emphasizes the concept of healing-centered engagement that respects the individual's cultural and contextual experiences as storytellers. It captures the importance of establishing the person's right to define oneself within the trauma narrative inclusive of environment, social justice and other factors that impact traumatic stress. It also shows that the process of modifying that narrative takes into consideration the individual's unique cultural and contextual challenges that affect outcome and capacity for change in both the short and long term.

Transforming Narratives through Expressive Arts

In most expressive arts therapy sessions, I witness trauma-laden stories communicated through movement, music, imagery, enactment and play as well as listening to them. When I first read Herman's explanation of the importance of telling one's story, I interpreted her observation through a lens of arts-based approaches in which storytelling would be amplified through the multiple levels of nonverbal sensory and affective expression. With most individuals, the type of expressive art I introduce to tell and transform stories is unique because each individual responds differently to media. However, two media are particularly suited to storytelling. One is dramatic enactment that is the focus of the latter part of this chapter. The other is visual art because it is a natural way to communicate stories through symbols and chronology. If visual art is introduced with the specific purpose of transforming trauma-laden stories, it is helpful to introduce relevant metaphors that naturally imply growth beyond the present or open up possibilities for envisioning the future in some way. While there are many approaches to this, the following is one arts-based strategy that works well within a narrative therapy framework and with children, adults, and families.

Tree of Strength/Tree of Life ·

Because a tree conveys the idea of growth and change over time, I frequently use this metaphor in sessions when I want to support transformative storytelling. I first started to use it in work with children of military and their parents as a way to explore resilience-based themes and how each person contributes to the strengths of the family. In order to make these trees "come alive," I introduce ways to construct them three-dimensionally out of large brown paper bags (Figure 10.1) that can be easily manipulated to create a trunk and branches. The process involves making decisions about how to embellish the tree with collage—paper, magazine images, text, or other items. Because I often see multiple groups of families at the same time when working in military settings, I offer some specific directives such as "think about the roots as who and what in your family gives you strength. What images would you place on your roots to depict that?" And "think about branches as what things your family has been able to do or accomplish because of your roots. Pretend the foliage or fruits on the tree can tell that story in images and words." A third question I sometimes ask is, "If your leaves and fruit could tell a story about what you will leave behind— like legacies, messages for others or good deeds—what would they look like?" If I am working with one family, I may respond with other relevant questions while the participants create their tree.

What I quickly found out from listening to stories about these images when I first introduced this process is that creating the simple brown paper bag tree as a family unit generated more than just stories about strengths. The metaphor of a tree tends to stimulate thinking about past (roots), present (trunk and branches), and future (what is growing or in some cases, changing about the tree). In other words, the tree takes on a chronology for many individuals and families, becoming something like a life story with beginnings, current experiences, and future possibilities.

Case Example. Tim: Altering the Narrative of Family Violence

Tim is the 9-year-old son of two parents in the military. Tim's father has been deployed overseas on at least five occasions and has been in active combat three times. His parents recently separated because Tim's father became

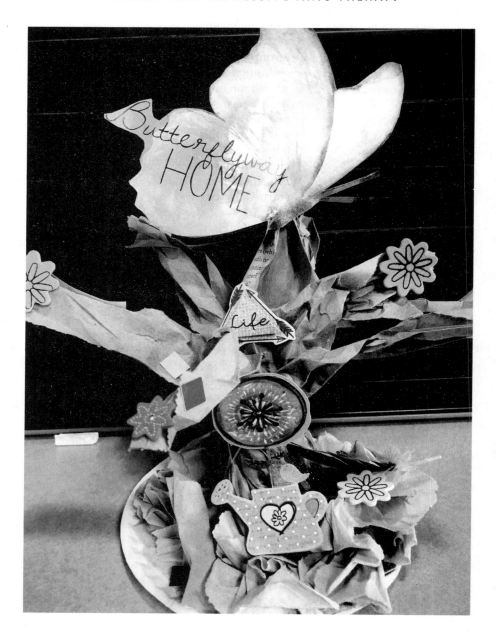

FIGURE 10.1. A family's "tree of strength" created from a paper bag.

violent toward his mother. During one incident Tim's mother had to go to a hospital emergency room because of serious injuries. Tim was referred to a children's resiliency-building group designed to support military families who were experiencing stress and interpersonal violence. His mother also insisted on individual treatment with me because he had responded well to arts- and play-based activities in the past. When I first met with Tim, he worried about "more hitting" and his teacher reported that he was becoming more withdrawn and anxious at school. His pediatrician also told me that she was worried about Tim because he had a higher than normal blood pressure for his age range, which she attributed to the stress he experienced at home. Like other children with similar profiles, he was hyperalert to his surroundings and was easily startled by environmental triggers. He had also developed a sleep disorder.

I introduced Tim to many different safety and self-regulatory practices during the children's group and also through individual expressive arts sessions. After several weeks in both the resiliency group and individual sessions, with Tim's permission I invited his mother to attend the next three meetings that were planned. During one session, I explained to Tim and his mother that it might be interesting to create a "strength tree" together, explaining the process of storytelling through the metaphors of roots, trunk, branches, and foliage. They quickly worked together to fashion a large tree from the brown paper bag and told many stories about Tim's grandparents who supported them during episodes of domestic violence, adding images representing them on the roots. They also decided to add colorful leaves and apples with positive words and statements about each other. One in particular stood out visually—a large leaf on which Tim wrote the word "BRAVE MOM" in large letters. When I asked Tim if he had anything specifically to say about his mother's bravery, he quickly volunteered, "She kept me safe when dad got scary. My dad is brave when he fights for our country, but my mom is just as brave as him." Hearing this statement caused Tim's mother to begin to cry, and she said, "Well, I am not the only one who has been brave. Tim had a lot of courage when my husband hit me over the last 2 years. I am so proud to be Tim's mother."

While these feelings were shared by both mother and son, this narrative never was articulated until that point. It was such a powerfully reparative moment that I asked if they could tell me the narratives of bravery again so I could write it down for them in the form of a short story. As they carefully repeated details, I also prompted them to give me clearer details so that I could "thicken" the story, a common approach in narrative work. I also thickened the sensory experience of their story by having them both show, through posture, gesture, and movement, what these experiences of bravery felt like in their bodies. In a sense, I was helping them practice what felt reparative and contributed to their somatosensory experience of strength, mastery, and self-efficacy (see the next section for additional discussion).

Fortunately, this session was the start of an even more reparative process, leading to a new narrative for Tim's mother and father. His parents eventually entered a relationship-building program for couples at the military base. Tim's father started treatment for anger management and for the post-traumatic stress reaction that contributed to his violence. After many months of intensive work, the couple reunited. Tim's father was reassigned to duty in the United States, which relieved the family of the stress of further multiple deployments for the short term. Tim continued to participate in groups for military children, and although he still experienced some learning difficulties, both his teachers and his doctor reported that he was generally less anxious and more outgoing.

Cases involving interpersonal violence are never easy to address, particularly when the therapist is trying to facilitate reparative narratives. Narrative therapists at the Dulwich Centre (Denborough, 2016) use a similar task called the "Tree of Life" and have added a unique metaphor to the process in working with violence. Like the Tree of Strength, it has roots, ground, branches, leaves, and fruits. Denborough explains the idea of introducing "compost" at the base of the tree, which becomes particularly relevant when working with individuals who have been physically or sexually assaulted by caregivers. When violent caregivers are part of one's roots, a compost heap at the base of the tree is a way for some individuals to transform what is often "rotten stuff" into fertilizer that helps the tree survive. This metaphor may not work or make sense to everyone. What is essential is to facilitate stories that help to reframe what has happened as well as support the capacity to generate a meaningful narrative to replace the trauma-laden ones.

REJOINING COMMUNITY

As I emphasized throughout this book, especially in Chapter 4, relationship is the central component of reparation and healing when it comes to trauma. Ideally, the expressive art therapy psychotherapeutic relationship lays a foundation for necessary transformational moments to occur and provide individuals with an implicit sense of safety, regulation and resilience. But there is another relational experience that is key to effectively addressing and altering memories of traumatic stress in the brain and body—revising one's relationship to others and the environment in a new way.

Ray's transformation into a working artist is just one example of this as well as another concept described by Herman that is part of the third stage of reparation—rejoining a community in a new way. For Ray, expressive arts took his recovery beyond the psychotherapeutic relationship and the clinic; he initiated his own actions leading to health and well-being in the long term. Re-entering a community or becoming part of a new one is a key element both in finding new meaning and, as many trauma specialists would agree, in the process of trauma integration. Ray also may be a good example of how individuals who use active task-focused and emotion-focused coping strategies generally do better and are more likely to report improvement in the long term. Toby, whose case was described in Chapter 9, showed signs of resilience, despite 15 years of multiple incidents of interpersonal violence. She became active in her reparation through her commitment to arts-based expression and exploration of intergenerational resilience in her Native American background. Her Native roots eventually connected her to a larger community of survivors through which she felt connected to other individuals who shared similar historical references and events.

Herman was one of the first to propose that individuals take identifiable steps toward self-determination within their relationships and environment as they begin to integrate trauma. At this stage, some individuals even find a mission that supports the process of meaning making post-adversity. Herman refers to this as a "survivor's mission," which is the need to transform meaning in the wider world through a political, spiritual, or social justice dimension. In this sense, redemption can be found through creating something in a larger context. I believe Herman is also referring to what we now call "post-traumatic growth" (Calhoun & Tedeschi, 2013), post-traumatic success, or adversarial growth. It is a process of reauthoring one's trauma narrative into a story that leads to a higher level of psychological functioning than before negative events occurred.

One goal of expressive arts therapy as a form of trauma-informed practice and healing-centered engagement is to help individuals return to their communities as individuals capable of directing their own journey of health and well-being. It can also be a way to re-enter the world using the arts as a form of post-traumatic growth for both oneself and others who have survived similar traumatic events or conditions. This experience often expands beyond personal reparation into social action and social justice. As Herman notes, even when there is no way to compensate for atrocity, there may be ways to transcend it through a mission or shared purpose.

As explained in Chapter 2, expressive arts grew in part from the work and vision of practitioners who were involved in advocacy in various social action and justice issues of the time period. As a result, work in communities became an important piece of the work and brought therapeutic applications of the arts to neighborhoods and culturally focused groups. This history is still very much alive today, and it is what I believe sets expressive arts aside from other therapeutic approaches, particularly within the context of trauma reparation. The following example describes one such program that brings soldiers together in art studios to help them transform and transcend the impact of combat and military service.

Combat Veterans Rejoining Community through the Arts

Although we have a long way to go in addressing traumatic stress among military personnel, there is a growing movement to facilitate recovery outside of clinics and offices. In many cases, this effort has been driven by the veterans themselves. Combat veterans have a long history of developing arts programs for both self-expression and rehabilitation. In the United States in 1981, a group of veterans established the National Vietnam Veterans Museum, a collection of art by those who served in the war in Vietnam. Although the works in this exhibit illustrate historical events and experiences of war, they also demonstrate how veterans themselves have discovered that art communicates feelings about combat, human triumph, and suffering.

Veterans of more recent conflicts in Iraq and Afghanistan are using the arts to record memories, express feelings, and make commentary through performances on the nature of war. One such program, called the Combat Paper Project (CPP; *www.combat-paper.org*), was founded by Iraq War veteran Drew Cameron and papermaking artist Drew Matott to provide a transformational experience to soldiers. Cameron personally experienced a need for catharsis and reconciliation after his tour of duty, believing that it was critical to bear witness to the soldiers' side of the story. The CPP approach centers on combat uniforms that usually sit in closets, boxes, or attics, remaining associated with feelings of subordination, battle and unacknowledged service to country. Soldiers are invited to take these uniforms and shred and pulp them to make paper for art, drawing, creative writing, and personal journals (Figures 10.2 and 10.3). Many of the soldiers who have participated in CPP either exhibit and speak about their work to public audiences or use creative writing as part of performances and readings, thus using dramatic enactment as a form of expression. In essence, the process transforms the experience of warfare into art and the warrior into an artist.

CPP is one of many programs that helps veterans re-enter community while confronting recurrent memories of trauma. Although clinics and hospitals provide psychotherapeutic treatment, for many soldiers, this type of community-based, soldier-run program is a key way to overcome the stigma of post-traumatic stress and moral injury. It is one of many arts-centered examples of what Herman envisioned as a mission not only to help oneself and others, but also to raise consciousness about the experience of trauma. (See another example of a veterans' program focusing on drama and theater later in this chapter.)

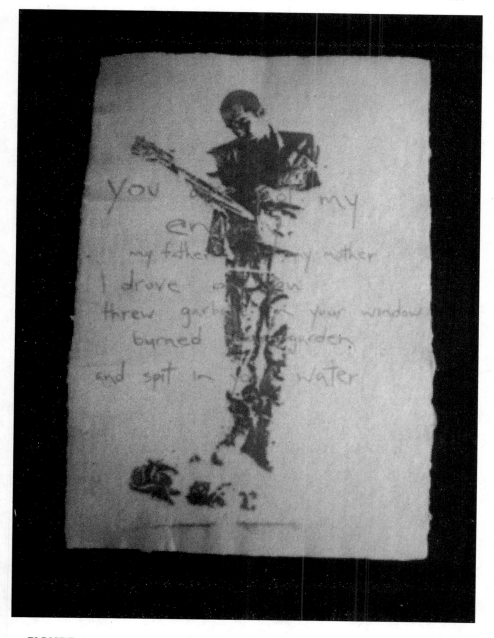

FIGURE 10.2. Example of paper art by Drew Cameron, military veteran and cofounder of the CPP. From Malchiodi (2012c). Copyright © 2012 The Guilford Press. Reprinted by permission.

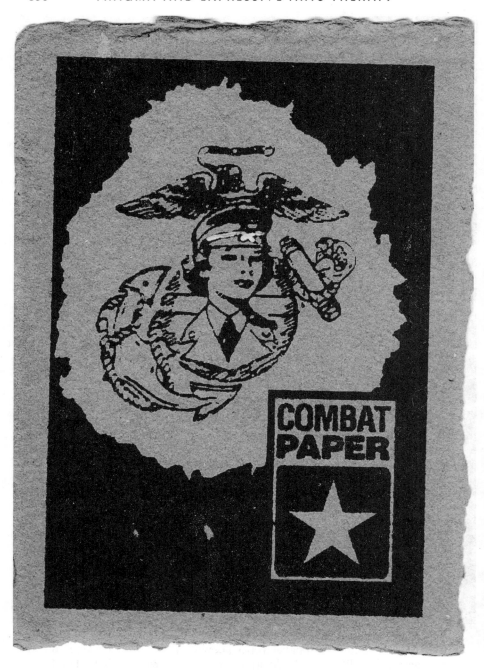

FIGURE 10.3. Example of paper art by Donna Perdue, veteran and participant in the CPP.

RESENSITIZING THE BODY

As emphasized throughout this book, Levine (1997, 2015) maintains that the body communicates the memory of trauma through posture, gesture, movement, breath, and other somatic responses. While not all individuals verbalize their experiences in each expressive arts therapy session, their bodies always tell a story of the traumatic stress they have experienced. This narrative is expressed in how the person enters the office, sits in a chair, and physically engages with me and through body-scan drawings when I say, "show me with colors, shapes, lines, or mark-making where you hold that emotion or sensation in your body." According to Levine, this somatic narrative is as important as the language-driven stories people tell. As their stories change over time, it is also observable in how people carry and move their bodies. While words convey the cognitive experience of meaning making, these deeper levels communicate important transformative stories. Similarly, Ogden and Fisher (2015) assert that body sensations and movements are constant sources of meaning making. Tronick and Reck (2009) echo this position, stating: "Meanings include anything from linguistic, symbolic, abstract realms, which we easily think of as forms of meaning, to the bodily, physiological, behavioral, and emotional structures and processes which we find more difficult to conceptualize as forms, acts, or actualizations of meaning" (p. 88).

Resensitizing the body is a focus that is missing from many current approaches that propose to help individuals decrease negative reactions to trauma memories, including popular methods such as memory reconsolidation. As explained in Chapter 8, trauma narratives do not just live in the brain as explicit stories; they are interoceptive experiences that include sensory and affective components. Also, in order to support the emergence of any type of reparative narrative, experiences that support safety, self-regulation and inhabiting the body in healthy and pleasurable ways are the foundation. Depending on the individual, these narratives may be expressed in movement, sound, enactment, or images or a combination of expressive arts. In Katja's case, a soldier described in earlier chapters, we unpacked that new narrative through movement and a playlist of music that eventually instilled a "good rhythm" in her body. Ultimately, when this shift happens, I see individuals like Katja start to become more playful and spontaneous, once again comfortable in their own sense of aliveness. However, for many a traumatized individual, this transformation can be difficult because the body has to reclaim its capacity for pleasure when long-held beliefs have convinced the person that this may not be possible for reasons of distress, shame, or guilt. The following example describes how one individual struggled with this challenge and reclaimed his body's aliveness through several of the practices described in earlier chapters.

Case Example. Anthony: Reclaiming Aliveness in the Body

Anthony was a 27-year-old Army medic who was referred to me because of post-traumatic stress responses including hyperactivation in the form of anxiety and anger and difficulty with relationships. He had already been in treatment with another psychologist for at least three sessions of EMDR and talk therapy, but his therapist could no longer see him because of her own medical issues. He was sent to the clinic for additional EMDR sessions because he felt he was making progress with this approach and needed some follow-up intervention.

As I took a brief history and we got to know each other, Anthony said something that shook me in the moment: "How can it be that my memories are more alive than me? I can't control my anxiety, yet my body feels hollow and lifeless." On a body outline, Anthony completed the image (Figure 10.4) in a way that many individuals who are numb to their body's sensory experiences depict their disconnection from sensations. While I have collected only informal clinical observations of how individuals with numbness or dissociation complete this task, there is emerging evidence that this form of psychological numbness is perceived as an empty space in the central torso of the body (Nummenmaa et al., 2018).

For those familiar with EMDR, a target memory that often has an associated image, negative belief, and body sensation is selected for the focus of a session. When I asked Anthony about his previous sessions, he reported that he and his psychologist focused mainly on his divorce from his wife of 5 years. This was a major source of stress for him because he also lost other relationships when his marriage dissolved. As our discussion continued, I started to notice what a tightly wound individual Anthony seemed to be, in both his rigid posture and the rapid cadence of his speech. When I asked him if we needed to continue to work on that memory or something else, Anthony once again surprised me, saying, "I think we need to work on the IED [improvised explosive device] explosion this time." I quickly realized that this was a memory, for whatever reason, that Anthony did not bring up in sessions with his previous psychologist. As he began to provide initial details about this event, I could easily see how his body responded with increasing tension and agitation.

In brief, the explosion caused the death of several soldiers because it was an unusual incident involving multiple devices and a series of mishaps. When I asked Anthony what his most vivid recollection during that time was, he responded that it was hearing that "the soldiers are gone" from the doctor on duty. When I asked him to isolate a word that might describe a negative belief that he had about himself now, without much hesitation he said, "Incompetent. We should have been quicker. We fucked up the mission and people died." At this point, we stopped for a moment, and I had Anthony once again show me on a body outline what sensations he was experiencing. Similar to his initial drawing, Anthony placed his negative

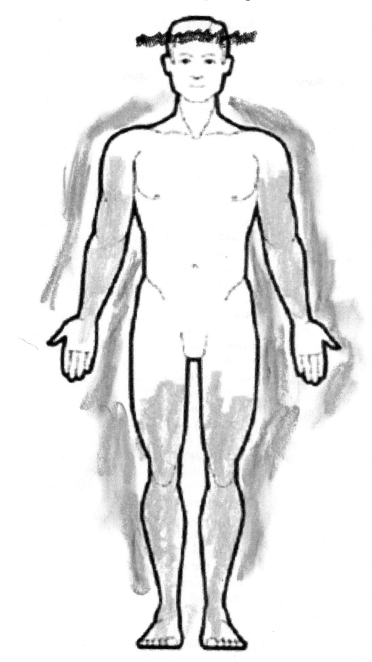

FIGURE 10.4. Anthony's "hollow and lifeless" body outline drawing. From the collection of Cathy A. Malchiodi (not to be reproduced without permission from the author).

association, this time that of stabbing sensations, all around the outside of the outline (Figure 10.5). In EMDR, individuals are also asked for a positive cognition, a statement that captures the belief the person would like to have about himself. Anthony took a long time to verbalize, "That I am competent and that I did the best in the moment. But I did fail these men." He was resistant to this positive belief but finally agreed to it, indicating that he felt it was impossible to accept at this point.

Using a series of eye movements to desensitize the negative sensations helped Anthony to more readily accept that he did the best he could under the circumstances. He reported feeling less tension and agitation, but understandably he still retained a sadness, saying, "I still have a numbness inside me. Good men died on that day." For Anthony, letting go of the body sensations associated with this memory was a necessary first step in dealing with the trauma. But just letting go of that sensation does not address the body's need for a new narrative. For Anthony, remaining numb to sensations and feelings had become his dominant somatic narrative; he could talk about releasing his anxiety and anger, but he continued to feel hollow and empty inside and unable to socially engage with others. Two approaches I introduced to him in previous sessions were particularly helpful to support the process of "resensitizing." Practicing self-compassion (Chapter 9) and trauma-sensitive mindfulness to accept his felt sense from moment to moment (Chapter 6) helped Anthony not only to allow himself to begin grieving the deaths of the soldiers, but also to slowly and carefully re-engage with sensations and emotions in his own body.

My other recommendation to Anthony was to take up a more physical practice like martial arts, tai chi, or yoga to continue maintaining a healthy focus on his body. Often this recommendation particularly resonates with soldiers who have trained their bodies for active duty but usually can benefit from a different way to experience physicality. Anthony decided to join a regular Bikram yoga (also known as hot yoga because the room is kept at a high temperature during poses) class and, combined with self-compassion practices, was able to slowly allow his body to begin the grieving process. He rediscovered a new body narrative that facilitated a sense of mastery, pleasure, and satisfying relationships with others. Like many trauma survivors, getting back into one's body is a process that is more potent if it extends beyond sessions in the psychotherapy office or clinic. Whatever the method, gradually bringing back the sensation of "aliveness" is a reparative process that inevitably helps to generate a new sense of self.

IMAGINING NEW NARRATIVES

Of all the concepts relevant to meaning making after traumatic events, imagination is possibly the most relevant to expressive arts therapy. The key ingredient of imagination is the capacity for mental flexibility that

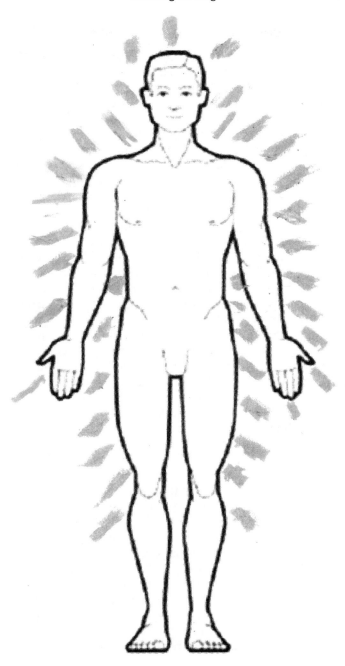

FIGURE I0.5. Anthony's "stabbing sensations" all around the outside of the body outline. From the collection of Cathy A. Malchiodi (not to be reproduced without permission from the author).

allows one to fantasize and create novel perceptions and thoughts and to envision new visions and outcomes—all of which are processes at the core of arts-based approaches. It is particularly significant for the process of meaning making because the ability to imagine something better than what has transpired is a necessary component of reparation. The various forms of meaning making presented throughout this chapter are, in part, predicated on the capacity to conceive of new outcomes.

Imagination is essential to making new meaning, post-trauma. However, I have often struggled with the role of imagination in my work with traumatized children and adults because of the impact of distress on the capacity to internally generate images, sensations, or ideas. If imagination is not accessible, it also can prevent or, at the very least, slow down the process of meaning making. This is supported by van der Kolk's research on military veterans (van der Kolk, 1994, 1996, 2014; van der Kolk & Ducey, 1989). Over half of the veterans had flashbacks of traumatic experiences when viewing a Rorschach test. The responses of a quarter of the group were even more interesting; these individuals could not see anything in the images and simply saw ink blots. Normally, a response to this type of stimulus is the use of imagination to make meaning through a story about the image. van der Kolk (2014) went on to reason that traumatized individuals may be more inclined to superimpose trauma on their day-to-day experiences and that indeed trauma impacts imagination in some way. This explains much of what I was seeing in children and adults who had significant traumatic stress and were struggling with using their imagination to play, move, draw, or role play.

From both personal experience and my work with children and adults, I believe that the ability to "pretend" is an important factor in changing negative stories about oneself. I have imagined my way through many difficulties throughout my life by pretending a different outcome or scenario. I can recall doing this even as a young child through the arts and play, and with the encouragement of my parents, to see beyond limitations. In order for anyone to mentally escape the more challenging moments of life, one has to be able to imagine pleasurable events such as travel, adventure, love, or whatever helps one to "feel better" in the moment. My pretend scenarios did not miraculously change my mood or my body's sense of distress overnight, but through imagination I gradually came to believe in something beyond a loss or setback. In part, my own artistic expressions—whether visual, movement, improvisation, or performance—are moments of envisioning new experiences that generally lead to eventual change.

As noted in the beginning of this book, the effectiveness of expressive arts therapy is often predicated on the individual's capacity for imagination. McNiff (2004) proposes that "art heals by activating the medicines of the creative imagination. Yet we know very little about the intelligence of the creative imagination, for the subject has been overlooked and even disparaged by many" (p. 221). Fortunately, this is becoming less true as imagination is now finding its place as an essential capacity not only for cognitive abilities, but also for social–emotional skills such as empathy, curiosity, sense of purpose, confidence, envisioning the future and meaning making (Kaufman, 2013a, 2013b; Kaufman et al., 2015). There is also emerging evidence that the brain's default mode network, a distributed system found in the frontal and parietal regions along the midline of the brain as well as the temporal and parietal areas, plays a significant role in the ability to imagine. Of interest to expressive arts, this system seems to support the ability to generate imaginative thoughts and facilitate creative responses (Beaty et al., 2014; Beaty, Benedek, Kaufman, & Silvia, 2015).

When we talk about trauma integration within the expressive arts, we ultimately are referring to the possibility of imagining new stories through arts-based experiences in order to become whole again. This goes beyond simply making meaning; it is the process of imagining a new self-concept of who we are as individuals and within our relationships and environments. In order to harness imagination in service of traumatized individuals, psychotherapists can use the expressive arts as a way to actively redirect attention away from the internalized experience of the world as a place of threat and other environmental cues that result in traumatic stress. The story of one early art therapy practitioner, Friedl Dicker-Brandeis, whose actions made a difference in the lives of hundreds of children, demonstrates the importance of imagination even in the most adverse conditions.

Imagination as an Antidote to Adversity

Many years ago, I was invited to study an unusual collection of drawings created by children at Theresienstadt, a hybrid concentration camp and ghetto built by the Nazi SS during World II, as well as the story of their teacher, artist Friedl Dicker-Brandeis. Friedl was born in Vienna in 1898 and studied art at the Weimar Bauhaus with the well-known artists Johannes Itten and Paul Klee. The Bauhaus philosophy embodies not only design, but also the aesthetics of empathy. Students like Friedl were taught to not merely depict an object in drawing or paint; they were encouraged to become one with their subject, to see it both inside and out, and to empathize with it. This philosophy influenced Friedl's own artwork and subsequently how she taught art to children at Theresienstadt.

In 1942, Friedl and her husband, Pavel Brandeis, were living in Czechoslovakia when they were deported to Theresienstadt. I was surprised to learn that, when Friedl was deported, she used most of her 50-kilo weight allowance to bring art supplies to this ghetto. While others were understandably focused on self-preservation and packed items needed for survival, Friedl obviously had a different intention in mind—to have what was necessary to teach art to hundreds of traumatized children. At the camp, she encountered over 600 children who were taken from their homes, communities, and routines and forcibly separated from their parents and families. They were placed in unspeakable conditions and sent to live in overcrowded houses. Because boys and girls were separated, even brothers and sisters no longer were allowed to stay together. This trauma of separation was compounded by starvation and illness.

As I reviewed these stories and records of the brutality of Theresienstadt, I realized that Friedl Dicker-Brandeis gave these children more than just a purpose or a way to cope. She purposively gave them the power of imagination to help them endure the atrocities of daily life. She realized that art could be a form of therapy for misery, fear, and uncertainty and encouraged her young students to create in the style of the Bauhaus philosophy. Using collage, watercolor painting, and drawing, she taught the children to look below the surface of a flower, person, or still life and become absorbed with the feeling of the object or individual. In witnessing dozens of these children's art works, I came to believe her goal was not only to stimulate the imagination of these children, but also to redirect them to internalize what existed far beyond the walls of Theresienstadt.

Like so many interned during the Holocaust, Friedl watched as her husband was deported from Thereseinstadt; as a result, she voluntarily signed up for the next possible transport to follow him. On October 6, 1944, Friedl and approximately 60 of her students were sent on transport number EO 167 to Auschwitz–Birkenau where they were either murdered on arrival or died of illness or starvation shortly after. What became of the children's art expressions and a few of her own drawings and paintings still sends chills throughout my body. In the hope that others would eventually see what they had created, she placed approximately 4,500 pieces of artwork in her two suitcases and hid them before she left on the transport to Auschwitz. Friedl did not sign most of the work she created during this time, but she had the children sign their artworks with their name and age.

While I am emphasizing the role of imagination in Friedl's work with these children, her deliberate action to make sure that each artwork had an identity also resonates with Herman's emphasis on the voice of the individual and reconnection to community. Although most of the children who created these works were murdered by the Nazis, I was able to meet with some of the few who did survive and remembered their art teacher. The consensus among these survivors—at the time in their 70s—was simple and profound. They believed Friedl redirected each of them to embody the beauty of life through their art expressions rather than depict the daily horror that surrounded them at Theresienstadt. I believe that imagining and re-creating that beauty surely sustained these survivors while they were experiencing the most abysmal, oppressive, and extreme conditions. As survivor Eva Dorian said of Friedl, "I believe that what she wanted from us was not directly linked to drawing, but rather to the expression of different feelings, to the liberation from our fears . . . these were not normal lessons, but lessons in emancipated meditation" (Wix, 2009, p. 154).

Imagination and the Capacity for Positive Change

The story of Friedl Dicker-Brandeis is a dramatic example of the power of imagination in the face of extremely traumatic and adverse conditions. The core of her approach to work with children underscores a principle that has been verified by research in the arts. In the field of art therapy, art making has traditionally been used to discharge negative emotions through self-expression (Kramer, 1993). But when it comes to stimulating new narratives with reparative capacities, this may not be the most optimal strategy. Research demonstrates that drawing what is negative may not be the best use of imaginative powers. In fact, using drawing as a distraction from negative emotions is more helpful in regulating mood (Drake & Winner, 2012). As it turns out, "drawing a picture of happiness" is improved by distracting oneself away from negative thoughts and is more effective in repairing mood than either venting negative feelings or simply allowing time to pass for the mood change. Drawing also was a more effective means of immediate mood repair than writing; both activities repaired mood more effectively through distraction than through venting (Drake, Coleman, & Winner, 2011).

The kinds of cognition, emotions, and somatosensory experiences we want to make "stick" in clients when we are using arts-based approaches are key to helping them imagine new narratives, post-trauma. In other words, if we do not eventually help individuals move away from distress, we will leave them with thoughts, feelings, and sensations that will not support new narratives of pleasure, confidence, and hope. This premise is also emphasized within somatic approaches, including sensorimotor psychotherapy (Ogden & Fisher, 2015), that underscore supporting new narratives and the capacity for positive emotion through playful engagement between client and therapist. Within the field of expressive arts, dramatic enactment is one particular approach that integrates multiple pathways for imagining novel and reparative stories.

Dramatic Enactment as Performative Change

Dramatic enactment is a form of expressive arts that helps individuals find reparation through *performative change*; that is, individuals are engaged in multilayered, action-oriented process that taps multiple levels of expression. Whether improvisation, role play, theatrical reading, or actual performance on stage, dramatic enactment generally integrates movement, sound, visual experiences, and storytelling. Pretend and imagination are central to drama and, when experienced as part of a group of actors, there are the added elements of relationships as well as proprioception of the body in the environment. Most importantly, dramatic enactment calls on individuals to take risks through pretend roles and novel identities. Dramatic enactment also provides the opportunity to try out new narratives not only through language, but also through embodiment of a character. When an audience is part of the dynamic, the element of being witnessed is an additional part of the experience for both the individuals playing roles and the viewers.

Bloom (2005) captures the challenge of making meaning after trauma.

> The traumatized person becomes possessed, haunted by the theater of the mind. He cannot control the intrusive images, feelings, sensations. He comes into consciousness unbidden, terrifying, vivid, producing a vicious cycle of helpless self-revictimization and even the victimization of others. Any efforts he took to protect himself or others at the time of trauma were a failure, and yet images of what he could have done— failed enactment—continue to obsess him. (p. xvi)

Bloom, a proponent of expressive therapies, notes that drama therapy can be one way to address the complex mind, body, and spiritual issues that traumatic stress entails and that is not easily ameliorated by medications or cognitive forms of intervention. Similarly, Landy (2005) explains dramatic enactment within the context of role play and storytelling, framing it as the "doubleness of all human life." When enacting a role then, the individual has to be more than one entity simultaneously playing one's own role and the pretend role. This dynamic naturally allows people to experience and act out multiple perspectives.

Johnson (2009b) proposed that drama and theater have the basic structure and purpose needed to integrate the communal aspects of traumatic experience. Some of this evidence comes from the consistent use of theater as a form of public communication to raise consciousness, "public confession," coming out as survivors of tragedy or as a rite of passage. Like the arts programming described in the previous section, there is a long tradition of veterans and people with disabilities or mental illness performing before public audiences, focusing on themes and issues related to their lives. Emunah and Johnson (1983) note:

> Transformation of self-image is heightened in these self-revelatory performances. Self-revelation by cast members affects the misconceived image a public audience often has of mental patients, presuming their problems are foreign and bizarre. A kinship is established between the audience and actors. For group members, who perceived themselves as alien, the audience's identification with their struggles brings about a sense of belonging to the larger community rather than exclusion from it. The self, already part of a small group, now becomes part of the world. (p. 238)

As previously mentioned, what is unique about dramatic enactment in any form is the element of witness in the form of audience. In an expressive arts therapy session, the psychotherapist becomes the audience. But in many cases, the witnessing takes place by groups and communities. Enactments also involve many individuals playing roles that include interaction and response to others. If you have ever worked with expressive arts groups, you have probably experienced how creative sparks move among participants, igniting new ideas and output. This is particularly helpful for traumatized individuals who may not be able to easily articulate thoughts or feelings. The proximity and interaction experienced through drama naturally stimulates ideas and insights. This is why groups are often more effective for many people whose distress may related to alexithymia or for those who benefit from hearing common experiences and stories of others.

Although many expressive arts programs capitalize on the value of theater as a pathway to reparation through imagination, one particular program demonstrates key principles that psychotherapists can apply in work with traumatized individuals. The DE-CRUIT program has had consistent success and positive research to support the many reasons why drama is a potent form of expressive arts when dealing with traumatic stress. The program is predicated on the human capacity for imagination as a psychotherapeutic element (Ali & Wolfert, 2019) as well as standard acting techniques to support performative change.

DE-CRUIT: Repairing Traumatic Stress in the Military

The DE-CRUIT program was developed by the Veterans Center for the Performing Arts (VCPA) as part of its mission to support veterans with traumatic stress. The programming captures what I have encountered with many of the military veterans I see in treatment, that is, symptoms and behavior that go beyond the typical diagnostic labels of post-traumatic stress and mood disorders. The program considers the context of military recruitment and how the indoctrination of young adults through training essentially "wires" them to combat. In order to function in combat, they become progressively more numb to violence. Once home, many of these soldiers continue to respond as warriors because there are few resources designed to undo their combat indoctrination. So while specific events may contribute to traumatic stress, veterans are also extremely vulnerable to the challenges of reintegration into civilian life.

DE-CRUIT uses principles found in classical actor training, including engagement in spoken verse and breathing and voice techniques that support recitation and performance. It also integrates empirically established psychotherapeutic methods such as narrative therapy and cognitive processing therapy to address post-traumatic stress (Ali & Wolfert, 2016). The program includes writing trauma monologues that are performed by the group and uses Shakespeare's verse to help veterans with articulation, sharing and processing trauma (Ali, Wolfert, Lam, & Rahman, 2018).

DE-CRUIT is a detailed process and has many components that make it successful as a reparative experience that capitalizes on making meaning and imagination. For the purpose of understanding how this expressive arts programming relates to the use of enactment in psychotherapy, two core processes (Ali et al., 2018) are described below.

Aesthetic Distance

Aesthetic distance is a key therapeutic element in drama-based approaches and is part of the "doubleness of human life" that Landy explained. It is the emotional expression that exists between what Landy called "under distancing" (overly emotional) and "over distancing" (removal from feeling). The optimum aesthetic distance is one in which the individual can identify with a narrative through enactment while not being overtaken by it. This concept echoes the window of tolerance model presented in Chapter 5, a framework that is used to keep the individual in a place that is slightly challenging, yet not overactivating or hypoarousing.

In DE-CRUIT, participants use Shakespeare as a form of distancing, and thus the words used are not the participants' words. The monologues are selected through the program's unique process that reflect the participants' experiences of trauma. Aesthetic distance is also supported by seeing and hearing one's narrative performed by other veterans, and the performance is also witnessed by an audience of friends and family. All of these principles form not only the principal components of DE-CRUIT, but also any form of dramatic enactment within the framework of expressive arts therapy.

Mimetic Induction

Mimetic induction is the use of "theater to provoke positive psychological change" involving "immersion in a fictional world that approximates the client's own world, thereby mimicking, revealing and eventually transforming their actions, responses and real-life behaviors" (Ali & Wolfert, 2016, p. 60). As an approach within drama and theater, it allows the individual to experience self-referential imagination (Oatley, 2016) or to view a dramatic performance while imagining him- or herself in the story. For example, Shakespeare's plays can stimulate strong universal emotions in those reading the verse or in those watching, but they also depict a world that is removed from current reality.

Aesthetic distance and mimetic induction are important processes that can support reparative narratives. While I recommend drama in the form of acting and performance as a potent form of expressive arts to support reparation and the formation of healing stories, it may not be practical for every psychotherapist to apply the principles found in DE-CRUIT and other forms of acting with traumatized individuals. However, there is one concept central to drama and acting that is applicable with most individuals—improvisation.

Improvisation and Imagination

Improvisation is the practice of acting, dancing, singing, playing musical instruments, and creating images with spontaneity and is the capacity to react in the moment. Improvisation is essentially a form of intuition in motion (Nachmanovitz, 1991). As a fine arts student, I gravitated to performance art as a minor in my education. Most of this training involved improvisation—a performing arts method that has no specific or scripted preparation. It is often referred to as "ad lib," "playing it by ear," or "making it up as we go along." I found that these improvisation skills could be applied to a wide variety of endeavors, including encouraging imagination in expressive arts. Family art therapist Shirley Riley (2004) later taught me another important reason for psychotherapists themselves to engage in improvisation. Riley participated in acting and improv classes with professional actors for many decades and applied this experience to her work with couples and families. In particular, she believed that stage performance and improvisation helped her to react more effectively in the moment as a psychotherapist, enhancing her spontaneity in working with clients to develop creative solutions to their challenges. Improvising with clients also begins the imaginative process often called "brainstorming," in which any ideas or solutions are expressed, regardless of how practical they seem in the moment. The point is to help individuals invent new thought patterns, practices, and ways to "act" and "improv" new ways of being and revising stories that, as Riley would say, are "now getting in the way."

It can be difficult for traumatized individuals to trust in spontaneous invention; especially in early sessions, improvisation can be a threatening skill to master. For reasons of hyperarousal or dissociation, responding in the moment is difficult and can even bring on reactions similar to freeze reactions, especially in those who are easily triggered by sensory cues. Fortunately, once judgment is suspended, expressive arts and play-based activities provide opportunities to practice what Csikszentmihalyi (2014) refers to as "flow"—a state of participation that brings pleasure in the "doing" in the moment and in losing one's sense of time and space.

One early mentor, Gestalt art therapist Janie Rhyne, taught me some simple approaches to improvisation that could be applied to expressive arts in psychotherapy. Rhyne encouraged her students to use chalk pastels or charcoal sticks to make bold movements, lines, and shapes on large paper and then respond to these images with movements, sounds, music, or performance. The goal was to become spontaneous and to learn to improvise by mirroring and amplifying the lines and shapes in images through other art forms.

If you haven't experienced or applied this type of exercise, I suggest that you experiment with this practice by creating several spontaneous pastel chalk images on large paper (at least 18″ × 24″) just using lines, shapes, and colors or mark-making. When making these images, try to use your entire arm and shoulder in your mark-making; you can also use both hands (bilateral drawing, Chapter 7) to create these images. Choose one image and lay it on the floor or tack it to a wall. Rather than analyze what you have created, simply be with the image in a mindful way—contemplate it without determining what you are going to do next. While you can choose to respond to the image with music, vocalization, or a performance, it is easiest to start with movement. Just start to move your body while looking at your image, using the lines, shapes and/or colors as inspiration for your movements. You can also just make a simple gesture. For example, if you have made a series of vertical lines, you might respond with thrusting both of your arms into the air. If you find one gesture that feels right, then try continuing to make that gesture over and over and let it develop into a rhythm. Otherwise, just stay focused on your image and move your body for a few minutes.

In adapting this exercise for use with clients, it is important to emphasize to them that no one can fail by just moving and that all improvisations are equal. While this approach to improvisation can be used in an expressive arts therapy session, it is often even more effective within a group where safety and self-regulatory practices have been established. In a group, a variation of this process can be introduced by inviting another participant to respond to a person's movement through movement, vocalization, or performance. In other words, that individual may be coached to respond with a gesture to support or simply communicate a felt sense.

PLAY AND DRAMATIC ENACTMENT: FACILITATING PERFORMATIVE CHANGE IN CHILDREN

Although I learned a great deal about imagination from a fine arts education, much of what I have learned came from a year of work as a preschool teacher. Working with young children is an excellent training ground for witnessing the emergence of imagination and the value of pretend behavior. From the age of 3 to 4 years, most of us develop and explore the capacity to be imaginative through play, creative activities, and storytelling. I was treated to seeing young children pretend, move, and dance without inhibition, boldly sharing statements like "I want to show you how to be a tiger. It's very easy to be a tiger" and "Now there's two things happening in my pants." Statements like "I just made a circtangle!" demonstrate how easily imagination is accessed by young children who have experienced positive and secure attachment and trust adults as helpers, teachers, and nurturers.

In Chapter 8, I explained how a set of expressive arts strategies helped Josh change his trauma narrative about witnessing an accident from a repetitive and stagnant story to a more reparative one. Josh was able to move through stages of recovery somewhat quickly because of secure attachment and other factors that allowed him to eventually imagine new outcomes. But the majority of the children I see in expressive arts therapy come from more challenged situations. When I started to work with children who had developmental trauma and experienced repeated interpersonal violence, I began to notice a sharp contrast in how imagination was expressed. For example, some simply did not know how to interact with toys, art materials, drums, or puppets because they never had the experience early in life to do so, nor did they have the guidance from a supportive adult caregiver. Many children were just too fearful of repercussions or punishment to freely play or make art. I quickly realized that it would be a challenge for these young clients to engage in the very experiences that I believed would bring about reparation and a sense of well-being because their ability to imagine was essentially impaired.

Despite these challenges, using drama and pretend play are, in my experience, the most effective ways to work with children stuck in unproductive trauma stories and in need of the "magical moment of change" that Terr underscored in her psychotherapeutic work. With regard to dramatic enactment and children, it is impossible to separate play from drama or acting from play; they are essentially partners in work with traumatized children. Both enable children to embody various characters, use distancing to pretend, provide opportunities to personify others, and, most of all, imagine new scenarios. They are key approaches that support the transformative work necessary to help young clients make sense and eventually make meaning and transform meaning in their lives.

Some of the toughest child client cases I have described throughout this book are those I have encountered who have witnessed domestic violence. These children come face to face with the horrors of watching a parent being controlled and abused; this often includes hitting, shoving, and yelling and may involve seeing weapons such as knives or guns. Watching one's parent be injured leaves children with at least two dominant narratives; on one hand, children want to protect their parent from harm, and on the other, they simultaneously need to feel protected from violence by the parent. When an altercation between a parent and a partner is reported, there are also other narratives, including leaving home and being brought to a community facility like a safe house or shelter.

While children who witness or are subjugated to interpersonal violence bear stories that often require additional support throughout their lives, there are opportunities to help them find islands of relief through play, especially dramatic enactment due to the action-oriented nature of these approaches. These approaches also provide windows for meaning making through the multi-sensory ways discussed throughout this chapter.

Case Example. Daniel: Supporting Imagination and Meaning Making with a Child from a Violent Home

I first met Daniel when he was 6 years old at a domestic violence shelter where I saw children for individual sessions several times a week. Theresa and her son, Daniel, were brought to the facility by the police late one night after a neighbor called an emergency hotline because she believed Theresa and her son were in danger. Theresa reported on intake to the shelter that she had been physically assaulted by her husband on numerous occasions but was afraid to report the incidents because she feared that her spouse "would end me in front of my son." She also reported that Daniel had witnessed most of these physical assaults and often "collapsed in a corner crying uncontrollably."

In the first session I worked with Daniel, it was apparent that he had many memories of what happened during the times he witnessed his father's brutality to his mother. Unlike many children I have worked with after witnessing violence, Daniel was immediately forthcoming through drawings that vividly illustrated the details of his experiences of seeing his mother assaulted. He was very hesitant, however, to verbalize details. At the time I surmised that he was experiencing a speechless state due to the horror of what he had witnessed. During the few sessions I met with Daniel, he remained frozen in a fear-laden posture that reminded me of someone who wanted desperately to hide or become invisible.

Unfortunately, as in many cases at shelter programs, my time with Daniel was cut short, when he and his mother were moved from the facility to long-term housing for safety and additional treatment. Two years later, like many survivors of domestic violence, Theresa returned to the shelter with Daniel because of more physical assaults, including one that was so severe she had to be hospitalized. During that time, Daniel was placed in foster care until his mother sufficiently recovered and could take care of him again. On this stay at the facility, I was able to arrange three sessions each week with Daniel. At this point, I simply wanted to help him begin to learn some self-regulatory and co-regulatory practices on his own and with his mother and to develop a relationship with him.

During our first session, I once again witnessed the little boy I had seen when we first met 2 years before—a young client with a posture and movements that communicated how unsafe he felt in his body. At age 8, Daniel was still clinging to his mother when she brought him to my art and playroom; when Theresa left, he seated himself in a far corner of the room with his head and shoulders slumped forward. It would take a while for him to make eye contact with me and when he did, it was tentative and fearful for the first several minutes. He continued to draw images similar to those I had seen 2 years before, depicting family violence, especially threats to his mother. But fortunately, after several sessions, Daniel also began to become more relaxed with me and the playroom, occasionally moving from his seat to explore some of the toys and materials.

At this point, I was able to encourage Daniel to work with miniatures and objects in the sandtray in an effort to engage him in something a little more interactive and dynamic than drawing. When I asked him to tell me about his sandtray scenes, he generally told stories about danger without hope or escape. When I suggested possibilities for help or protection, he still could not conceptualize those outcomes even with my support. This seemed to reflect Daniel's lack of a course of action for when he was threatened, especially during the incidents he witnessed at home. His dominant narrative was one of cowering in a corner, unable to move or escape and trying to become invisible. While a freeze response is certainly a common reaction in child witnesses to violence, it is one body-based narrative that must be transformed in order to help support a sense of self-efficacy and reduce the likelihood of post-traumatic stress reactions. To learn alternative ways to respond to fear or danger and to overcome situations where immobility dominates, children like Daniel literally have to practice enacting a different reaction.

Therapists who work in domestic violence shelters generally have a limited amount of time to effect change. They therefore have to consider what interventions might have maximum impact in the short term. Mask making is one strategy that will quickly engage even the most withdrawn or fearful children. While there are various ways to create masks with anything from a paper plate to a brown paper bag, I like to use premade paper mâché masks that are life-like, enticing to decorate, and very easy to wear for the purpose of dramatic enactment.

Although drama is more impactful within a group, most psychotherapists are in session with a single individual. To make up for that missing interaction, I often become part of the drama. In the tradition of approaches like Playback Theatre (Gil & Dias, 2014), I also try to create a stage within my office. This can simply mean draping a colorful sheet or fabric over something tall like an existing curtain rod or bookcase to identify a space where the "drama" will take place. Also, in the tradition of Playback Theatre, I might act as the host, announcing the beginning of the performance, welcoming the young "actor" to the stage, and making closing remarks at the end of the performance. I may also improvise a re-enactment of the story told by the child, similar to how a narrative therapist might retell a story and ask the individual for feedback on accuracy.

In addition to simply going with the story the individual develops, there are several simple techniques practitioners can try with young clients like Daniel.

Mirroring

Mirroring is a body-based form of reflection and is a key response to affirm children's enactments. One common group approach is to have children stand in a circle; each comes forward, one at a time, making a gesture or movement based on a theme. Then the entire group mirrors that movement. A sound or word can be added to each movement, and the group can also "mirror" that back to the individual. While this type of approach is more effective in groups, in individual sessions the therapist can do the mirroring of movements and repetition of sounds or words. With children like Daniel, the point is to reinforce acceptance and "being seen" through implicit communications.

Strike a Pose

"Strike a pose" is just what it says—children are asked to move around a space, and the therapist calls out a word like "happy" or "worried," asking the participants to freeze in their steps. The children then stop and create a pose or gesture for that word; the therapist can vary the activity by inviting the participants to walk around the space while embodying that word or feeling. At this point, the facilitator can provide feedback, noting, "I see a lot of you have your heads held high and are swinging your arms" or "Some of you are walking really slowly with your shoulders slumped over."

In Daniel's case, this simple activity was an initial turning point for him while wearing a paper mâché mask of a "superhero" we decorated together. The mask made all the difference in his participation, which became more and more animated as I called out various suggestions for poses. Wearing his mask (we also fashioned a cape from some fabric and a pole became a "laser gun"), he experienced some aesthetic distance. But Daniel may have also felt hidden behind the mask, able to spontaneously enact various scenarios. This was an important step forward from his tendency to want to remain invisible due to dominant freeze response to one of action and efficacy.

Big–Bigger–Biggest

Gil and Dias (2014) cite Playback Theater as a source for a simple drama technique that focuses on the senses and emotion. This technique involves three "actors" who stand side by side while the therapist or another group member calls out an emotion. Each actor comes forward and uses movement and gesture to show the emotion, with increasing intensity; a static pose can also be used instead of movement. In Playback Theater, the audience always enthusiastically applauds the actors for their efforts. As with the other approaches described, this one seeks to convey implicit sensations and emotions and to be seen and accepted by others for what is communicated. I varied this process to adapt to working with Daniel as the sole participant. In his case, as I described previously, I set the stage for his performance with a special curtain in my office and he acted out words and emotions as "small, medium and large." I was the announcer and audience that enthusiastically applauded his performances, occasionally challenging him to "give a repeat performance" or "take an extra curtain call and bow." As with any dramatic enactment with children, the therapist becomes part of the theater as either a supporting cast member or a master of ceremony to enliven and "thicken" the story and performance.

When working with narratives in the form of play and particularly dramatic enactment, I try to make short films that children can watch and actually witness what they look like when acting and improvising. I used to use simple digital cameras, but now tablet technology permits immediate playback. For Daniel, this experience was another effective strategy to help him transform his story from helpless to one of empowerment. Simply seeing himself on film playing and later with his mask enacting his superpowers began to help him learn new ways of moving and gesturing with more confidence and assertiveness.

While making meaning of what Daniel witnessed during childhood will likely be a longer process, he was able to change some of his story in the short term. For Daniel, using simple drama techniques enhanced his capacity to enact new ways of moving and thus "play out" new stories for himself that gave him more confidence. Unfortunately, children who witness assault to a parent often repeatedly encounter interpersonal violence, despite protective services or foster care. Even though my ultimate goal was to help Daniel develop an internal sense of safety, I also used drama and play as forms of performative change to support his self-efficacy when presented with distressful situations he might face in the future.

IMAGINATION REFRAMES TRAUMA INTO HOPE AND HEALING

Seeing individuals like Daniel manifest a new way of being through imagination is a moment of personal gratification for any therapist. It is impossible not to feel deep satisfaction when a child or an adult shows the first spark of imagination and creates reparative stories during a session. Over decades of work with trauma, each experience has had a lasting impact on me, not only in hearing transformative narratives but also in witnessing expressive work that signifies reparation and healing.

In closing this chapter and this book, I share the story of an individual whose meaning-making process taught me how truly reparative the expressive arts within the context of psychotherapy can be. It captures how expressive arts can become a central component of meaning making, going far beyond what any words can convey. It is also not often that a therapist is able to witness the entirety of an individual's confrontation with trauma and adversity through the most difficult junctures of self-reflection. These encounters form the most profound moments of our work. Working with this exceptional person also showed me without a doubt that even when "bad things happen to good people," the human spirit will prevail and can make meaning. This final example demonstrates how the expressive arts play a role in pivotal moments of change, in the reparative experience of expressing one's story, and ultimately in how imagination reframes tragedy into hope and healing.

Case Example. Shannon: Making Meaning in the Context of Overwhelming Life Events

At age 45, Shannon was diagnosed with ovarian cancer. For most of her adult life she had been a triathlete and a self-proclaimed "health nut" who was very careful about her diet and health. She was also a physician's assistant who worked in an adult oncology unit and assisted doctors at a university teaching hospital. Because of her medical background, Shannon knew in great detail what a diagnosis of ovarian cancer meant and the challenges that were ahead of her, including treatment that would be physically exhausting and often toxic in order to rid her body of the cancer. When I met her for our first few sessions, Shannon explained that she wanted to include art making, creative writing, and music as part of her treatment. She jokingly referred to her illness as "cancer schmancer," trying to maintain a positive attitude during what were months of chemotherapy's debilitating side effects and fatigue resulting from radiation. From the outset, Shannon committed herself to do whatever possible not only to treat the disease, but also to explore the social–emotional and spiritual effects of the illness on mind and body with everything available, including expressive arts therapy.

Like many of the people I see, Shannon had never considered herself to be a particularly creative person. But she said she was "all in" to take the risk of expressing herself in art, writing, and music as ways to cope with her diagnosis, medical interventions, medications, and changes in her life. Although Shannon was not diagnosed with PTSD, her level of hyperactivation about cancer was consistent with traumatic stress and, as she observed, her body's felt sense was constantly "off balance each day." When I asked her to identify one word that best described this body sensation, Shannon was quick to say "precarious" because everything in "my body feels out of whack and unpredictable." To begin to address this sensation, we focused on safety and self-regulatory practices in initial sessions to address her overwhelming feelings about her illness through modified chair yoga and trauma-sensitive mindfulness. We also used chakra drumming (a small metal drum that is easy to play and is known for soothing tones), a practice she eventually continued at home with her own drum. Because I wanted her to have the best possible experiences with music, I arranged for a music therapist to see her at the university hospital for supplemental sessions that provided additional relaxation and self-regulatory experiences during her work day.

During the third session, Shannon felt comfortable enough to begin to confront some of the feelings that were creating stress in her body and contributing to her felt sense of instability. One of the first images (Figure 10.6) she created was a drawing of her resentment at this felt sense. For the first time in her life, she was deeply angry and even questioned and blamed herself for her illness, despite her own medical knowledge about her form of ovarian cancer. Shannon was embarrassed about expressing this anger to even her closest family members and friends but drawing and writing

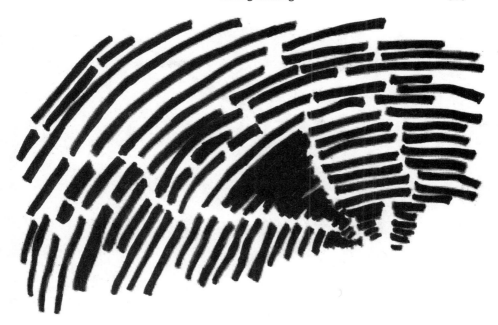

FIGURE 10.6. Shannon's felt sense of anger. From the collection of Cathy A. Malchiodi (not to be reproduced without permission from the author).

about her feelings provided a way to put her emotions into perspective. As we explored just where the anger was experienced in her body, she realized that it mostly stayed "in my head and heart" as the locations of where she obsessively felt the frustrations of being a patient for the "first time in my life." When I suggested that she stay with this sensation and see where it might go or possibly transform, Shannon quickly acknowledged a sense of growing depression (Figure 10.7), a condition she hid from others, including her colleagues at the hospital. Unlike anger, this experience was held deep in her "gut," well hidden from even those closest to her and protected by defined boundaries. As we continued to explore those somatic experiences and the characteristics of the drawing, it was easy for Shannon to see how the lines in this drawing were connected to her image of anger and essentially another component of her body's "story" about the challenges of a life-threatening illness.

A year after surgery, chemotherapy, and radiation treatments, Shannon's cancer went into remission. She began long-distance running again, took on more responsibilities at work, and became more hopeful about her prognosis because there was no evidence of cancer according to tests. Shannon continued working with me and decided she wanted to share something of her expressive arts experiences with other patients with cancer. She used

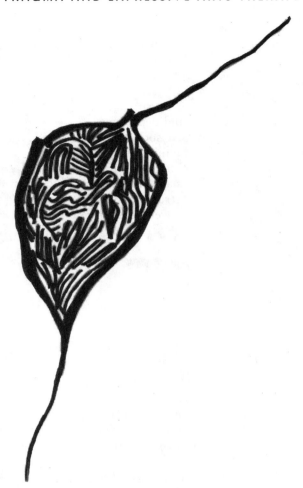

FIGURE 10.7. Shannon's drawing of depression. From the collection of Cathy A. Malchiodi (not to be reproduced without permission from the author).

the simple felt pen feelings drawings she created and her journal entries from early sessions as the basis for a series of larger drawings and paintings, which were eventually exhibited at the local Gilda's Club (a community-based program for cancer patients and their families) where she also would read from her writing journals, sharing her experiences as a patient. While this captures the "rejoining community" that Herman explained, it also reflects Herman's initial contention in *Trauma and Recovery* that stories of atrocities must be told. As much as any assault or incident of violence, cancer is an atrocity, and Shannon was telling the story of its abuse to her body through art and public performances of her journal entries.

Unfortunately, Shannon's remission was short-lived; less than a year later, her cancer returned in an inoperable Stage 4 form in her liver and lungs. Right after her remission came to an end, Shannon's husband of 13 years decided that he did not want to remain in a marriage to a terminally ill wife and filed for divorce. As Shannon explained to me, "things have really hit rock bottom now," and she subsequently experienced a month of severe grief reactions, anxiety, and depression due to the divorce and her prognosis. While she had extensive social support from family and friends as well as the Gilda's Club community, this was by far the most devastating period for her. Our sessions focused on the inevitable progression of her cancer, the shock and trauma of the loss of a primary relationship, and what Shannon called the "struggle between life and death" (Figure 10.8). I admit these conversations were existentially powerful for me while

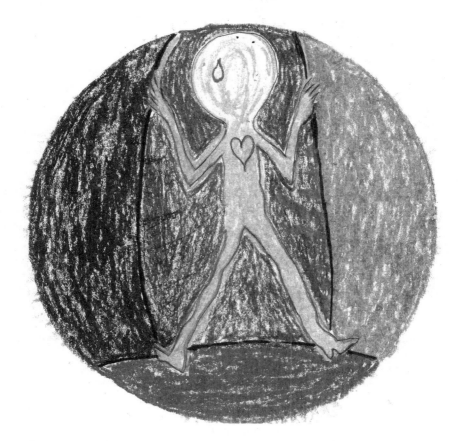

FIGURE 10.8. Shannon's depiction of "between life and death." From the collection of Cathy A. Malchiodi (not to be reproduced without permission from the author).

we explored the most fundamental questions we all inevitably face—the possibility of an afterlife, a soul or spirit that lives on after death, and speculations about what the process of dying will be like. We also discussed the differences between "cure," an outcome that was now impossible, and "healing," the potential for finding peace and wholeness. In tackling these topics, to my amazement Shannon strengthened her resolve to find peace from any lingering anger and sadness about cancer and her husband's abandonment of their relationship.

As Shannon became more physically debilitated, visits to my office became too exhausting, so I made home visits at her apartment. In these final sessions and before she became too ill to participate, I helped Shannon organize her writing journals and create colorful binders for them while we continued our conversations. The trauma-sensitive mindfulness she practiced in earlier sessions with me now focused on self-compassion, and she continued to make art, working on what she called an "inner sense of love" for herself, similar to the Dharma practices described in Chapter 9. In a final art expression, a small mixed-media collage, "Buddha Blossom," captured all that Shannon had reframed from the experience of terminal illness and subsequent losses (Figure 10.9). The brilliantly colored flower in the center was placed on a background that she said represented the cancer cells overtaking her body. With regard to this image, Shannon quoted lines from "*Saint Francis and the Sow*," a poem by Galway Kinnell (1980): "to reteach a thing its loveliness, / to put a hand on its brow / of the flower / and retell it in words and in touch / it is lovely until it flowers again from within, of self-blessing" (p. 9).

Through this simple art image and quote, I watched Shannon transform herself into someone who was no longer a medical patient, but the essence of spirit that embodied her discovery of meaning and beauty amidst the cruelty of cancer. While all the art that Shannon created during our sessions was left to her family and friends, she wanted me to have this image as a memory of our work together. I have displayed it on my office wall as an exceptional example of what meaning making can be, even in the face of death; it marks my encounter with an extraordinary individual who transformed into the Buddha in body, mind, and spirit before my eyes.

Shannon's story may seem like a heartbreaking one on which to end a book, but hers is a rich and multifaceted story that continues to guide my work as an expressive arts therapist. It captures the essence of arts-based approaches and their role in repairing not only trauma, but also individuals on many levels, including mind, body, and spirit. Not all clients reach these depths of transformation when facing life's most profound and defining moments, and they may not meet it as gracefully or fully as Shannon did. Nor may every trauma survivor, particularly those who have survived complex events that impact individuals in unspeakable ways, achieve the same degree of healing that Shannon did. But she did gracefully teach me

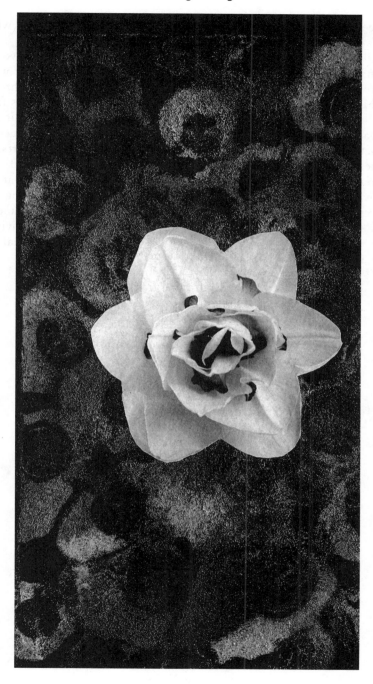

FIGURE 10.9. "Buddha blossom." From the collection of Cathy A. Malchiodi (not to be reproduced without permission from the author).

the deeper meaning of what it means to become whole, no matter what a story's ending turns out to be.

Ultimately, it is that experience of becoming whole that I have been fortunate to witness countless times through how individuals risk communicating through the arts and come to use the practices described throughout this book. There are, of course, many ways to help our clients find a sense of wholeness, and expressive arts therapy is one of many. It is an approach that has never been clearly categorizable because it bridges two distinct domains that support wholeness—psychotherapy and the arts. Psychotherapy is an established tradition with empirically established methods to resolve trauma. In contrast, the latter—the expressive arts—are still somewhat unknown to many therapists and are based on emerging data. But expressive arts are one of few ways that the capacity to imagine and create new narratives is not only manifested, but also helps individuals begin to live more fully and recover the core of what it means to heal from trauma and once again become whole.

Resources

CHILDREN AND TRAUMA

ACEs Connection. One of the most active communities on the topic of ACEs and trauma-informed practices. See *www.acesconnection.com.*

ACEs Too High News. This site provides regularly updated news on ACE information and research. See *https://acestoohigh.com.*

Centers for Disease Control and Prevention: Violence Prevention. This site explains the development of the Centers for Disease Control and Prevention–Kaiser Permanente ACE study, one of the largest investigations of childhood abuse and neglect and household challenges and later-life health and well-being. See *www.cdc.gov/violenceprevention/childabuseandneglect/acestudy/index.html.*

National Child Traumatic Stress Network (NCTSN). The NCTSN is an American organization whose mission is to raise the standard of care and improve access to services for traumatized children, their families, and communities throughout the United States. This site provides a wide range of information, including best practices and effective treatments for children, reviews of instruments and measures for evaluating child trauma, and resources for trauma training. See *www.nctsn.org.*

The Neurosequential Network®. The Neurosequential Model of Therapeutics is a developmentally sensitive, neurobiology-informed approach to clinical problem solving. The model, developed by Bruce D. Perry, MD, PhD, is not a specific therapeutic technique or intervention. It is an approach that integrates core principles of neurodevelopment and traumatology to inform work with children, families, and the communities in which they live. For more information, see *www.neurosequential.com.*

ADULTS AND TRAUMA

American Psychological Association (APA). The APA has a guide for traumatized individuals at *www.apa.org/topics/trauma.*

International Society for the Study of Trauma and Dissociation (ISSTD). The ISSTD advances clinical, scientific, and societal understanding about the prevalence and consequences of chronic trauma and dissociation. See *www.isst-d.org.*

International Society for Traumatic Stress Studies (ISTSS). The ISTSS is dedicated to sharing information about the effects of trauma and the discovery and dissemination of knowledge about policy, program, and service initiatives that seek to reduce traumatic stressors and their immediate and long-term consequences. See *www.istss.org.*

Sidran Institute. Sidran helps people cope with, and heal from, their negative experiences by directing them to specialized trauma treatment centers, therapists, support groups, and reading materials. See *www.sidran.org.*

EXPRESSIVE ARTS AND TRAUMA

Arts and Health on Psychology Today. For a wide variety of articles on expressive arts, creative arts therapies, arts in health care, and psychotherapy- and trauma-related topics, see *www.psychologytoday.com/us/blog/arts-and-health.*

Association for Play Therapy (APT). The APT is a national professional society established in 1982 to foster contact among mental health professionals interested in exploring and, when developmentally appropriate, applying the therapeutic power of play to communicate with and treat clients, particularly children. See *www.a4pt.org.*

DE-CRUIT®. DE-CRUIT is an integrative, veteran-created, performing arts-based treatment program to help veterans transition from military service to civilian life. See *www.decruit.org.*

Express Yourself (EXYO). EXYO provides programming that immerses young people in the arts, where they find a powerful tool for self-expression, uncover inner strength, and deepen connection with others. See *www.exyo.org.*

Florence Cane. Florence Cane's innovative work as an art educator contributed to the foundations of bilateral drawing and other sensory-based methods of art expression. See *https://everyoneanartist.weebly.com/florence-cane.html.*

Focusing and Expressive Arts Institute® (FOAT). FOAT is a mindfulness-based approach developed by Laury Rappaport that integrates renowned psychologist and philosopher Eugene Gendlin's focusing with the expressive arts. See *www.focusingarts.com.*

Guided Drawing, Clay Field®, and Sensorimotor Art Therapy. To learn more about Cornelia Elbrecht's work and these arts-based, bilateral processes and available training, see *www.sensorimotorarttherapy.com.*

International Expressive Arts Therapy Association® (IEATA). The IEATA is a nonprofit professional organization founded in 1994 to encourage the creative spirit. This organization supports expressive arts therapists, artists, educators, consultants, and others using integrative, multimodal arts processes for personal and community growth and transformation. IEATA also provides a credentialing process for becoming a Registered Expressive Arts Therapist (REAT) and a Registered Expressive Arts Consultant Educator (REACE). See *www.ieata.org.*

Person-Centered Expressive Arts Therapy. To learn more about the history and work of Natalie Rogers, see *www.personcenteredexpressivearts.com.*

Theraplay®. Theraplay is a child and family therapy for building and enhancing attachment, self-esteem, trust in others, and joyful engagement. Sessions create an active, emotional connection between the child and parent or caregiver, resulting in a changed view of the self as worthy and lovable and of relationships as positive and rewarding. See *www.theraplay.org/index.php.*

Trauma-Informed Practice and Expressive Arts Therapy Institute. This organization provides resources and training in Trauma-Informed Expressive Arts Therapy®, an integrative approach to applying movement, music, storytelling, dramatic enactment, art making, and mindfulness practices. It also provides education through certificate programs to mental health professionals and expressive arts facilitators throughout the United States and internationally. See *www.trauma-informedpractice.com.*

SOMATIC APPROACHES TO TRAUMA

American Dance Therapy Association (ADTA). The ADTA was founded in 1966 to support the emerging profession of dance/movement therapy and is dedicated to promoting the practice and training of dance/movement therapists. See *https://adta.org.*

Sensorimotor Psychotherapy Institute. The Sensorimotor Institute provides training in Sensorimotor Psychotherapy® that draws from somatic therapies, neuroscience, attachment theory, and cognitive approaches, as well as from the Hakomi method. See *www.sensorimotorpsychotherapy.org/about.html.*

Somatic Experiencing®. The Somatic Experiencing method is a body-oriented approach to the healing of trauma and other stress disorders developed by Peter Levine. The approach releases traumatic shock, which is key to transforming posttraumatic stress and the wounds of emotional and early developmental attachment trauma. See *https://traumahealing.org.*

MINDFULNESS

Mindfulness-Based Stress Reduction (MBSR). For a history, journal articles, and research on MBSR, see the University of Massachusetts website at *www.umassmed. edu/cfm/mindfulness-based-programs/mbsr-courses/about-mbsr/history-of-mbsr.*

Mindfulness Meditations. For an introduction to specific practices, see Jack Kornfield's website at *https://jackkornfield.com/meditations.*

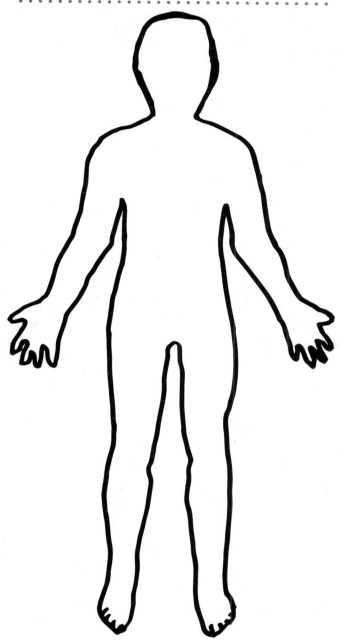

369

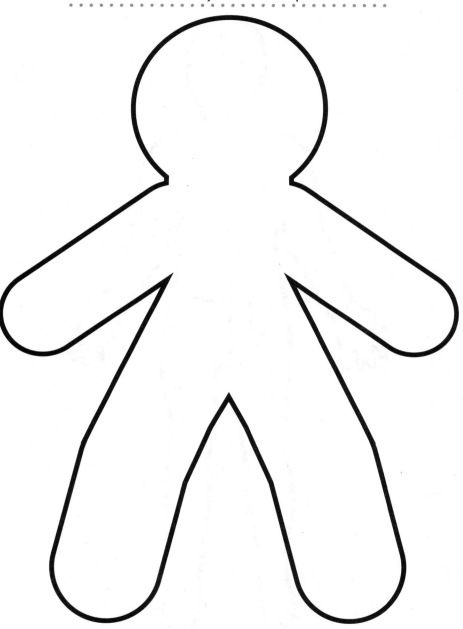

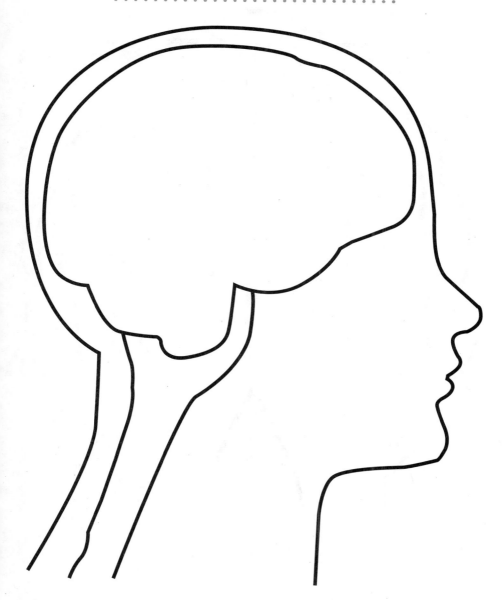

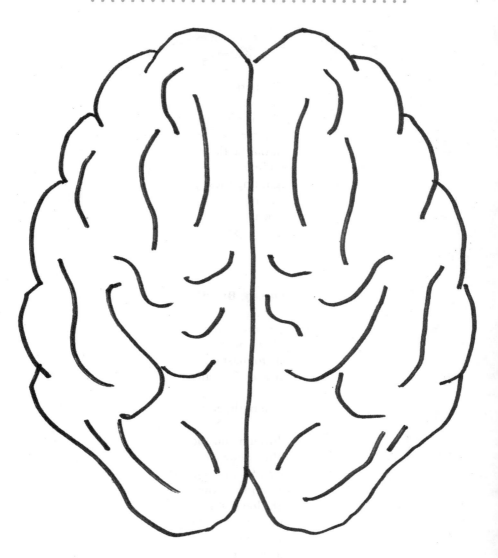

The following breathing prompts are based on extensive evidence that structured, rhythmic breathing patterns are key to calming the autonomic nervous system (ANS). These practices can often improve mood and decrease stress in children and adults experiencing traumatic stress.

I have included three of the more popular intentional breathing routines here because no one style of breathing is effective for everyone. Before introducing any breathing prompts, be sure the individual is seated upright, if possible, in a comfortable chair with feet flat on the floor. Breathing should always be comfortable for the person in holding breaths and exhaling breaths. Deep breaths are not necessary when beginning these practices. Always ask the individual to breathe as deeply as feels comfortable when using these prompts. The shapes included in this section can be used as visual aids for counting breaths; children in particular benefit from tracing the shapes with a finger while practicing breathing.

Four-Square Breathing

Square breathing, also known as box breathing or four-square breathing, is a technique used when practicing rhythmic breathing. A standard technique in hospital settings, it is an easy one to master and is particularly useful with individuals who are experiencing distress or panic.

1. Slowly exhale through your mouth, getting all the oxygen out of your lungs.
2. Inhale slowly and deeply through your nose to the count of four. If comfortable, feel the air filling your lungs a little at a time until they are completely full and the air seems to move into your abdomen.
3. Next, hold your breath for another slow count of four.
4. Exhale through your mouth slowly for the same count of four, expelling the air from your lungs and abdomen. If comfortable, be aware of the feeling of the air leaving your lungs.
5. Hold your breath again for the same slow count of four.
6. Repeat the entire process several times.

(continued)

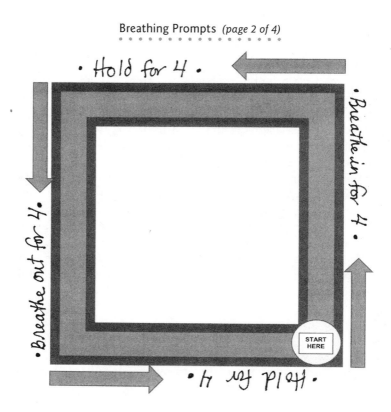

Star Breathing

Star breathing, another way to practice rhythmic breathing, uses a five-pointed star as a guide. Children like this technique because of the shape, and they enjoy using a finger to trace a side of the star while inhaling, holding, and exhaling. It can be used with adults too.

1. Slowly exhale through your mouth, getting all the oxygen out of your lungs.
2. Trace your finger over a "Breathe In" side of one point of the star. Inhale slowly and deeply through your nose to the count of four (or determine the count that is most comfortable for the individual). Feel the air filling your lungs a little at a time until they are completely full and the air seems to move into your abdomen.
3. Next, hold your breath for another slow count of four (or determine a count with the individual) at the tip of the star's point.

(continued)

374

4. While using your finger to trace the "Breathe In" side of the star for the same count, exhale through your mouth slowly for the same count, expelling the air from your lungs and abdomen. If comfortable, be aware of the feeling of the air leaving your lungs.

5. Hold your breath again for the same slow count at the tip of the star's point.

6. Repeat the process until you have completed five breathe-ins/breathe-outs.

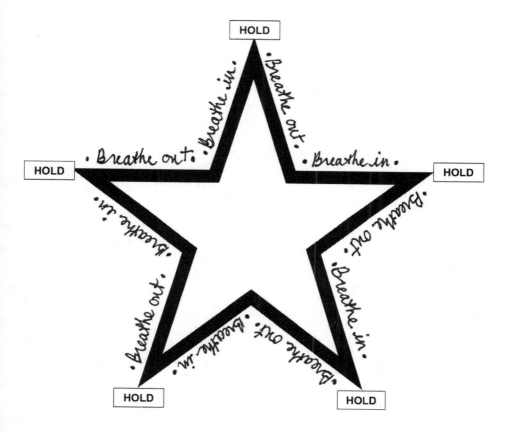

Figure-Eight Breathing

Figure-eight breathing is a third pattern that is an effective way to practice rhythmic breathing. I have modified this technique and created a "lopsided figure eight" to support and teach a specific breathing pattern. This particular version is useful with children who enjoy using a finger to trace the image while

(continued)

inhaling and exhaling. Because this breathing pattern is so effective, try introducing it to adults, too.

1. Slowly exhale through your mouth, getting all the oxygen out of your
   lungs.
2. Starting from the midpoint of the diagram (Start Here), trace your
   finger over the right side of the diagram to the count of four while
   breathing in. Inhale deeply through your nose and feel the air filling
   your lungs.
3. Continue using your finger to cross over the midpoint of the diagram
   and trace the left side for a count of eight while exhaling. Exhale
   through your mouth, expelling the air from your lungs and abdomen.
4. Repeat this process four more times.

This breathing pattern of breathing in for four counts and breathing out for
eight counts is believed to calm the vagal system and ANS. It is generally effective after five repetitions (approximately 1 minute of structured breathing),
although some individuals may benefit from several minutes of practice.

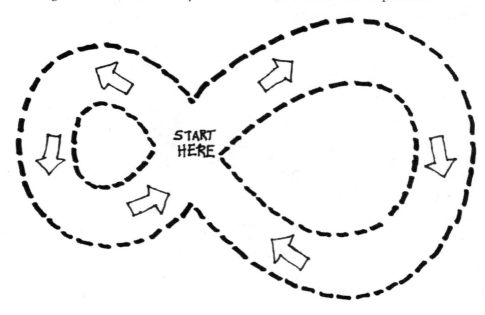

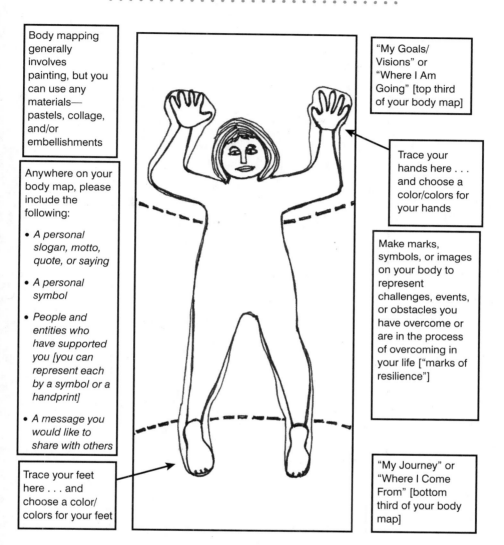

Body mapping generally involves painting, but you can use any materials—pastels, collage, and/or embellishments

Anywhere on your body map, please include the following:

• *A personal slogan, motto, quote, or saying*

• *A personal symbol*

• *People and entities who have supported you [you can represent each by a symbol or a handprint]*

• *A message you would like to share with others*

Trace your feet here . . . and choose a color/ colors for your feet

"My Goals/ Visions" or "Where I Am Going" [top third of your body map]

Trace your hands here . . . and choose a color/colors for your hands

Make marks, symbols, or images on your body to represent challenges, events, or obstacles you have overcome or are in the process of overcoming in your life ["marks of resilience"]

"My Journey" or "Where I Come From" [bottom third of your body map]

When you are finished, do whatever feels right to complete your body map. Fill in spaces, add elements, or emphasize parts.

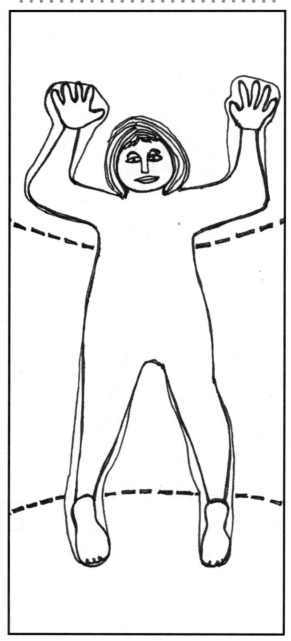

References

Adichie, C. (2009, July). The danger of a single story. Retrieved from *www.ted.com/ talks/chimamanda_adichie_the_danger_of_a_single_story?language=en.*

Adler, A. (2002). *The collected works of Alfred Adler* (Vol. 1). Bellingham: Alfred Adler Institute of Northwestern Washington.

Ali, A., & Wolfert, S. (2016). Theatre as a treatment for posttraumatic stress in military veterans: Exploring the psychotherapeutic potential of mimetic induction. *The Arts in Psychotherapy, 50*, 58–65.

Ali, A., & Wolfert, S. (2019). Treating trauma through the imagination: Therapeutic effects of simulation and mimetic induction. In L. Green & K. Obozoh (Eds.), *We've been too patient: Voices from radial mental health* (pp. 163–169). Berkeley, CA: North Atlantic Books.

Ali, A., Wolfert, S., Lam, I., Fahmy, P., & Chaudhry, A. (2018). Psychotherapeutic processes in recovery from military and pre-military trauma in veterans: The effects of theatre as a mental health treatment. *Journal of Applied Arts and Health, 9*(3), 337–350.

Ali, A., Wolfert, S., Lam, I., & Rahman, T. (2018). Intersecting modes of aesthetic distance and mimetic induction in therapeutic process: Examining a theatre-based treatment for military-related traumatic stress. *Drama Therapy Review, 4*(2), 153–165.

All-Party Parliamentary Group on Arts, Health and Wellbeing. (2017). Creative health: The arts for health and wellbeing. Retrieved from *www.art-shealthandwellbeing.org.uk/appg-inquiry/Publications/Creative_Health_Inquiry_Report_2017.pdf.*

Allen, J. G., Fonagy, P., & Bateman, A. W. (2008). *Mentalizing in clinical practice.* Arlington, VA: American Psychiatric Publishing.

American Dance Therapy Association. (2019). What is dance/movement therapy? Retrieved from *https://adta.org/faqs.*

American Music Therapy Association. (2019). What is music therapy? Retrieved from *www.musictherapy.org/about/musictherapy.*

American Psychiatric Association. (2013). *Diagnostic and statistical manual of mental disorders* (5th ed.). Arlington, VA: Author.

Anthony, E., & Cohler, B. (Eds.). (1987). *The invulnerable child.* New York: Guilford Press.

Arom, E. (2017, June 29). Saved by art: How one man's skill got him through seven Nazi camps and the difficult years that followed. *Jewish Journal.* Retrieved from *https://jewishjournal.com/culture/221086/saved-art-one-mans-skill-got-seven-nazi-camps-difficult-years-followed.*

Arrien, A. (2013). *The four-fold way.* New York: Harper.

Atkinson, J. (2003). *Trauma trails, recreating song lines: The transgenerational effects of trauma in indigenous Australia.* Brisbane, Australia: Gnibi Papers.

Ayres, J. (1976). *Sensory integration and learning disorders.* Torrance, CA: Western Psychological Services.

Badenoch, B. (2008). *Becoming a brain-wise therapist.* New York: Norton.

Badenoch, B. (2018). *The heart of trauma: Healing the embodied brain in the context of relationships.* New York: Norton.

Bai, Y., Maruskin, L., Chen, S., Amie, M., Stellar, J., McNeil, G., et al. (2017). Awe, the diminished self, and collective engagement: Universals and cultural variations in the small self. *Journal of Personality and Social Psychology, 113*(2), 185–209.

Bateman, A., & Fonagy, P. (2006). Mentalizing and borderline personality disorder. In J. G. Allen & P. Fonagy (Eds.), *The handbook of mentalization-based treatment* (pp. 185–200). Hoboken, NJ: Wiley.

Bayles, D., & Orland, T. (2001). *Art and fear: observations on the perils (and rewards) of artmaking.* Santa Cruz, CA: Image Continuum Press.

Beaty, R. E., Benedek, M., Kaufman, S. B., & Silvia, P. J. (2015). Default and executive network coupling supports creative idea production. *Nature Scientific Reports, 5,* 10964.

Beaty, R. E., Benedek, M., Wilkins, R. W., Jauk, E., Fink, A., et al. (2014). Creativity and the default network: A functional connectivity analysis of the creative brain at rest. *Neuropsychologia, 64,* 92–98.

Bennink, F. (2014). *Posttraumatic success: Positive psychology and solution-focused strategies to help clients survive and thrive.* New York: Norton.

Benson, H., & Kipper, M. (2000). *The relaxation response.* New York: Harper.

Bloom, S. (2005). Foreword. In A. M. Weber & C. Haen (Eds.), *Clinical applications of drama therapy in child and adolescent treatment* (pp. xv–xviii). New York: Brunner-Routledge.

Bloom, S. (2016). Advancing a national cradle-to-grave-to-cradle public health agenda, *Journal of Trauma and Dissociation, 17*(4), 383–396.

Bonanno, G. A. (2004). Loss, trauma, and human resilience: Have we underestimated the human capacity to thrive after extremely aversive events? *American Psychologist, 59*(1), 20–28.

Bonanno, G. A. (2009). *The other side of sadness: What the new science of bereavement tells us about life after loss.* New York: Basic Books.

Botton, A. D., & Armstrong, J. (2013). *Art as therapy.* London: Phaidon Press.

Bowlby, J. (1988). *A secure base: Parent–child attachment and healthy human development.* New York: Basic Books.

Bräuninger, I. (2012). The efficacy of dance movement therapy group on improvement of quality of life: A randomized controlled trial. *The Arts in Psychotherapy, 39*(4), 296–303.

Braveheart, M. Y. H. (2003). The historical trauma response among natives and its relationship with substance abuse: A Lakota illustration. *Journal of Psychoactive Drugs, 35*(1), 7–13.

Brett-MacLean, P. (2009). Body mapping: Embodying the self while living with HIV/AIDS. *Canadian Medical Association Journal, 19*(7), 140–141.

Bronson, H., Vaudreuil, R., & Bradt, J. (2018). Music therapy treatment of active duty military: An overview of intensive outpatient and longitudinal care programs. *Music Therapy Perspectives, 36*(2), 195–206.

Brooks, R. (2010). The power of mindsets: A personal journey to nurture dignity, hope and resilience in children. In D. Crenshaw (Ed.), *Reverence in healing: Honoring strengths without trivializing suffering* (pp. 19–40). Lanham, MD: Jason Aronson.

Brooks, R., & Goldstein, R. (2015). The power of mindsets: Guideposts for a resilience-based treatment approach. In D. A. Crenshaw, R. Brooks, & S. Goldstein (Eds.), *Play therapy interventions to enhance resilience* (pp. 3–31). New York: Guilford Press.

Bruscia, K. (1998). *Defining music therapy.* Philadelphia: Barcelona.

Calhoun, L. G., & Tedeschi, R. G. (2013). *Posttraumatic growth in clinical practice.* New York: Routledge.

Campbell, J. (2011). *The power of myth.* New York: Anchor.

Cane, F. (1951). *The artist in each of us.* London: Thames and Hudson.

Cannon, W. B. (1932). *The wisdom of the body.* New York: Norton.

Carlson, L., Speca, M., Patel, K., & Goodey, E. (2004). Mindfulness-based stress reduction in relation to quality of life, mood, symptoms of stress and levels of cortisol, dehydroepiandrosterone sulfate (DHEAS) and melatonin in breast and prostate cancer outpatients. *Psychoneuroendocrinology, 29*(4), 448–474.

Centers for Disease Control and Prevention. (2019). Adverse childhood experiences. Retrieved from *www.cdc.gov/violenceprevention/childabuseandneglect/acestudy/index.html.*

Chapman, L. (2014). *Neurobiologically informed trauma therapy with children and adolescents: Understanding mechanisms of change.* New York: Norton.

Cloitre, M., Stolbach, B. C., Herman, J. L., van der Kolk, B., Pynoos, R., Wang, J., et al. (2009). A developmental approach to complex PTSD: Childhood and adult cumulative trauma as predictors of symptom complexity. *Journal of Traumatic Stress, 22,* 399–408.

Cohen, J. A., Deblinger, E., & Mannarino, A. (2017). Trauma-focused cognitive behavioral therapy for children and families. *Psychotherapy Research, 28*(1), 47–57.

Collingwood, J. (2018). The power of music to reduce stress. *Psych Central.* Retrieved July 24, 2019, from *https://psychcentral.com/lib/the-power-of-music-to-reduce-stress.*

Crawford, A. (2010). If the body keeps the score: Mapping the dissociated body in trauma narrative, intervention, and theory. *University of Toronto Quarterly, 79*(2), 702–719.

Creative Forces. (2018). *Summary report from the Creative Forces Clinical Research Summit.* Washington, DC: National Endowment for the Arts.

Crenshaw, D. A. (2006). *Evocative strategies in child and adolescent psychotherapy.* Lanham, MD: Jason Aronson.

Crenshaw, D. A. (2008). *Therapeutic engagement of children and adolescents: Play, symbol, drawing and storytelling strategies.* New York: Jason Aronson.

Crenshaw, D. A., & Stewart, A. L. (Eds.). (2016). *Play therapy: A comprehensive guide to theory and practice*. New York: Guilford Press.

Csikszentmihalyi, M. (2014). *Flow and the foundations of positive psychology*. New York: Springer.

Dalebroux, A., Goldstein, T. R., & Winner, E. (2008). Short-term mood repair through art-making: Positive emotion is more effective than venting. *Motivation and Emotion, 32*, 288–295.

Damasio, A. (1999). *The feeling of what happens: Body and emotion in the making of consciousness*. Fort Worth, TX: Harcourt College.

Dayton, T., & Moreno, J. (2004). *The living stage: A step-by-step guide to psychodrama, sociometry and group psychotherapy*. Deerfield Beach, FL: Health Communications.

Denborough, D. (2016). *Retelling the stories of our lives*. New York: Norton.

Devine, C. (2008). The moon, the stars, and a scar: Body mapping stories of women living with HIV/AIDS. *Border Crossings, 27*, 58–65. Retrieved from *www.catie.ca/pdf/bodymaps/BC_105_BodyMapping.pdf*.

Dieterich-Hartwell, R. (2017). Dance/movement therapy in the treatment of post-traumatic stress: A reference model. *The Arts in Psychotherapy, 54*, 38–46.

Diliberto-Macaluso, K. A., & Stubblefield, B. L. (2015). The use of painting for short-term mood and arousal improvement. *Psychology of Aesthetics, Creativity, and the Arts, 9*(3), 228–234.

Dissanayake, E. (1995). *What is art for?* Seattle: University of Washington Press.

Drake, J. E., Coleman, K., & Winner, E. (2011). Short-term mood repair through art: Effects of medium and strategy. *Art Therapy, 28*(1), 26–30.

Drake, J., & Hodge, A. (2015). Drawing versus writing: The role of preference in regulating short-term affect. *Art Therapy, 32*(1), 27–33.

Drake, J. E., & Winner, E. (2012). Confronting sadness through art-making: Distraction is more beneficial than venting. *Psychology of Aesthetics, Creativity, and the Arts, 6*, 251–261.

Elbrecht, C. (2014). Being touched through touch: Trauma treatment through haptic perception at the Clay Field: A sensorimotor art therapy. *International Journal of Art Therapy 19*(1), 19–30.

Elbrecht, C. (2015). The clay field and developmental trauma in children. In C. A. Malchiodi (Ed.), *Creative interventions with traumatized children* (2nd ed., pp. 191–212). New York: Guilford Press.

Elbrecht, C. (2018). *Healing trauma with guided drawing*. Berkeley, CA: North Atlantic Books.

Ellis, A., & Dryden, W. (1987). *The practice of rational-emotive therapy (RET)*. New York: Springer.

Emerson, D. (2015). *Trauma-sensitive yoga in therapy: Bringing the body into treatment*. New York: Norton.

Emerson, D., Sharma, R., Chaudhry, S., & Turner, J. (2009). Trauma-sensitive yoga: Principles, practice, and research. *International Journal of Yoga Therapy, 19*(1), 123–128.

Emunah, R., & Johnson, D. R. (1983). The impact of theatrical performance on the self-images of psychiatric patients. *The Arts in Psychotherapy, 10*(4), 233–239.

Estrella, K. (2006). Expressive therapy: An integrated arts approach. In C. A. Malchiodi (Ed.), *Expressive therapies* (pp. 183–209). New York: Guilford Press.

Etcherling, L. (2017). *Crisis intervention.* San Diego, CA: Cognella Academic.

Fancourt, D., Perkins, R., Asceno, S., Carvalho, L., Steptoe, A., & Williamon, A. (2016). Effects of group drumming interventions on anxiety, depression, social resilience and inflammatory immune response among mental health service users. Retrieved from *https://doi.org/10.1371/journal.pone.0151136.*

Feldenkrais, M. (2010). *Embodied wisdom: The collected papers of Moshe Feldenkrais.* Berkeley, CA: North Atlantic Books.

Felitti, V. J., Anda, R. F., Nordenberg, D., Williamson, D. F., Spitz, A. M., Edwards, V., et al. (1998). Relationship of childhood abuse and household dysfunction to many of the leading causes of death in adults: The Adverse Childhood Experiences (ACE) Study. *American Journal of Preventive Medicine, 14*(4), 245–258.

Fisher, J. (2017). *Healing the fragmented selves of trauma survivors.* New York: Routledge.

Fivush, R., Sales, J., & Bohanek, J. (2008). Meaning making in mothers' and children's narratives of emotional events. *Memory, 16,* 579–594.

Foa, E. B., Keane, T. M., Friedman, M. J., & Cohen, J. A. (Eds.). (2009). *Effective treatments for PTSD: Practice guidelines from the International Society for Traumatic Stress Studies* (2nd ed.). New York: Guilford Press.

Forgeard, M. J. C. (2013). Perceiving benefits after adversity: The relationship between self-reported posttraumatic growth and creativity. *Psychology of Aesthetics, Creativity, and the Arts, 7*(3), 245–264.

Frankl, V. (1997). *Man's search for meaning: An introduction to logotherapy.* Boston: Beacon Press. (Original work published 1963)

Freud, S. (1954). Beyond the pleasure principle. In J. Strachey (Ed. & Trans.), *Standard edition of the complete psychological works of Sigmund Freud* (Vol. 3). London: Hogarth Press. (Original work published 1920)

Gallese, V., Eagle, M., & Migone, P. (2007). Intentional attunement: Mirror neurons and the neural underpinnings of interpersonal relations. *Journal of the American Psychoanalytic Association, 55,* 131–176.

Gardner, H. (1993). *Multiple intelligences: The theory in practice.* New York: Basic Books.

Gardstrom, S., & Sorel, S. (2016). Music therapy methods. In B. L. Wheeler (Ed.), *Music therapy handbook* (pp. 116–127). New York: Guilford Press.

Gaskill, R. L., & Perry, B. D. (2014). The neurobiological power of play: Using the neurosequential model of therapeutics to guide play in the healing process. In C. A. Malchiodi & D. A. Crenshaw (Eds.), *Creative arts and play therapy: Creative arts and play therapy for attachment problems* (pp. 178–194). New York: Guilford Press.

Gaskill, R. L., & Perry, B. D. (2017). A neurosequential therapeutics approach to guided play, play therapy, and activities for children who won't talk. In C. A. Malchiodi & D. A. Crenshaw (Eds.), *What to do when children clam up in psychotherapy: Interventions to facilitate communication* (pp. 38–66). New York: Guilford Press.

Gastaldo, D., Magalhaes, L., Carrasco, C., & Davy, C. (2012). Body-map storytelling as research: Methodological considerations for telling the stories of undocumented workers through body mapping. Retrieved from *www.migrationhealth.ca/undocumented-workers-ontario/body-mapping.*

Gendlin, E. T. (1982). *Focusing.* New York: Bantam Books.

Gendlin, E. T. (1996). *Focusing-oriented psychotherapy: A manual of the experiential method.* New York: Guilford Press.

Gerity, L. (Ed.). (2000). *Art as therapy: Collected papers.* London: Jessica Kingsley.

Ghetti, C. M., & Whitehead-Pleaux, A. M. (2015). Sounds of strength: Music therapy for hospitalized children at risk of traumatization. In C. A. Malchiodi (Ed.), *Creative interventions for traumatized children* (pp. 324–341). New York: Guilford Press.

Gil, E. (2010). *Working with children to heal interpersonal trauma: The power of play.* New York: Guilford Press.

Gil, E. (2011). *Helping abused and traumatized children: Integrating directive and nondirective approaches.* New York: Guilford Press.

Gil, E. (2016). *Play in family therapy* (2nd ed.). New York: Guilford Press.

Gil, E. (2017). *Posttraumatic play in children: What clinicians need to know.* New York: Guilford Press.

Gil, E., & Dias, T. (2014). The integration of drama therapy and play therapy in attachment work with traumatized children. In C. A. Malchiodi & D. A. Crenshaw (Eds.), *Creative arts and play therapy for attachment problems* (pp. 100–120). New York: Guilford Press.

Ginwright, S. (2018, May 31). The future of healing: Shifting from trauma informed care to healing centered engagement. Retrieved from *https://medium.com/@ginwright/the-future-of-healing-shifting-from-trauma-informed-care-to-healing-centered-engagement-634f557ce69c.*

Goffney, D. (2002). Seasons of grief: Helping children grow through loss. In J. Loewy & A. Hara (Eds.), *Caring for the caregiver: The use of music therapy in grief and trauma* (pp. 54–26). Silver Spring, MD: American Music Therapy Association.

Goleman, D. (2012). *Emotional intelligence: Why it can matter more than IQ.* New York: Bantam.

Graves-Alcorn, S., & Kagin, C. (2017). *Implementing the expressive therapies continuum: A guide for clinical practice.* New York: Routledge.

Gray, A. E. (2015). Dance/movement therapy with refugee and survivor children: A healing pathway is a creative process. In C. A. Malchiodi (Ed.), *Creative interventions with traumatized children* (2nd ed., pp. 169–212). New York: Guilford Press.

Gray, A. E., & Porges, S. (2017). Polyvagal-informed dance/movement therapy with children who shut down: Restoring core rhythmicity. In C. A. Malchiodi & D. A. Crenshaw (Eds.), *What to do when children clam up in psychotherapy: Interventions to facilitate communication* (pp. 102–136). New York: Guilford Press.

Greenberg, M. S., & van der Kolk, B. (1987). Retrieval and integration of traumatic memories with the "painting cure." In B. A. van der Kolk (Ed.), *Psychological trauma* (pp. 191–215). Washington, DC: American Psychiatric Press.

Gross, J., & Haynes, H. (1998). Drawing facilitates children's verbal reports of emotionally laden events. *Journal of Experimental Psychology, 4,* 163–179.

Guber, T. (2005). *Yoga pretzels.* Cambridge, MA: Barefoot Books.

Haen, C. (2015). Vanquishing monsters: Group drama therapy for treating trauma. In C. A. Malchiodi (Ed.), *Creative interventions with traumatized children* (2nd ed., pp. 235–257). New York: Guilford Press.

Halprin, D. (2003). *The expressive body in life, art, and therapy: Working with movement, metaphor and meaning.* London: Jessica Kingsley.

Hanh, T. N. (2011). *Planting seeds: Practicing mindfulness with children*. Berkeley, CA: Parallax Press.

Harel-Shalev, A., Huss, E., Daphna-Tekoah, S., & Cwikel, J. (2017). Drawing (on) women's military experiences and narratives—Israeli women soldiers' challenges in the military environment. *Gender, Place and Culture: A Journal of Feminist Geography, 24*(4), 499–514.

Hass-Cohen, N., Bokoch, N., Findlay, J., & Witting, A. (2018). A four-drawing art therapy trauma and resiliency protocol study. *The Arts in Psychotherapy, 61,* 44–56.

Heinonen, T., Halonen, D., & Krahn, E. (2018). *Expressive arts for social work and social change*. New York: Oxford University Press.

Heller, L., & LaPierre, A. (2012). *Healing developmental trauma*. Berkeley, CA: North Atlantic Books.

Herman, J. (1992). *Trauma and recovery*. New York: Basic Books.

Hill, A., & Ardau, A. (2013). The politics of drawing: Children, evidence, and the Darfur conflict. *International Political Sociology, 7*(4), 369–387.

Hillman, J. (2013). *The essential James Hillman: A blue fire*. New York: Routledge.

Hinz, L. (2009). *Expressive therapies continuum: A framework for using art in therapy*. New York: Routledge.

Hölzel, B., Carmody, J., Vangel, M., Congleton, C., Yerramsetti, M., Gard, T., et al. (2011). Mindfulness practice leads to increases in regional brain gray matter density. *Psychiatry Research: Neuroimaging, 191*(1), 36.

Humphrey, C. (2011). *Shoot for the moon: Lessons on life from a dog named Rudy*. San Francisco: Chronicle Books.

Huppert, F. A., & Johnson, D. M. (2010). A controlled trial of mindfulness training in schools: The importance of practice for an impact on well-being. *Journal of Positive Psychology, 5,* 264–274.

Interlandi, J. (2014). A revolutionary approach to treating PTSD. Retrieved from *www.nytimes.com/2014/05/25/magazine/a-revolutionary-approach-to-treating-ptsd.html*.

Israel Center for the Treatment of Psychotrauma. (2014). Building resilience intervention (BRI). Retrieved July 3, 2014, from *www.traumaweb.org/content. asp?PageId=477&lang=En*.

Jackson, L., Jackson, Z., & Jackson, F. (2018). Intergenerational resilience in response to the stress and trauma of enslavement and chronic exposure to institutionalized racism. *Journal of Clinical Epigenetics, 4,* 15.

James, B. (1989). *Treating traumatized children: New insights and creative interventions*. Lexington, MA: Lexington Books.

Johnson, D. R. (2009a). Commentary: Examining underlying paradigms in the creative arts therapies of trauma. *The Arts in Psychotherapy, 36*(2), 114–120.

Johnson, D. R. (2009b). *Current approaches in drama therapy*. Springfield, IL: Charles C Thomas.

Johnson, D. R., Lahad, M., & Gray, A. E. (2009). Creative arts therapies for adults. In E. B. Foa, T. M. Keane, M. J. Friedman, & J. A. Cohen (Eds.), *Effective treatments for PTSD: Practice guidelines from the International Society for Traumatic Stress Studies* (2nd ed., pp. 470–490). New York: Guilford Press.

Jones, J., Walker, S., Drass, J. M., & Kaimal, G. (2018). Art therapy interventions for active duty military service members with post-traumatic stress disorder and traumatic brain injury. *International Journal of Art Therapy, 23*(2), 70–85.

Joseph, S., & Linley, P. A. (2008). Psychological assessment of growth following adversity: A review. In S. Joseph & P. A. Linley (Eds.), *Trauma, recovery, and growth: Positive psychological perspectives on posttraumatic stress* (pp. 21–38). Hoboken, NJ: Wiley.

Jung, C. G. (1989). *Memories, dreams, reflections*. New York: HarperCollins.

Jung, C. G. (2009). *The red book* (S. Shamdasani, Ed.). New York: Norton.

Kabat-Zinn, J. (2013). *Full catastrophic living: How to cope with stress, pain and loss using mindfulness meditation*. New York: Bantam.

Kabat-Zinn, J., Lipworth, L., & Burney, R. (1985). The clinical use of mindfulness meditation for the self-regulation of chronic pain. *Journal of Behavioral Medicine, 8*(2), 163–190.

Kagin, S., & Lusebrink, V. (1978). The expressive therapies continuum. *The Arts in Psychotherapy, 5*, 171–180.

Kaimal, G., Ayaz, H., Herres, J. M., Makwana, B., Dieterich-Hartwell, R. M., Kaiser, D. H., et al. (2017). fNIRS assessment of reward perception based on visual self expression: Coloring, doodling and free drawing. *The Arts in Psychotherapy, 55*, 85–92.

Kandel, E. (2012). *The age of insight: The quest to understand the unconscious in art, mind, and brain, from Vienna 1900 to the present*. New York: Random House.

Kaufman, S. B. (2013a). Opening up openness to experience: A four-factor model and relations to creative achievement in the arts and sciences. *Journal of Creative Behavior, 47*, 233–255.

Kaufman, S. B. (2013b). *Ungifted: Intelligence redefined*. New York: Basic Books.

Kaufman, S. B., Quilty, L. C., Grazioplene, R. G., Hirsh, J. B., Gray, J. R., Peterson, J. B., et al. (2015). Openness to experience and intellect differentially predict creative achievement in the arts and sciences. *Journal of Personality, 84*(2), 248–258.

Kestly, T. A. (2014). *The interpersonal neurobiology of play: Brain-building interventions for emotional well-being*. New York: Norton.

Kinnell, G. (1980). Saint Francis and the sow. In *Mortal acts, mortal words* (p. 9). Boston: Houghton Mifflin.

Knill, P., Barba, N., & Fuchs, M. (1995). *Minstrels of soul: Intermodal expressive therapy*. Toronto: Palmiston Press.

Knill, P., Barba, H., & Fuchs, M. (2004). *Principles and practices of expressive arts therapy*. London: Jessica Kingsley.

Kossak, M. (2008). Attunement and free jazz. In *Voices: A world forum for music therapy* [online]. Retrieved from *https://voices.no/index.php/voices/article/view/1784/1545*.

Kossak, M. (2015). *Attunement in expressive arts therapy: Toward an understanding of embodied empathy*. Springfield, IL: Charles C Thomas.

Krahula, B. (2012). *One Zentangle a day*. Minneapolis, MN: Quarry Books.

Kramer, E. (1986). The art therapist's third hand: Reflections on art, art therapy and society at large. *American Journal of Art Therapy, 24*, 71–86.

Kramer, E. (1993). *Art as therapy with children*. Chicago: Magnolia Street.

Kross, E., Bruehlman-Senecal, E., Park, J., Burson, A., Dougherty, A., Shablack, H., et al. (2014). Self-talk as a regulatory mechanism: How you do it matters. *Journal of Personality and Social Psychology, 106*(2), 304–324.

Kruk, K. A., Aravich, P. F., Deaver, S. P., & deBeus, K. (2014). Comparison of brain activity during drawing and clay sculpting: A preliminary qEEG study. *Art Therapy, 31*(2), 52–60.

Lambert, K. (2010). *Lifting depression. A neuroscientist's hands-on approach to activating your brain's healing power.* New York: Basic Books.

LaMothe, K. (2015). *Why we dance: A philosophy of bodily becoming.* New York: Columbia University Press.

Lamott, A. (1994). *Bird by bird: Some instructions on writing and life.* New York: Anchor.

Landgarten, H. (1981). *Clinical art therapy.* New York: Brunner Mazel.

Landis-Shack, N., Heinz, A. J., & Bonn-Miller, M. O. (2017). Music therapy for posttraumatic stress in adults: A theoretical review. *Psychomusicology: Music, Mind, and Brain, 27*(4), 334–342.

Landy, R. (2005). *Drama therapy: Concepts, theories and practices* (2nd ed.). London: Jessica Kingsley.

Lanius, R., Bluhm, R. L., Coupland, N. J., Hegadoren, K. M., Rowe, B., & Theberge, J. (2005). Functional connectivity of dissociative responses in posttraumatic stress disorder: A functional magnetic resonance imaging investigation. *Biological Psychiatry, 57*(8), 873–884.

Leavy, P. (2009). *Method meets art: Art-based research practice* (2nd ed.). New York: Guilford Press.

LeDoux, J. (2015). *Anxious: Using the brain to understand and treat fear and anxiety.* New York: Viking.

Lev-Weisel, R., & Liraz, R. (2007). Drawings versus narratives: Drawing as a tool to encourage verbalization in children whose fathers are drug abusers. *Clinical Child Psychology and Psychiatry, 12*(1), 65–75.

Levine, E., & Levine, S. (Eds.). (2011). *Art in action: Expressive arts therapy and social change.* London: Jessica Kingsley.

Levine, P. (1997). *Waking the tiger: Healing trauma.* Berkeley, CA: North Atlantic Books.

Levine, P. (2015). *Trauma and memory: Brain and body in a search for the living past: A practical guide for understanding and working with traumatic memory.* Berkeley, CA: North Atlantic Books.

Levine, S. (1992). *Poesis: The language of psychology and the speech of the soul.* Toronto: Palmerston Press.

Levitan, D. (2006). *This is your brain on music: The science of a human obsession.* New York: Plume/Penguin.

Linehan, M. M. (2014). *DBT skills training manual* (2nd ed.). New York: Guilford Press.

Loumeau-May, L., Seibel-Nicol, E., Hamilton, M. P., & Malchiodi, C. A., (2015). In C. A. Malchiodi (Ed.), *Creative interventions with traumatized children* (2nd ed., pp. 94–125). New York: Guilford Press.

Lowen, A. (2012). *The voice of the body.* Burlington, VT: Alexander Lowen Foundation.

Lusebrink, V. (1990). *Imagery and visual expression in therapy.* New York: Plenum Press.

Lusebrink, V. (2010). Assessment and therapeutic application of the expressive therapies continuum: Implications for brain structures and functions. *Art Therapy: Journal of the American Art Therapy Association, 27*(4), 168–177.

MacGregor, N. H. (2009). Mapping the body: Tracing the personal and the political dimensions of HIV/AIDs in Khayelitsha, South Africa. *Anthropology and Medicine, 16*(1), 85–95.

Macy, R., Macy, D., Gross, S., & Brighton, P. (2003). Healing in familiar settings:

Support for children and youth in the classroom and community. *New Directions for Youth Development, 98,* 51–79.

Malchiodi, C. A. (1990). *Breaking the silence: Art therapy with children from violent homes.* New York: Brunner Mazel.

Malchiodi, C. A. (1997). *Breaking the silence: Art therapy with children from violent homes* (2nd ed). New York: Taylor & Francis.

Malchiodi, C. A. (1998). *Understanding children's drawings.* New York: Guilford Press.

Malchiodi, C. A. (2003). Art therapy and the brain. In C. A. Malchiodi (Ed.), *Handbook of art therapy* (pp. 17–26). New York: Guilford Press.

Malchiodi, C. A. (2006). Expressive therapies: History, theory and practice. In C. A. Malchiodi (Ed.), *Expressive therapies* (pp. 1–15). New York: Guilford Press.

Malchiodi, C. A. (2007). *The art therapy sourcebook.* New York: McGraw-Hill.

Malchiodi, C. A. (2008, September 26). Telling without talking: Breaking the silence of domestic violence. Retrieved from *www.psychologytoday.com/us/blog/arts-and-health/200809/telling-without-talking-breaking-the-silence-domestic-violence.*

Malchiodi, C. A. (2011). Trauma-informed art therapy. Retrieved January 31, 2011, from *www.cathymalchiodi.com.*

Malchiodi, C. A. (2012a). Art therapy and the brain. In C. A. Malchiodi (Ed.), *Handbook of art therapy* (2nd ed., pp. 17–25). New York: Guilford Press.

Malchiodi, C. A. (2012b). Expressive arts therapy and multi-modal approaches. In C. A. Malchiodi (Ed.), *Handbook of art therapy* (2nd ed., pp. 130–140). New York: Guilford Press.

Malchiodi, C. A. (Ed.). (2012c). *Handbook of art therapy* (2nd ed.). New York: Guilford Press.

Malchiodi, C. A. (2012d). Trauma-informed art therapy and sexual abuse. In P. Goodyear-Brown (Ed.), *Handbook of child sexual abuse* (pp. 341–354). Hoboken, NJ: Wiley.

Malchiodi, C. A. (2013). Introduction to art therapy in health care settings. In C. A. Malchiodi (Ed.), *Art therapy and health care* (pp. 1–12). New York: Guilford Press.

Malchiodi, C. A. (2014a). Art therapy, attachment and parent–child dyads. In C. A. Malchiodi & D. A. Crenshaw (Eds.), *Creative arts and play therapy for attachment problems* (pp. 52–66). New York: Guilford Press.

Malchiodi, C. A. (2014b). Creative arts therapy approaches to attachment issues. In C. A. Malchiodi & D. A. Crenshaw (Eds.), *Creative arts and play therapy for attachment problems* (pp. 3–18). New York: Guilford Press.

Malchiodi, C. A. (2015a). Calm, connection and confidence: Using art therapy to enhance resilience in traumatized children. In D. A. Crenshaw, R. Brooks, & S. Goldstein (Eds.), *Play therapy interventions to enhance resilience* (pp. 126–145). New York: Guilford Press.

Malchiodi, C. A. (2015b). Creative interventions and childhood trauma. In C. A. Malchiodi (Ed.), *Creative interventions with traumatized children* (2nd ed., pp. 3–21). New York: Guilford Press.

Malchiodi, C. A. (2015c). Neurobiology, creative interventions, and childhood trauma. In C. A. Malchiodi (Ed.), *Creative interventions with traumatized children* (2nd ed., pp. 3–23). New York: Guilford Press.

Malchiodi, C. A. (2016, December 29). Creativity and emotional well-being: Recent research. Retrieved from *www.psychologytoday.com/us/blog/arts-and-health/201612/creativity-and-emotional-well-being-recent-research.*

Malchiodi, C. A. (2018). Creative arts therapies and arts-based research. In. P. Leavy (Ed.), *Handbook of arts-based research* (pp. 68–87). New York: Guilford Press.

Malchiodi, C. A. (2019). Kindling the spark: The healing power of expressive arts. *Psychotherapy Networker, 43*(2), 40–45.

Malchiodi, C. A., & Crenshaw, D. A. (Eds.). (2014). *Creative arts and play therapy for attachment problems.* New York: Guilford Press.

Malchiodi. C. A., & Crenshaw, D. A. (Eds.). (2017). *What to do when children clam up in psychotherapy: Interventions to facilitate communication.* New York: Guilford Press.

Marks-Tarlow, T. (2018). *Play and creativity in psychotherapy.* New York: Norton.

Martin, L., Oepen, R., Bauer, K., Nottensteiner, A., Mergheim, K., Gruber, H., et al. (2018). Creative arts interventions for stress management and prevention: A systematic review. *Behavioral Sciences (Basel, Switzerland), 8*(2), E28.

Marvasti, J. (1997). Eriksonian play therapy. In K. O'Connor & L. Braverman (Eds.), *Play therapy theory and practice* (pp. 285–309). New York: Wiley.

Masten, A. (2001). Ordinary magic: Resilience process in development. *American Psychologist, 56,* 227–228.

Maté, G. (2011). *When the body says no: The cost of hidden stress.* Toronto: Vintage Canada.

May, R. (1994). *The courage to create.* New York: Norton.

McGilchrist, I. (2009). *The master and his emissary: The divided brain and the making of the Western world.* New Haven, CT: Yale University Press.

McGoldrick, M., Gerson, R., & Petry, S. (2008). *Genograms: Assessment and intervention* (3rd ed.). New York: Norton.

McNiff, S. (2004). *Art heals: How creativity cures the soul.* Boston: Shambhala.

McNiff, S. (2009). *Integrating the arts in therapy: History, theory and practice.* Springfield, IL: Charles C Thomas.

Meichenbaum, D. (2004). *Stress inoculation training.* New York: Prentice Hall.

Mercer, A., Warson, E., & Zhao, J. (2010). Visual journaling: An intervention to influence stress, anxiety and affect levels in medical students. *The Arts in Psychotherapy, 37* (2), 143–148.

Meyburgh, T. (2006). *The body remembers: Body mapping and narratives of physical trauma.* Unpublished master's thesis, University of Pretoria, Pretoria, South Africa.

Mithoefer, M. C., Feduccia, A. A., Jerome, L., Mithoefer, A., Wagner, M., Walsh, Z., et al. (2019). MDMA-assisted psychotherapy for treatment of PTSD: Study design and rationale for phase 3 trials based on pooled analysis of six phase 2 randomized controlled trials. *Psychopharmacology, 236*(9), 273–274.

Monti, D. A., Peterson, C., Kunkel, E. J., Hauck, W. W., Pequignot, E., Rhodes, L., et al. (2006). A randomized, controlled trial of mindfulness-based art therapy (MBAT) for women with cancer. *Psycho-Oncology, 15,* 363–373.

Moore, K. (2013). A systematic review on the neural effects of music on emotion regulation: Implications for music therapy practice. *Journal of Music Therapy, 50*(3), 198–242.

Moser, J. S., Dougherty, A., Mattson, W. I., Katz, B., Moran, T. P., Guevarra, D., et al. (2017). Third-person self-talk facilitates emotion regulation without engaging cognitive control: Converging evidence from ERP and fMRI. *Scientific Reports, 7*(1), 4519.

Nachmanovitz, S. (1991). *Free play: Improvisation in life and art.* New York: Putnam.

National Association for Poetry Therapy. (2019). History of NAPT. Retrieved from *https://poetrytherapy.org/index.php/about-napt/history-of-napt*.

National Center for Trauma-Informed Care. (2019). Purpose and mission statement. Retrieved from *https://tash.org/nctic*.

National Drama Therapy Association. (2019). What is drama therapy? Retrieved from *www.nadta.org/what-is-drama-therapy.html*.

National Organization for Arts in Health. (2019). About NOAH. Retrieved from *https://thenoah.net/about*.

Neff, K. D. (2012). The science of self-compassion. In C. Germer & R. D. Siegel (Eds.), *Wisdom and compassion in psychotherapy: Deepening mindfulness in clinical practice* (pp. 79–92). New York: Guilford Press.

Neff, K. D. (2019). Definition of self-compassion. Retrieved from *https://self-compassion.org/the-three-elements-of-self-compassion-2*.

Nummenmaa, L., Hari, R., Hietanen, J. K., & Glerean, E. (2018). Maps of subjective feelings. *Proceedings of the National Academy of Sciences of the USA, 115*(37), 9198–9203.

Oaklander, V. (2015). *Windows to our children: A Gestalt therapy approach to children and adolescents*. Highland, NY: Gestalt Journal Press.

Oatley, K. (2016). Imagination, inference, intimacy: The psychology of pride and prejudice. *Review of General Psychology, 20*(3), 236–244.

Ogden, P., & Fisher, J. (2015). *Sensorimotor psychotherapy: Interventions for trauma and attachment*. New York: Norton.

Ogden, P., Minton, K., & Pain, C. (2006). *Trauma and the body: A sensorimotor approach to psychotherapy*. New York: Norton.

Panskepp, J. (2004). *Affective neuroscience: The foundations of human and animal emotions*. New York: Oxford University Press.

Payne, P., Levine, P., & Crane-Godreau, M. (2015). Somatic experiencing: Using interoception and proprioception as core elements of trauma therapy. *Frontiers in Psychology, 6*, 93.

Pelletier, C. (2004). The effect of music on decreasing arousal due to stress: A meta-analysis. *Journal of Music Therapy, 41*(3), 192–214.

Pennebaker, J. W., & Chung, C. K. (2011). Expressive writing and its links to mental and physical health. In H. S. Friedman (Ed.), *Oxford handbook of health psychology* (pp. 417–437). New York: Oxford University Press.

Pennebaker, J. W., & Smyth, J. M. (2016). *Opening up by writing it down: How expressive writing improves health and eases emotional pain* (3rd ed.). New York: Guilford Press.

Perry, B. (2006). The neurosequential model of therapeutics: Applying principles of neuroscience to clinical work with traumatized and maltreated children. In N. B. Webb (Ed.), *Working with traumatized youth in child welfare* (pp. 27–52). New York: Guilford Press.

Perry, B. (2009). Examining child maltreatment through a neurodevelopmental lens. *Journal of Trauma and Loss, 14*, 240–255.

Perry, B. D. (2015). Foreword. In C. A. Malchiodi (Ed.), *Creative interventions with traumatized children* (2nd ed., pp. ix–xi). New York: Guilford Press.

Perry, B. D., & Szalavitz, M. (2017). *The boy who was raised as a dog*. New York: Basic Books.

Piaget, J., & Inhelder, B. (1969). *The psychology of the child*. New York: Basic Books.

Pipher, M. (2019). *Women rowing north: Navigating life's currents and flourishing as we age.* New York: Bloomsbury.

Porges, S. (2004). Neuroception: A subconscious system for detecting threats and safety. *ZERO TO THREE, 24*(5), 19–24.

Porges, S. (2010). Music therapy and trauma: Insights from the polyvagal theory. In K. Stewart (Ed.), *Music therapy and trauma: Bridging theory and clinical practice* (pp. 3–15). New York: Satchnote Press.

Porges, S. (2012). *The polyvagal theory.* New York: Norton.

Progoff, I. (1992). *At a journal workshop: Writing to access the power of the unconscious and evoke creative ability.* New York: Tarcher Perigee.

Pynoos, R., & Eth, S. (1986). Witness to violence: The child interview. *Journal of the American Academy of Child Psychiatry, 25,* 306–319.

Rakoff, V., Sigal, J. J., & Epstein, N. B. (1966). Children and families of concentration camp survivors. *Canada's Mental Health, 14,* 24–26.

Rappaport, L. (2009). *Focusing-oriented art therapy.* London: Jessica Kingsley.

Rappaport, L. (Ed.). (2013). *Mindfulness and the arts therapies: Theory and practice.* London: Jessica Kingsley.

Rappaport, L. (2015). Focusing-oriented expressive arts therapy and mindfulness with children and adolescents experiencing trauma. In C. A. Malchiodi (Ed.), *Creative interventions with traumatized children* (2nd ed., pp. 301–323). New York: Guilford Press.

Reich, W. (1994). *Beyond psychology: Letters and journals 1934–1939.* New York: Farrar Straus & Giroux.

Repke, M. A. (2018). How does nature exposure make people healthier?: Evidence for the role of impulsivity and expanded space perception. *PLOS ONE, 13*(8), e0202246.

Reynolds, D., & Reason, M. (Eds.). (2012). *Kinesthetic empathy in creative and cultural practices.* Bristol, UK: Intellect.

Rhodes, A., Spinazzola, J., & van der Kolk, B. A. (2016). Yoga for adult women with chronic PTSD: A long-term follow-up study. *Journal of Alternative and Complementary Medicine, 22*(3), 189–196.

Rhyne, J. (1973). *The Gestalt art therapy experience.* Pacific Grove, CA: Brooks/Cole.

Riley, S. (2004). *Integrative approaches to family art therapy.* Chicago: Magnolia Street.

Rockliff, H., Karl, A., McEwan, K., Gilbert, J., Matos, M., & Gilbert, P. (2011). Effects of intranasal oxytocin on "compassion focused imagery." *Emotion, 11*(6), 1388–1396.

Rogers, C. (2012). *On becoming a person: A therapist's view of psychotherapy.* Boston: Houghton Mifflin.

Rogers, N. (1993). *The creative connection: Expressive arts as healing.* Palo Alto, CA: Science & Behavior Books.

Rolf, I. (1990). *Rolfing and physical reality.* New York: Simon & Schuster.

Rothschild, B. (2000). *The body remembers.* New York: Norton.

Rothschild, B. (2011). *Trauma essentials: The go-to guide.* New York: Norton.

Sacks, O. (2007). *Musicophilia: Tales of music and the brain.* New York: Random House.

Sänger, J., Müller, V., & Lindenberger, U. (2012). Intra- and interbrain synchronization and network properties when playing guitar in duets. *Frontiers in Human Neuroscience, 6,* 312.

Savage, B., Lujan, H., Thipparthi, R., & DiCarlo, S. (2017). Humor, laughter, learning, and health: A brief review. *Advances in Physiology Education, 41*(3), 341–347.

Schäfer, T., Sedlmeier, P., Städtler, C., & Huron, D. (2013). The psychological functions of music listening. *Frontiers in Psychology, 4*, 511.

Schore, A. (2003). *Affect regulation and the repair of the self.* New York: Norton.

Schore, J. R., & Schore, A. N. (2008). Modern attachment theory: The central role of affect regulation in development and treatment. *Clinical Social Work Journal, 36*(1), 9–20.

Schroder, D. (2015). *Exploring and developing the use of art-based genograms in family of origin therapy.* Springfield, IL: Charles C Thomas.

Seligman, M. (2007). *The optimistic child.* Boston: Houghton Mifflin.

Selye, H. (1976). *The stress of life.* New York: McGraw-Hill.

Shapiro, F. (2012). *Getting past your past.* New York: Rodale.

Shapiro, F. (2018). *Eye movement desensitization and reprocessing (EMDR) therapy: Basic principles, protocols, and procedures* (3rd ed.). New York: Guilford Press.

Shultis, C., & Gallagher, L. (2016). Medical music therapy for adults. In B. L. Wheeler (Ed.), *Music therapy handbook* (pp. 441–453). New York: Guilford Press.

Siegel, D. (2010). *Mindsight.* New York: Norton.

Siegel, D. (2011). *The whole-brain child: 12 revolutionary strategies to nurture your child's developing mind.* New York: Delacorte Press.

Siegel, D. (2012). *The developing mind: How relationships and the brain interact to shape who we are* (2nd ed.). New York: Guilford Press.

Siegel, D. (2014). *Brainstorm: The power and purpose of the teenage brain.* New York: Jeremy Tarcher/Penguin.

Siegel, D., & Hartzell, M. (2003). *Parenting from the inside out.* New York: Jeremy Tarcher/Penguin.

Sinha, J. W., & Rosenberg, L. B. (2013). A critical review of trauma interventions and religion among youth exposed to community violence. *Journal of Social Service Research, 39*(4), 436–454.

Solomon, J. (2002). *"Living with X": A body mapping journey in time of HIV and AIDS. Facilitator's Guide.* Johannesburg, South Africa: REPSSI.

Solomon, J. (2007). *"Living with X": A body mapping journey in time of HIV and AIDS. Facilitator's guide.* Johannesburg, South Africa: REPSSI.

Southwick, S. M., Bonanno, G. A., Masten, A. S., Panter-Brick, C., & Yehuda, R. (2014). Resilience definitions, theory, and challenges: Interdisciplinary perspectives. *European Journal of Psychotraumatology, 5.*

Spiegel, D., Malchiodi, C. A., Backos, A., & Collie, K. (2006). Art therapy for combat-related PTSD: Recommendations for research and practice. *Art Therapy, 23*(4), 157–164.

Spinazzola, J., van der Kolk, B. A., & Ford, J. D. (2018). When nowhere is safe: Interpersonal trauma and attachment adversity as antecedents of posttraumatic stress disorder and developmental trauma disorder. *Journal of Traumatic Stress, 5*, 631–642.

Steele, W., & Malchiodi, C. A. (2011). *Trauma-informed practices with children and adolescents.* New York: Routledge.

Steele, W., & Raider, M. (2001). *Structured sensory intervention for children, adolescents and parents: Strategies to alleviate trauma.* Lewiston, NY: Edwin Mellen Press.

Stellar, J. E., John-Henderson, N., Anderson, C. L., Gordon, A. McNeil, G. D., & Keltner, D. (2015). Positive affect and markers of inflammation: Discrete positive emotions predict lower levels of inflammatory cytokines. *Emotion, 15*(2), 129–133.

Substance Abuse and Mental Health Services Administration. (2019). Trauma-informed care in behavioral health services. Retrieved from *https://store.samhsa.gov/system/files/sma14-4816.pdf.*

Teicher, M. H. (2000). Wounds that won't heal: The neurobiology of child abuse. *Cerebrum, 2*(4), 50–62.

Terr, L. (1981). Forbidden games: Post-traumatic child's play. *Journal of the American Academy of Child Psychiatry, 20,* 741–760.

Terr, L. (1990). *Too scared to cry: Psychic trauma in childhood.* New York: Harper & Row.

Terr, L. (2008). *Magical moments of change: How psychotherapy turns kids around.* New York: Norton.

Thoma, M. V., La Marca, R., Brönnimann, R., Finkel, L., Ehlert, U., & Nater, U. M. (2013). The effect of music on the human stress response. *PLOS ONE, 8*(8), e70156.

Thomson, P., & Jaque, S. V. (2017). *Creativity and the performing artist.* San Diego, CA: Academic Press.

Treleavan, D. (2018). *Trauma-sensitive mindfulness: Practices for safe and transformative healing.* New York: Norton.

Tronick, E. (2007). *The neurobehavioral and social-emotional development of infants and children.* New York: Norton.

Tronick, E., & Reck, C. (2009). Infants of depressed mothers. *Harvard Review of Psychiatry, 17*(2), 147–156.

Urhausen, M. T. (2015). Eye movement desensitization and reprocessing and art therapy with traumatized children. In C. A. Malchiodi (Ed.), *Creative interventions with traumatized children* (2nd ed., pp. 45–74). New York: Guilford Press.

van der Kolk, B. A. (1994). The body keeps the score: Memory and the evolving psychobiology of posttraumatic stress. *Harvard Review of Psychiatry, 1*(5), 253–265.

van der Kolk, B. A. (1996). The complexity of adaptation to trauma: Self-regulation, stimulus discrimination, and characterological development. In B. A. van der Kolk, A. C. McFarlane, & L. Weisaeth (Eds.), *Traumatic stress: The effects of overwhelming experience on mind, body, and society* (pp. 182–213). New York: Guilford Press.

van der Kolk, B. A. (2000). Posttraumatic stress disorder and the nature of trauma. *Dialogues in Clinical Neuroscience, 2*(1), 7–22.

van der Kolk, B. A. (2005). Developmental trauma disorder: Towards a rational diagnosis for children with complex trauma histories. *Psychiatric Annals, 35,* 401–408.

van der Kolk, B. A. (2006). Clinical applications of neuroscience research in PTSD. *Annals of the New York Academy of Science, 1071*(4), 277–293.

van der Kolk, B. A. (2014). *The body keeps the score.* New York: Penguin.

van der Kolk, B. A., & Ducey, C. P. (1989). The psychological processing of traumatic experience: Rorschach patterns in PTSD. *Journal of Traumatic Stress, 2*(3), 259–274.

van der Kolk, B. A., Stone, L., West, J., Rhodes, A., Emerson, D., Suvak, M., & Spinazzola, J. (2014). Yoga as an adjunctive treatment for posttraumatic stress disorder: A randomized controlled trial. *Journal Clinical Psychiatry, 75*(6), 550–565.

van der Kolk, B. A., Pelcovitz, D., Roth, S., Mandel, F., McFarlane, A., & Herman, J. L. (1996). Dissociation, somatization, and affect dysregulation: The complexity of adaptation to trauma. *American Journal of Psychiatry, 153*(7), 83–93.

Verfaille, M. (2016). *Mentalizing in the arts therapies.* New York: Routledge.

Voigt, V., Neufeld, F., Kaste, J., Bühner, M., Sckopke, P., Wuerstlein, R., et al. (2017). Clinically assessed posttraumatic stress in patients with breast cancer during the first year after diagnosis in the prospective, longitudinal, controlled COGNICARES study. *Psycho-Oncology, 26*, 74–80.

Wammes, J. D., Meade, M. E., & Fernandes, M. A. (2016). The drawing effect: Evidence for reliable and robust memory benefits in free recall. *Quarterly Journal of Experimental Psychology, 69*(9), 1752–1776.

Warson, E. (2013). Healing across cultures: Arts in health care with American Indian and Alaska Native cancer survivors. In C. A. Malchiodi (Ed.), *Art therapy and health care* (pp. 162–183). New York: Guilford Press.

Warson, E., & Lorance, J. (2013). Physiological measures in evidence-based art therapy research. In C. A. Malchiodi (Ed.), *Art therapy and health care* (pp. 363–375). New York: Guilford Press.

Wheeler, B. (Ed.). (2016). *Music therapy handbook.* New York: Guilford Press.

White, M., & Epston, D. (1990). *Narrative means to therapeutic ends.* New York: Norton.

Whitehouse, M. (1995). The Tao of the body. In D. H. Johnson (Ed.), *Bone, breath, and gesture: Practices of embodiment.* Berkeley, CA: North Atlantic Books & California Institute of Integral Studies.

Willard, C. (2010). *Child's mind: Mindfulness practices to help our children be more focused, calm and relaxed.* Berkeley, CA: Parallax Press.

Winner, E. (1982). *Invented worlds: The psychology of the arts.* Cambridge, MA: Harvard University Press.

Winnicott, D. (1971). *Playing and reality.* New York: Routledge.

Wix, L. (2009). Aesthetic empathy in teaching art to children: The work of Friedl Dicker-Brandeis in Terezin. *Art Therapy, 26*(4), 152–158.

Woodyard, C. (2011). Exploring the therapeutic effects of yoga and its ability to increase quality of life. *International Journal of Yoga, 4*(2), 49–54.

Wright, M. O. D., Masten, A. S., & Narayan, A. J. (2013). Resilience processes in development: Four waves of research on positive adaptation in the context of adversity. In S. Goldstein & R. B. Brooks (Eds.), *Handbook of resilience in children* (2nd ed., pp. 15–37). New York: Springer.

Wylie, M. S. (2004). The limits of talk. *Psychotherapy Networker, 28*(1), 30–46.

Yehuda, R., & Bierer, M. (2007). Transgenerational transmission of cortisol and PTSD risk. *Progress in Brain Research, 167*, 121–135.

Yehuda, R., & Lehrner, A. (2018). Intergenerational transmission of trauma effects: Putative role of epigenetic mechanism. *World Psychiatry, 17*, 243–257.

Index

Note. *f* or *t* following a page number indicate a figure or a table.